The 18 Korean Masters in Plastic Surgery
한국 미용성형의 고수 18

International Special Edition

Must-read with regard to plastic surgery
introduced by the 18 Korean Masters in Plastic Surgery!

The 18 Korean Masters in Plastic Surgery
한국 미용성형의 고수 18

International Special Edition

M&C Korea

실패하지 않고 더 나은 아름다움을 보장받을 수 있는 한국미용성형 고수를 단박에 만나실 수 있습니다.

한국의 미용성형 수준은 이미 전 세계적으로 높게 평가되고 있습니다.

과거부터 다양한 수술 방법뿐만 아니라 기술과 장비, 재료까지 아주 다양하게 개발되어 안전하고 높은 수준의 수술과 시술을 제공하고 있기 때문에 세계 각지에서 많은 환자들이 한국을 찾아오고 있습니다.

한국 성형외과는 선진국들과 비교해도 기술적인 수준이 높은 편이며, 최근에는 개인 맞춤형 수술과 최소 침습 수술 등을 중심으로 보다 안전하고 회복이 빠르며, 효과적인 수술 방법이 개발되고 있습니다. 또한 K-뷰티와 K-팝 등의 문화적인 요소가 미용성형 산업의 전반에까지 큰 영향을 미치고 있으며, 실제로 수많은 세계인들이 한국의 연예인들처럼 보이고 싶어하고, 또한 이러한 요소들이 미용성형 수술의 방향성과 트렌드를 결정하는 경우도 많습니다.

이러한 한류 열풍으로 한국이 성형 강국으로 인정받고, 의료관광의 메카가 되었지만, 그 한편엔 과도하게 미용성형 수술이 행해지고 있는 것은 아닌가 걱정과 염려와 시선이 있는 것도 사실입니다. 미용성형 수술은 항상 부작용과 위험성이 존재하기 때문에 환자들은 신중하게 선택하고 전문적인 상담을 받아야 합니다.

그렇다면 성형수술을 잘 받기 위해 고려해야할 사항은 어떤 것이 있을까요?

첫째로 전문성이 있고, 수술 경험이 많은 안전한 병원과 의사를 선택하는 것이 중요합니다.

둘째는 수술 전 수술을 할 선생님에게 자세한 상담을 받아야 합니다. 본인이 왜 수술을 하고 싶은지, 이 수술이 본인에게 왜 필요한지 그리고 수술 방법, 부작용 등에 대해서도 구체적으로 듣고, 충분히 이해하고 난 뒤에, 수술을 결정 해야 합니다.

셋째는 음주, 흡연 등을 하지 않고 컨디션을 최상으로 유지해야하고, 수술 후에도 빠르게 회복될 수 있도록 의사의 지시에 정확히 잘 따라야 합니다.

넷째로 다방면의 인터넷 검색이나 실제 환자의 소개, 평가 등을 듣고, 여러 개의 병원을 선택한 후에 방문 상담을 받아야 합니다.

이 책은 그 누구보다 경험이 많은 고수들에게 듣는 미용성형에 대한 모든 것이 담겨져 있습니다. 성형에 관심이 있으신 분들이라면 직접 발품을 팔지 않고 이 책 하나로 모든 궁금증이 해결할 수 있으며, 지금 성형을 준비하고 계시다면 실패하지 않고 더 나은 아름다움을 보장받을 수 있는 미용성형 고수를 단박에 만나실 수 있습니다.

"한국 미용성형 고수 18" 책이 발간되는 이유가 바로 여기에 있습니다.

2023년 12월
CDU 청담유성형외과의원 원장 양동준
성형외과 전문의

You can immediately meet a Korean cosmetic plastic surgery expert who will guarantee better beauty without failure.

South Korea's plastic surgery standards are already highly regarded worldwide. Over the years, a wide variety of surgical techniques, as well as advancements in technology and materials, have been developed. This has enabled the provision of safe and high-quality surgical and cosmetic procedures. As a result, many patients from all around the world are choosing to come to South Korea for these procedures.

Korean plastic surgery is known for its advanced techniques when compared to many other countries. Recently, there has been a focus on personalized and minimally invasive surgeries, which are not only safer but also offer quicker recovery times and more effective results.

Cultural factors such as K-beauty and K-pop have had a significant influence on the beauty and cosmetic surgery industry as a whole. In fact, numerous people from around the world aspire to look like Korean celebrities. Additionally, these cultural factors often shape the direction and trends in the field of cosmetic surgery.

Thanks to the Hallyu wave, South Korea has gained recognition as a cosmetic surgery powerhouse and a hub for medical tourism. However, on the other side, there are concerns about the excessive use of cosmetic surgery. Since cosmetic surgery always carries the risk of side effects and dangers, patients should make careful choices and seek professional advice.

Here are some important considerations for receiving cosmetic surgery successfully

Choose a Qualified and Experienced Surgeon: It's crucial to select a reputable hospital and a surgeon with a strong track record and extensive experience in the specific procedure you desire. Ensure they have the necessary certifications and licenses.

Thorough Consultation : Schedule a detailed consultation with the surgeon who will perform the procedure. During this consultation, discuss why you want the surgery, the specific goals you hope to achieve, and gain a comprehensive understanding of the procedure, including potential risks and complications.

Preparation and Lifestyle: Prior to the surgery, maintain a healthy lifestyle. Avoid smoking and alcohol consumption, as these can negatively impact your ability to heal. Follow the surgeon's pre-operative instructions to optimize your condition for surgery.

Research and Multiple Consultations: Conduct comprehensive research online, read patient reviews, and ask for recommendations from trusted sources. Consider consulting with multiple hospitals or surgeons before making a final decision.

This book contains everything about cosmetic surgery, heard from experts with more experience than anyone else. If you have an interest in plastic surgery, you can solve all your questions with just this book without wasting time. If you are planning for plastic surgery now, you can meet a cosmetic surgery expert who guarantees a better beauty without failure through this book.

This is reason for the publication of the book 'Korean Cosmetic Surgery Experts 18' is right here.

Dong-Jun Yang (Plastic Surgery Specialist)
Director of CDU Cheongdam U Plastic Surgery Clinic
December 2023

목차

쌍꺼풀 수술(Double eyelid surgery)
상안검 · 눈썹거상술 (Upper eyelid/brow lift surgery)
하안검/눈밑지방재배치(Lower eyelid/under eye fat relocation)

마음과 마음을 여는 미학 눈성형

Eye-contact Aesthetic eyelid surgery that opens the heart

사람의 눈은 서로의 공감대를 형성할 수 있고 호감과 비호감을 느낄 수 있는 첫인상의 포인트로 상대방에게 나의 첫 이미지를 전달하는 마음의 창이다.

A person's eyes are the window to the heart that conveys one's first image to the other person as a point of first impression through which one can form a consensus and feel likes or dislikes.

에이블리 성형외과
Ably Plastic Surgery

ablyps.com

이진규(Lee Jin-gyu)

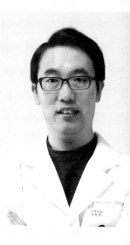

- 성형외과 전문의(Regular member of the Korean Society of Plastic Surgery)
- 대한성형외과학회 정회원(Regular member of the Korean Society of Aesthetic Plastic Surgery)
- 대한미용성형외과학회 정회원(Regular member of the Korean Society of Hand Surgery)
- 대한두부안면성형외과 정회원(Regular member of Korean Craniofacial Plastic Surgery)
- 대한성형외과학회 눈성형연구회 학술위원
(Academic member of the Oculoplastic Research Society of the Korean Society of Plastic Surgery)
- 대한미용성형외과학회 상임이사(Executive Director, Korean Society of Aesthetic Plastic Surgery)

01-1 눈만 예뻐도 미인이 될 수 있다!

다른 이의 시선을 끄는 또렷하고 시원한 눈

사랑에 빠진 연인들이 주로 하는 말이 "첫눈에 반했어"라고 하는 것처럼 눈은 중요한 감정을 표현하는 창으로써 첫 만남에서 보여지는 상대방의 눈매는 첫인상을 어떻게 남기는가에 매우 중요한 요소가 된다.

마음에 드는 이성과 마주해서 눈을 마주쳤을 때 심장 박동이 빨라지고 동공이 확장되는 느낌을 느껴본 경험은 아마 적지 않을 것이다.

반대로 눈매가 무서운 사람을 마주했을 때는 불편한 감정을 느끼기도 하고 눈이 작고 눈동자를 가려 보이는 눈을 가진 사람에게는 답답함을 느끼는 경우도 없지 않다. 첫인상이 호감 가는 인상이 아니라 해서 안 좋은 것은 아니겠지만 첫눈에 반하진 않더라도 좋은 인상을 남기는 것은 상대방에게 호감을 줄 수 있는 방법이기 때문이다.

이처럼 사람의 눈은 상대방에게 전달하는 마음의 창이 되기도 하고 첫인상에서 호감과 비호감을 주는 가장 큰 요소이기도 하다.

쌍꺼풀 수술

쌍꺼풀 수술은 성형의 시작이라고 말할 정도로 쌍꺼풀 수술 하나만으로 인상의 변화를 크게 줄 수가 있다. 각자 개성에 어울리는 쌍꺼풀 수술로 좀 더 크고 또렷한 눈매와 라인으로 더 예뻐진 눈을 기대할 수 있다.

매몰법

눈꺼풀 피부에 직경 1mm의 창을 통해 봉합사를 피부로부터 결막으로 넣은 후 다시 다른 구멍으로 빼내 근육과 피부가 붙도록 매듭을 만들어 줌으로써 구멍을 연결한 가상 선에 맞춰 쌍꺼풀이 생기게 하는 방법이다.

매몰법은 절개법에 비하여 수술시간이 짧고, 수술 후 붓기가 적어서 며칠 안에 자연스러운 모양을 나타내기 때문에 선호도가 높다. 다만 피부 절개가 필요 없고 눈꺼풀이 얇은 눈에는 효과적이나 눈꺼풀이 두껍고 지방이 많은 사람의 경우 쌍꺼풀이 풀릴 경우가 많으므로 이런 사람들에게는 절개법이 효과적이다.

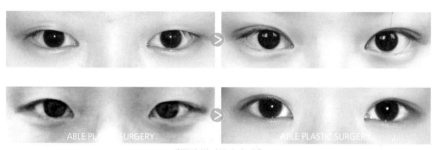

매몰법 쌍꺼풀 수술전후

부분절개

절개식 방법과 매몰식 방법의 장점들을 절충한 방법으로 최소한의 절개로 흉을 최소화하여 자연스럽고 시원한 눈매로 연출하는 방법이다. 또한 매몰법과 절개법

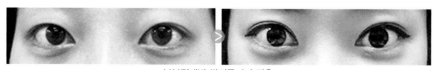

부분절개법 쌍꺼풀 수술전후

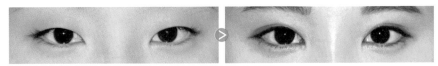

부분절개법 쌍꺼풀 수술전후

의 장점만을 절충한 형태의 수술법으로 붓기와 흉터가 적고 절개법과 비교해 회복이 빠르다. 쉽게 풀리지 않고 지방이 많은 두터운 눈도 에이블 성형외과만의 노하우로 자연스럽고 원하는 라인의 쌍꺼풀을 원할 때 사용된다.

절개법

매몰법에 비해 수술 후 자연스러워질 때까지 오래 걸리는 단점에도 불구하고 피부가 많이 늘어져 있거나 지방층이 두툼한 사람들에게 가장 보편적으로 시행되는 확실한 쌍꺼풀 수술법이다. 쌍꺼풀 수술 시 눈이 졸려 보이는 환자의 경우 눈매교정술을 같이 해줘야 보다 아름다운 눈을 만들어 줄 수 있게 된다.

절개법도 다이나믹 방법과 고정식 절개 방법이 있는데 이는 환자의 상태 등에 따라서 선택되어져 쓰일 수 있다. 에이블리 성형외과에서는 환자의 상태에 따라서 수술방법을 선택하여 시행하고 있다.

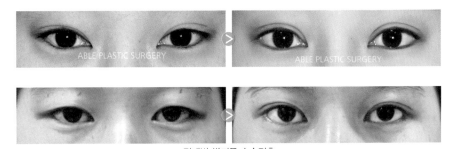

절개법 쌍꺼풀 수술전후

TIP_쌍꺼풀 수술 수술정보

수술시간	마취방법	입원여부	실밥제거	회복기간	체류기간
30분~1시간	국소마취	입원없음	3~6일 후	3~7일	3~7일

눈매교정술

눈꺼풀이 내려앉은 안검하수가 아니더라도 눈의 상하 폭이 작은 경우 눈이 답답해 보이고 힘이 없어 보인다. 에이블리 성형외과의 크리스탈 눈매교정술은 시야가 답답해 보이고 흐릿해 보이는 눈매를 교정하여 시원하고 또렷한 눈매로 바꾸어주는 수술이다. 눈꺼풀을 들어 올리는 상안검거근과 뮬러근을 조작하여 수술을 하게 되며, 이때 절개법을 이용한 쌍꺼풀 수술로 라인을 얇게 하는 방법이 동시에 이루어진다. 눈매교정술 시 자연스러운 눈의 모양을 맞추면서 눈이 너무 크지도 작지도 않게 얼굴의 조화를 맞추는 것이 중요하다.

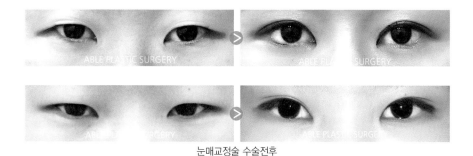

눈매교정술 수술전후

짝눈교정술

사람의 얼굴은 완벽하게 대칭일 수 없으며 누구나 자신의 눈 양쪽이 다른 짝눈이라는 것을 알 수 있다. 하지만 대부분의 사람이 짝눈을 교정할 정도가 아니지만 좌우 눈의 크기, 쌍꺼풀의 모양 그리고 안구의 돌출 정도, 안와 골의 모양과 좌우 폭의 차이가 짝눈의 원인이 될 수 있으며 가장 큰 원인은 눈이 떠지는 정도에 따른 검은 눈동자의 노출 비율에 따라 결정된다고 할 수 있다.

눈을 뜨게 하는 근육에 문제가 있거나 쌍꺼풀 수술 후 비대칭이 된 경우, 또는

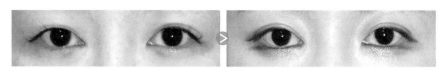

짝눈교정술 수술전후

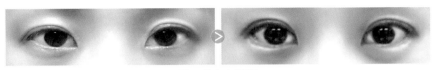

짝눈교정술 수술전후

복합적인 형태의 짝눈의 교정은 눈매교정과 쌍꺼풀 절개법 수술을 병행하여 교정하게 된다. 눈매교정으로 검은 눈동자의 노출 정도를 교정하여 눈의 크기도 시원하게 커 보이도록 하면서 쌍꺼풀 라인도 예쁘게 만들게 된다.

피부상태에 맞게 눈떠지는 정도가 적은 한쪽 눈의 안구 노출을 교정하는 방법도 있으며 쌍꺼풀이 한쪽 눈에만 있는 비대칭의 경우 디자인을 통해 쌍꺼풀을 동일한 크기로 만들어주면 된다.

다만 짝눈이라고 해서 한쪽 눈만 수술하기를 고집하기보다는 개인 취향과 트렌드, 전체적인 모양을 고려하여 양쪽 눈 모두를 같이 수술하는 것이 또 다른 비대칭을 예방할 수 있다.

TIP_눈매교정술 수술정보

수술시간	마취방법	입원여부	실밥제거	회복기간	체류기간
1시간	국소마취	입원없음	6~7일 후	7일	7일

상안검 · 눈썹거상술

처진 눈꺼풀로 인한 기능적 문제해결과 한층 어려 보이는 동안 효과까지 한번에 얻을 수 있는 수술이다.

상안검

노화로 인해 눈꺼풀이 처지게 되면 더 나이가 들어 보이게 되고 원래 있던 쌍꺼풀도 보이지 않고 심한 경우 눈꺼풀이 시야를 가리게 된다. 이와 더불어 눈썹이 처진 경우 눈썹거상술로 진행할 수도 있다.

눈의 처진 피부 양을 측정하여 제거하고 필요한 경우 상안검 거근이 분리된 경우 다시 원래의 위치에 되돌려 놓는 술식이 필요하다. 상안검수술로 눈꺼풀의 주름 없이 눈이 커지고 시원한 젊은 인상으로 변화를 줄 수 있다.

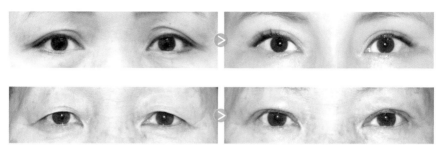

상안검 수술전후

눈썹거상술

눈썹거상술은 원하는 높이와 모양을 고려하여 제거할 피부의 양을 측정한 후에 눈썹 아래를 절개, 피부 및 근육을 제거하고 처진 근육을 끌어올린다. 골막에 고정하고 봉합하여 피부와 근육을 위로 끌어올려 고정함으로써 밝고 젊은 인상을 갖게 된다.

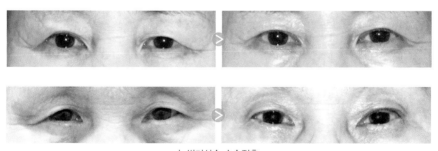

눈썹거상술 수술전후

TIP_상안검 / 눈썹거상술 수술정보					
수술시간	마취방법	입원여부	실밥제거	회복기간	체류기간
1시간	국소마취	입원없음	5~7일 후	7일	7일

하안검 / 눈밑지방재배치

눈 밑 나이 흔적을 감쪽같이! 주름은 물론 눈물고랑, 꺼진 눈매, 다크서클까지 한 번에 해결하는 매직!

하안검

처진 하안검은 눈 아래 지방을 싸고 있는 막이 느슨해져 지방이 돌출되어 눈 밑이 볼록해지고 골이져 보여 더 나이 들어 보이게 된다. 처진 지방을 단순히 제거하는 것이 아니라 보존하면서 눈 아래 골막밑이나 위에 깔아주게 되면 단순히 지방을 제거하는 것보다 더 좋은 결과를 얻을 수 있다.

속눈썹 가까이 절개해 튀어나온 지방을 이용해 골이 진 부위를 편편해지도록 메워 주고 남은 지방과 늘어진 피부를 제거한다. 피부와 근육을 위로 잡아당겨 고정해 아래 속눈썹에 가려지도록 봉합함으로써 주름은 물론 눈물고랑, 꺼진 눈매, 다크서클까지 한 번에 해결 가능하다.

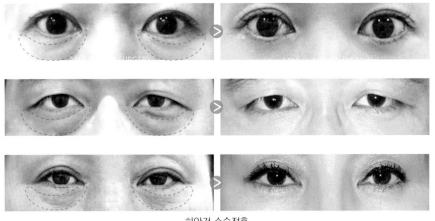

하안검 수술전후

스타 눈밑지방재배치

나이 들어 보이는 얼굴의 주범 눈 밑 지방, 스타 연예인에게서 검증된 이진규 원장의 눈밑지방재배치술은 최근 스타 연예인들이 눈밑지방재배치 수술 후 밝은 인상을 얻게 됨으로써 자연스레 동안성형으로 알려지게 된 수술이다.

눈 아래 지방을 싸고 있는 막이 느슨해져 생기는 눈 밑 지방을 눈 안쪽 결막을 통해 간단히 제거하거나 재배치하는 수술이다. 불룩한 눈 밑 지방은 다크서클의 원인이 되기도 하며, 나이 들어 보이게 만들고, 피곤해 보이는 인상을 줄 수 있다.

다크서클 경계부위 위쪽으로 지방이 불룩하게 돌출되었거나 다크서클 경계부위 아래쪽이 함몰되어 주름형태로 보이는 경우 눈 밑의 지방을 재배치해 밝은 눈매로 교정하는 수술이다.

비교적 간단한 수술이지만 수술경험과 술기가 필요한 수술방법으로 결막 안쪽을 통해 수술하기 때문에 흉터 없이 빠른 회복으로 젊어 보이고 인상이 밝아지는 효과를 얻을 수 있는 방법이다.

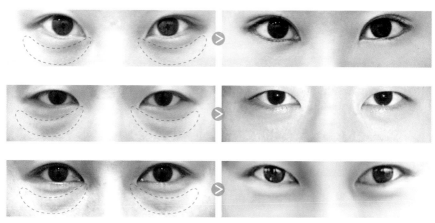

스타 눈밑지방재배치 수술전후

TIP_하안검 / 눈밑지방재배치 수술정보					
수술시간	마취방법	입원여부	실밥제거	회복기간	체류기간
1시간	국소마취	입원없음	5일/제거없음	3~7일	3~7일

01-1 You can be a beauty just by having pretty eyes

Clear, large eyes that attract others' attention

The most common thing couples in love say is, "I fell in love at first sight." In this way, eyes are a window that expresses important emotions, and the eyes of the other person during a first meeting are a very important factor in making a first impression.

Many people have probably experienced the feeling of their heartbeat speeding up and their pupils dilating when they make eye contact with the person they like.

On the other hand, it is not uncommon to feel uncomfortable when encountering a person with scary eyes, and to feel frustrated when faced with a person whose eyes are small and have obscured pupils.

Just because your first impression isn't a favorable one doesn't mean it's bad, but even if it's not love at first sight, leaving a good impression is a way to make the other person like you.

In this way, a person's eyes serve as a window to the other person's mind and are one of the most important factors in giving favorable or unfavorable feelings in first impressions.

| Double eyelid surgery

Double eyelid surgery can be said to be the beginning of plastic surgery and can greatly change one's appearance. With double eyelid surgery tailored to each individual, you can expect prettier eyes with larger, clearer eyes.

Non incisional method

The suture is inserted from the skin into the conjunctiva through a 1 mm long incision in the eyelid skin, and then pulled out through another hole, and this is repeated. This method causes the eye tissue and skin tissue to adhere to each other. This is a method of creating double eyelids according to the designed line.

The Non incisional method is preferred because the surgery time is shorter than the incision method, the swelling is less after surgery, and a natural appearance is achieved within a few days. It does not require a skin incision and is effective for eyes with thin eyelids. However, in people with thick eyelid skin and a lot of fat, the double eyelids often become loose, so the incision method is effective for these people.

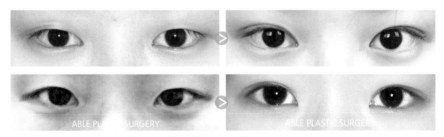

Non incisional method, Before and after double eyelid surgery

The partial incisional method

It is a method that compromises the advantages of the incision method and the non incisional method. This method creates natural double eyelids by minimizing scarring with minimal incisions.

In addition, it is a surgical method that compromises the advantages of the non incisional method and the incisional method, resulting in less swelling and scarring and quicker recovery compared to the incision method. It is used when you want double eyelids with a natural and desired line, thanks to Ably Plastic Surgery's unique know-how, even on thick eyelids that do not loosen easily and have a lot of fat.

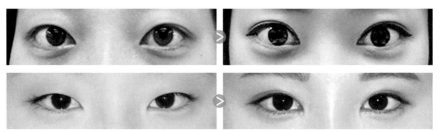

The partial incisional method, Before and after double eyelid surgery

The incision method

Despite the disadvantage that it takes longer to look natural after surgery compared to the burial method, it is a reliable double eyelid surgery method that is most commonly performed on people who have a lot of loose skin or a thick layer of fat.

For patients whose eyes look sleepy during double eyelid surgery, ptosis surgery must also be performed to create more beautiful eyes.

There are two types of incision methods: dynamic and fixed incision methods, which can be selected and used depending on the patient's condition. At Ably Plastic Surgery Clinic, we select and perform surgical methods depending on the patient's condition.

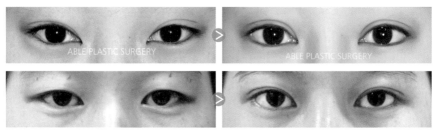

The incision method, Before and after double eyelid surgery

TIP_Double eyelid surgery surgery information						
Surgery time	Anesthetizing method	Hospitalization	Stitch removal	recovery time	length of stay
30 minutes ~1 hour	Local anesthesia	No hospitalization	After 3~6 days	3~7 days	3~7 days

Blepharoptosis surgery

Even if it is not severe ptosis where the eyelids are drooped, if the width between the top and bottom of the eyes is small, the eyes look stuffy and weak.

Ably Plastic Surgery Clinic's crystal Blepharoptosis surgery is a surgery that changes sleepy-looking eyes into wide-open, beautiful eyes.

The surgery is performed by manipulating the levator palpebrae superioris and Müller muscles, which lift the eyelids, and surgery to create double eyelids using an incision method is also performed at the same time.

When performing Blepharoptosis surgery, it is important to match the natural shape of the eyes and harmonize the face so that the eyes are neither too big nor too small.

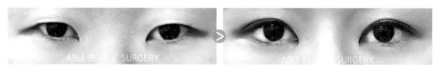

Blepharoptosis surgery,Before and after double eyelid surgery

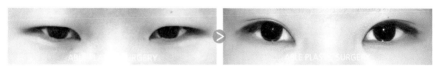

Blepharoptosis surgery,Before and after double eyelid surgery

The asymmetric eyelid correction

A person's face cannot be perfectly symmetrical, and everyone can see that both sides of their eyes are slightly asymmetrical.

However, most people cannot correct their asymmetrical eyes, but in severe cases, correction is necessary.

Differences in the size of the left and right eyes, the shape of the double eyelids, the degree of protrusion of the eyeball, and the shape and width of the orbital bone can cause asymmetric eyes. One of the biggest causes can be said to be determined by the degree of exposure of the pupil depending on the degree to which the eyes are opened.

If there is a problem with the muscles that open the eyes, if the eyelids become asymmetrical after double eyelid surgery, or if a complex type of double eyelid is corrected, ptosis correction and double eyelid incision surgery are performed simultaneously.

Ptosis correction corrects the degree of exposure of the pupils, making the eyes appear larger and creating a prettier double eyelid line.

There is also a method of correcting the eye exposure of one eye with less eye opening depending on the skin condition, and in the case of asymmetry where the double eyelid is only in one eye, the double eyelid can be made the same size through appropriate design before surgery.

However, rather than insisting on performing surgery on only one eye due to asymmetrical eyes, performing surgery on both eyes at the same time, taking into account personal preference, trends, and overall shape, can prevent further asymmetry.

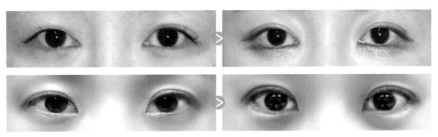

Before and after the asymmetric eyelid correction

TIP_Blepharoptosis correction surgery information					
Surgery time	Anesthetizing method	Hospitalization	Stitch removal	recovery time	length of stay
1 hour	Local anesthesia	No hospitalization	6~7 days later	7 days	7 days

Upper blepharoplasty Eyebrow lift sugery

This is a surgery that solves functional problems caused by sagging eyelids and provides the effect of making you look younger.

Upper blepharoplasty

Upper blepharoplasty When your eyelids sag due to aging, you will look older, your original double eyelids will not be visible, and in severe cases, your eyelids will block your vision. In addition, if the eyebrows are sagging, eyebrow lift surgery can be performed.

A procedure is needed to measure the amount of sagging skin in the eye, remove the upper eyelid skin appropriately, and, if necessary, return it to its original position if the levator palpebrae muscle is separated.

Upper eyelid surgery can enlarge your eyes without wrinkles in the eyelids and give you a fresh, youthful look.

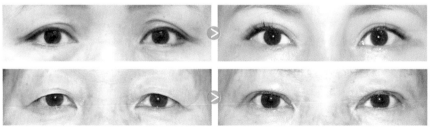

Before and after upper blepharoplasty

The eyebrow lift surgery

Eyebrow lift surgery measures the amount of skin to be removed in consideration of the desired eyelid shape, then makes an incision under the eyebrow, removes the skin and muscle, and pulls up the sagging muscle.

By pulling the skin and muscles upward and fixing them, you get a bright and youthful look.

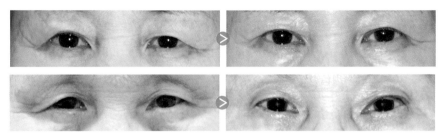

Before and after eyebrow lift surgery

TIP_Upper eyelid / eyebrow lift surgery information					
Surgery time	Anesthetizing method	Hospitalization	Stitch removal	recovery time	length of stay
1 hour	Local anesthesia	No hospitalization	5~7 days later	7 days	7 days

Lower eyelid surgery / Lower eyelid fat relocation

Remove signs of age under your eyes! A surgery that solves not only wrinkles, but also tear troughs, sunken eyes, and dark circles all at once!

Lower eyelid surgery

Sagging lower eyelids cause the membrane surrounding the fat under the eyes to loosen, causing the fat to protrude, causing the area under the eyes to become convex and ridged, making you look older.

If the sagging fat is preserved rather than simply removed and placed under or over the periosteum under the eyes, better results can be obtained than simply removing the fat.

An incision is made near the eyelashes, the protruding fat is used to fill in the furrowed area to make it flat, and the remaining fat and sagging skin are removed.

By pulling the skin and muscles upward, fixing them and suturing them, not only wrinkles but also tear troughs, sunken eyes, and dark circles can all be solved at once.

If the sagging under the eyes is severe, it may be necessary to correct it using a tissue called SOOF.

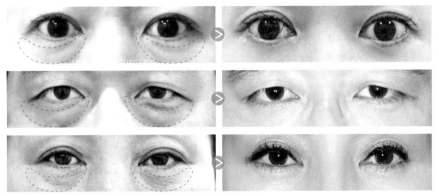

Before and after lower eyelid surgery

Star lower eyelid fat reposition surgery

Fat under the eyes, the cause of an older-looking face.

Dr. Jin-gyu Lee's lower eyelid fat reposition surgery, which has been proven on star celebrities, is a surgery that has recently become known as a plastic surgery that makes celebrities look naturally younger as they gain brighter impressions after lower eyelid fat reposition surgery. This is a surgery that simply removes or relocates the fat under the eyes, which occurs when the membrane surrounding the fat under the eyes becomes loose, through the conjunctiva inside the eye.

Bulging fat under the eyes can cause dark circles and make you look older and tired.

If the fat bulges above the border of the dark circle or the bottom of the border of the dark circle is depressed and looks like a wrinkle, this is a surgery to redistribute the fat under the eyes to brighten the eyes.

Although it is a relatively simple surgery, it requires surgical experience and skills. Because the surgery is performed through the inside of the conjunctiva, it is a method that allows you to look younger and have a brighter impression with quick recovery without scars.

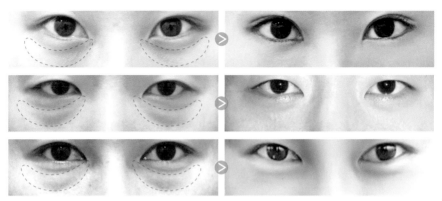

Before and after Lower eyelid fat relocation

TIP_Lower eyelid/lower eyelid fat reposition surgery information					
Surgery time	Anesthetizing method	Hospitalization	Stitch removal	recovery time	length of stay
1 hour	Local anesthesia	No hospitalization	No removal	3~7 days	3~7 days

눈이 커지기 위한 수술(Double eyelid surgery with canthoplasty)
눈재수술(Revision surgery)
중년 눈성형(Middle age eyelid surgery)
눈썹이 낮은 경우(Low eyebrows)

아름다운 눈을 그리다

Drawing Beautiful eyes with Surgery

매력적이게 보이는 눈빛은 다른 사람이 봤을 때 분위기는 물론이고 첫인상을 결정할 수 있는 필수 요소다. 본인의 외모에 대한 개선을 하고자 한다면 먼저 눈의 모양, 크기, 주름 등 눈에 변화를 주는 것이 필요하다.

Attractive eyes are an essential factor that can determine not only your mood but also the first impression when others see you. If you want to improve your appearance, you first need to change the shape, size, and wrinkles of your eyes.

그리다성형외과
Grida plastic surgery

www.gridaprs.com

김현수(Hyun-Soo Kim)

- 성형외과 전문의(Plastic surgery specialist)
- 가톨릭대학교 의과대학 졸업(Graduated from Catholic University School of Medicine)
- 가톨릭대학교 의과대학 성형외과 외래교수 및 자문의
(Adjunct Professor and Consultant of Plastic Surgery, Catholic University College of Medicine)
- 대한미용성형외과학회 정회원(Regular member of the Korean Society of Aesthetic Plastic Surgery)
- 대한성형외과학회 눈성형연구회 정회원
(Regular member of the Oculoplastic Research Society of the Korean Society of Plastic Surgery)

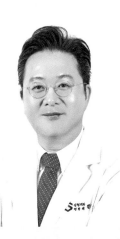

01-2

보다 젊게!
보다 자연스럽게!
성공적 눈 재수술을 위한 조건

눈 재수술 원인과 두번 실패하지 않기 위해서는 정확한 진단 중요

"눈이 커지고 시원해지고 싶다. 짝눈이다."

"이전에 눈 수술을 했는데 마음에 들지 않는다."

"눈이 처졌다. 눈 밑이 튀어나왔다."

"이마에 주름이 많고, 시야를 가린다."

눈 수술을 위해 성형외과를 방문하시는 분들을 상담하다 보면, 대부분 비슷한 이야기를 많이 듣게 된다. 눈 성형의 경우, 본인의 눈꺼풀의 피부의 두께, 피부의 처짐 정도, 눈썹의 높이, 안구의 돌출 정도 등에 필요로 하는 수술이 달라질 수 있으므로 이에 대한 정확한 분석이 우선이다.

재수술의 경우에는 첫 수술과는 다르게 과거에 수술받은 이력과 그로 인한 현재 눈꺼풀의 피부 및 연부조직의 상태에 따라 필요로 하게 되는 수술 및 결과가 달라질 수 있어 충분한 상담 및 진찰을 통해 수술을 계획하는 것이 좋다.

세월의 흐름으로 인한 처짐 등으로 눈 위 혹은 아래를 수술하는 경우, 가장 중요한 점은 인상이 최대한 변하지 않으며, 자연스럽게 처짐을 개선하는 것이라 할 수

있다. 이를 위해서는 단순히 남는 피부를 많이 잘라내는 것이 중요한 것이 아니고, 과하지 않은 적정한 눈꺼풀 피부의 제거 및 이와 동시에 피부 안 쪽의 연부조직 및 지방 등에 대한 조작을 통해 보다 더 젊게 보이는 눈을 만들 수 있다.

┃ 눈이 커지기 위한 수술

대부분의 젊은 사람들의 경우 눈이 커지기 위한 부분이 수술의 첫 번째 목적이 되는 경우가 많다.

눈이 커지기 위한 수술을 할 경우 얼굴 중앙선에서 가까운 속눈썹이 가리지 않고 드러나면서 쌍꺼풀을 만들게 되면 인, 인아웃, 아웃폴드에 관계없이 시원하고 아름다운 눈을 만드는데 도움을 줄 수 있다. 또한 눈가쪽도 트임 수술을 통해 눈꼬리가 좁거나 올라간 모양을 개선할 수 있다.

피부가 처짐이 별로 없으며, 피부가 두껍지 않고, 눈앞머리가 가려 있는 경우 앞트임을 통해서 앞트임을 통해서 앞머리를 노출시키며, 비절개 방법으로 쌍꺼풀을 만들어 시원하고, 또렷해 보이는 눈을 만들 수 있다.

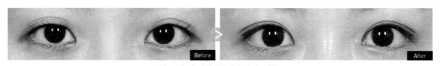

앞트임 비절개 쌍꺼풀 수술전후

비슷한 케이스로, 추가적으로 눈꼬리가 올라가 있는 경우, 듀얼트임(뒷트임, 밑트임)을 통해서 눈이 앞쪽뿐만 아니라 뒤쪽도 시원하고 큰 눈을 만들 수 있다.

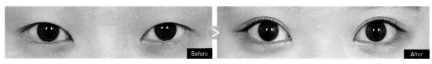

듀얼 트임 쌍꺼풀 수술전후

수술시간	마취방법	입원여부	실밥제거	회복기간	체류기간
1시간	수면 국소마취	입원없음	7일	1주일	1주일

| 눈재수술

재수술의 원인들을 살펴보면 쌍꺼풀 높이가 높거나 낮은 경우, 눈동자가 보이는 크기가 작거나 큰 경우, 양쪽 눈의 비대칭, 모양의 불만족, 기능적으로 불편한 경우들이 있다.

성공적인 수술을 위해서는 이전에 받은 수술에 대한 충분한 정보 및 현재 환자가 기대하는 정도에 대한 의견 교환 및 실제로 가능한 결과에 대한 자세한 설명을 통하여 수술을 준비함으로써 수술에 대한 만족도를 높일 수 있다.

쌍꺼풀 수술 및 앞트임 수술을 하였으나 오른쪽 쌍꺼풀(환자의 오른쪽 눈/왼편 사진)의 두꺼움은 물론 눈 앞쪽 라인 낮고 눈꼬리 쪽의 답답함 등으로 양쪽 비대칭을 이루고 있다. 앞트임 재수술을 통해서 눈 앞머리의 날카로운 각도를 보다 부드럽고, 시원하게 개선하였고, 절개법을 통하여 쌍꺼풀의 비대칭 교정, 눈꼬리 또한 뒤트임과 동시에 눈꼬리를 내려줌으로서 훨씬 부드러운 느낌으로 변모하였다.

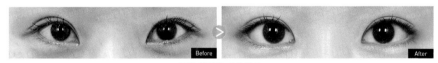

양쪽 비대칭 수술전후

쌍꺼풀 수술을 하였으나 한쪽이 더 낮고 두툼한 느낌이 있어, 절개법으로 눈두덩이를 가볍게 만들고 쌍꺼풀 라인 또한 시원하게 높이면서 비대칭을 맞추었다. 이와 더불어 소위 눈 밑 다크서클에 대하여 결막을 통한 눈 밑 지방 재배치 방법을 통하여 개선하였다.

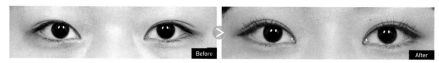

쌍꺼풀 재수술, 눈밑 지방 재배치 수술전후

쌍꺼풀 수술을 하였으나, 눈을 뜨는 근육의 힘이 전체적으로 부족하며, 양쪽 눈의 크기 및 쌍꺼풀의 두께가 다른 소위 '짝눈'인 경우이다. 이 경우에는 오른쪽 눈을 뜨는 힘이 더 약하여 오른쪽 눈이 더 작아 보이며, 보상 작용으로 오른쪽 눈썹을 보다 더 사용하고 이에 따라 쌍꺼풀은 더 두꺼워 보인다. 다만 눈꺼풀의 두께가 두껍지 않아 절개를 하지 않고 비절개를 통한 방법으로 눈 뜨는 힘을 개선하여 맞추어 주면, 비교적 간단한 방법으로 좋은 결과를 기대할 수 있다.

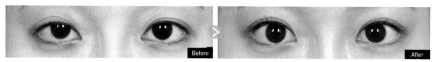

쌍꺼풀의 두께가 다른 짝눈, 수술전후

쌍꺼풀 수술을 하였으나, 한쪽 눈 위에 겹주름이 잡히며, 눈이 더 작아 보이고, 양쪽 눈 위에 눈 지방의 부족으로 인해 꺼짐이 관찰된다. 오른쪽 눈이 더 심하지만, 양쪽 눈 모두 눈을 뜨는 근육인 안검거근의 힘을 보강하였으며, 눈 지방의 부족으로 눈꺼풀이 꺼지고 이로 인한 눈을 뜨는 게 불편해지는 것을 개선하기 위하여 지방이식을 시행하였다. 수술 후 보기에도 또렷해 보이지만, 눈을 뜨는 게 매우 편해진 것을 관찰할 수 있었다.

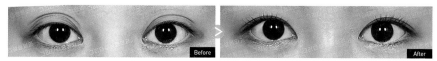

양쪽 눈위, 지방의 부족으로 인해 꺼짐 수술전후

TIP_눈 재수술정보

수술시간	마취방법	입원여부	실밥제거	회복기간	체류기간
1시간	수면 국소마취	입원없음	7일	1주일	1주일

중년 눈성형

세월이 흐르면 사람의 얼굴은 변한다. 눈꺼풀이 처지게 되면 쌍꺼풀 라인이 낮아지고, 눈 크기도 작아 보이게 된다.

인상이 변하지 않으면서, 인위적이지 않고, 자연스럽게 젊어지게 하는 게 중요하다. 필요에 따라 상안검수술, 눈썹하거상술, 하안검 수술 중에 적절한 방법을 선택한다.

윗 눈꺼풀의 피부가 얇으며 처짐이 심하지 않은 경우에는 간단히 피부를 제거하고 쌍꺼풀 라인을 올려 줌으로서 보다 젊어 보이는 눈매를 만들 수 있다.

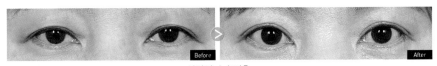

상안검 수술전후

눈밑 피부가 처지고, 눈밑 지방이 많이 튀어나온 경우로, 첫 번째로 개선해야 할 목표는 튀어 나온 눈밑 지방 및 지방 아래로 깊게 골이 진 부분이 되겠다. 단순히 피부를 자르고 지방을 많이 제거하는 방법으로 수술을 하는 것보다는, 전체적으로 눈밑 부위의 볼륨을 유지하면서, 볼륨을 위쪽으로 끌어올려 주며(거상) 수술을 해주는 것이 더욱 젊어 보이는 눈밑을 만들어 준다.

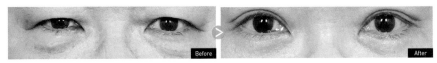

하안검 수술전후

눈 위아래의 처짐이 있으며, 특히 눈가 쪽의 처짐이 많고, 눈꺼풀 위쪽의 꺼짐, 눈밑 지방의 양은 많지 않아 보이나, 그 아래의 골이 강하게 보이는 경우이다. 우선 눈꺼풀 윗부분의 꺼진 부분을 본인의 원래 눈 지방을 내려서 개선함으로써 더욱 젊어 보이는 인상으로 변하며, 눈가 쪽 처진 피부의 경우 충분히 절제하여, 짓무름 등의 개선 및 표정을 지을 때에도 좋은 결과를 기대할 수 있다. 눈 밑의 경우, 눈 밑 지방 제거술이 아닌 지방을 재배치하여 하안검 수술을 함으로서 눈 밑의 볼륨을 유지하며 골진 부분을 개선하였다.

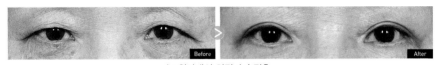

눈 위아래의 처짐 수술전후

TIP_중년 눈성형 수술정보					
수술시간	마취방법	입원여부	실밥제거	회복기간	체류기간
1시간	수면 국소마취	입원없음	7일	1주일	1주일

| 눈썹이 낮은 경우

이마와 눈썹의 위치가 낮은 경우에는 노화와 맞물려 더욱 답답한 인상을 줄 수 있는 만큼 이마거상술이 대안이 될 수 있다.

눈썹이 낮은 경우, 과거에는 두피를 횡으로 가로지르는 절개선을 넣어 수술을 하였으나, 최근에는 대부분의 경우 헤어라인 안쪽에 작은 구멍을 3~5군데 만들어 내시경을 활용한 이마거상술(눈썹거상술)을 활용하여 개선을 하고 있다. 눈썹이 낮은 경우, 이에 대한 개선 없이 원인을 잘 못 파악하여 과하게 눈꺼풀 피부를 제거하게 되면 처짐은 개선되나, 이마 주름을 만들 필요가 없어지며 오히려 눈썹의 위치가 내려가 부자연스러운 인상으로 변하게 된다.

이러한 경우에는 일반적으로 상담을 올 때, 눈 부위만 수술을 마음속으로 계획하고 오더라도 충분한 상담을 통해 수술의 범위를 넓혀 이마거상술과 눈 수술을 함께 하는 것이 훨씬 더 좋은 결과를 얻게 되는 경우가 많다.

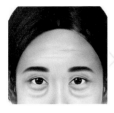
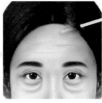
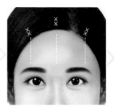
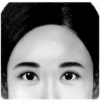

헤어라인 위쪽 두피에
1cm 정도의 작은 세로 절개

Full HD 내시경을 통해 신경과
혈관을 섬세하고 정확하게 박리

근육과 근막을 조절, 고정한 후
눈썹이나 이마 모양을 조절

수술 후

중년의 여성뿐만 아니라, 젊은 여성분들의 경우에도 눈썹의 위치가 낮은 경우가 있다. 내시경 이마거상술의 경우, 보통 중년들이 많이 하지만, 실제로 눈썹이 낮게 위치하는 경우가 중년 여성들이 많아서 중년 여성들이 수술을 받는 빈도 또한 높은 것이지, 젊은 경우에도 눈썹의 위치가 낮은 경우에는 수술의 적응증이 된다.

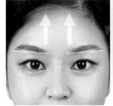
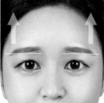
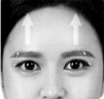
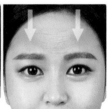

눈썹 위치와 각도 조절로
사나워 보이거나
피곤해 보이는 인상 개선

눈썹, 눈꺼풀 처짐에 의해
작고 답답해 보이는
눈매를 교정

눈썹뼈와 눈의 거리가 가까워
여색한 눈매를 교정

미간과 이마의 주름 해결로
동안 얼굴로 개선

젊은 여성의 경우로 사진상으로는 눈썹이 높아보이나, 실제로는 이마근육을 통하여 눈썹을 올리고 있는 것으로, 쌍꺼풀 수술을 할 경우 눈썹이 내려와 답답한 인상이 될 수 있다. 쌍꺼풀 수술과 이마거상술을 함께 시행함으로서 수술 전에 비해 시원하면서도 커진 눈을 관찰할 수 있다.

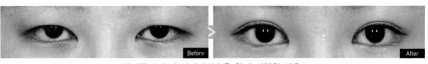

쌍꺼풀 수술과 이마거상술을 함께 시행한 경우

눈썹이 많이 낮으며, 눈꺼풀이 두꺼우면서 처짐이 있으며, 비대칭이 있다. 마찬가지로 이마 근육을 통하여 눈썹을 들어 올리고 있는게 사진상으로 관찰된다. 내시경을 통한 이마거상술을 통하여 눈썹의 위치가 내려가지 않게 올려줌과 동시에 상안검 수술을 통하여 두툼하던 눈꺼풀의 제거 및 쌍꺼풀 라인을 만들어 줌으로 젊어 보이는 눈으로 만들었다.

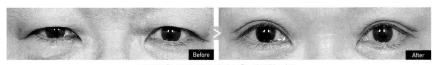

내시경을 통한 이마거상술을 시행한 경우

TIP_이마거상수술정보

수술시간	마취방법	입원여부	실밥제거	회복기간	체류기간
1시간	수면 국소마취	입원없음	10일	10일	10일

01-2 Drawing(GRIDA) beautiful eyes

Accurate diagnosis is important to understand the causes of revision surgery and to failure second time

When consulting with people who visit plastic surgery clinics for eye surgery, most of them say similar stories. In the case of eye plastic surgery, the required surgery may vary depending on the thickness of the eyelid skin, the degree of skin sagging, the height of the eyebrows, and the degree of protrusion of the eyeball, so an accurate analysis is necessary.

In the case of revision surgery, unlike the first surgery, the required surgery and results may vary depending on the previous surgical history and the resulting condition of the skin and soft tissue of the eyelid, so it is recommended to plan the surgery through sufficient consultation and examination.

When undergoing surgery above or below the eyes due to sagging due to age, the most important thing is to keep the impression as unchanged as possible and improve the sagging naturally. For this purpose, it is important not to simply cut off a lot of excess skin, but rather, remove an appropriate amount of eyelid skin and at the same time manipulate the soft tissue and fat inside the skin to create younger-looking eyes.

| For beautiful and bigger eyes

For most young people, enlarging the eyes is often the first goal of surgery. Double eyelid surgery with epicanthoplasty

When undergoing surgery to enlarge the eyes, creating double eyelids by exposing the eyelashes close to the center line of the face without covering them can help create cool and beautiful eyes regardless of whether they are in, in, or out fold. Additionally, the narrow or raised shape of the eye corners can be improved through canthoplasty.

If the skin is not thick, non-incisional blepharoplasty with medial epicanthoplasty is helpful to make a bigger looking eye.

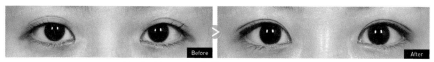

Non-incision method with medical canthoplasty

Similarly, if you have an additional upturned corner of the eye, lateral canthoplasty can be used to create a bigger looking eye.

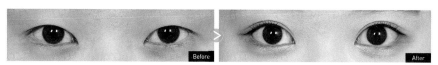

Double eyelid surgery surgery lateral canthoplasty

TIP_For beautiful and bigger eyes, surgery information					
Surgery time	Anesthetizing method	Hospitalization	Stitch removal	Recovery time	Length of stay
1 hour	sleep, Local anesthesia	No hospitalization	7 days	7days	7days

Revision surgery

Looking at the causes of reoperation, there are cases where the double eyelid height is high or low, the visible size of the iris is small or large, asymmetry of both eyes, dissatisfaction with the shape, and functional discomfort.

For a successful surgery, satisfaction with the surgery can be increased by preparing for the surgery through sufficient information about the previous surgery, exchanging opinions about the patient's current expectations, and providing detailed explanations about the actual possible results.

Steep angle on medial epicanthus, asymmetry in both folds, high fold on right side(the patient's right eye, left in the photo), low medial fold, and a steep angle at the lateral corner of the eye is noted. Through the revisional medial epicanthoplasty, the sharp angle of the front of the eye was softened, and the asymmetry of the eyelids was corrected through the incision method, and the corner of the eye was also lowered with canthoplasty at the same time resulting in a much softer look.

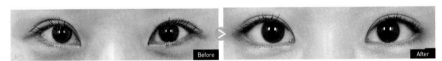

Asymmetry revision with canthoplasty

She had previous dobule eyelid sugery, but low uneven fold and puffy eyelid is still seen. With incision method, the fold was evenly raised, and the puffy eyelid was corrected with fat excision. Under-eye dark circles were improved through the method of repositiong the under-eye fat through the conjunctiva.

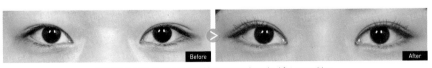

Double eyelid reoperation with transconjunctival fat reposition

Double eyelid surgery has been performed, but there is an overlapping crease over right eye, the eye appears smaller, The strength of the levator palpebrae, the muscle that opens the eyes was strengthened, and fat grafting was performed to improve the sunken of the eyelids due to the lack of eye fat and the discomfort while opening the eyes.

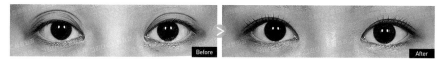

Sunken eyelid fat graft

If you have undergone double eyelid surgery, but are dissatisfied with the shape of the eyelid, you can improve it more naturally by revision surgery. The shape of the fold looks more natural by removing puffiness of the eyelid that causes the eyelid to loosen, and shape of medial epicanthus is improved with revisional epicanthoplasty.

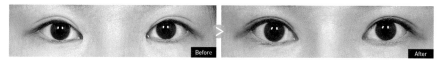

Fold Lowering surgery

In this case, the strength to open the right eye is weaker, making the right eye appear smaller. As a compensation, the right eyebrow is used more and the fold is higher. If your eyelids are thin enough, you may be able to improve eye opening force by using a non-incision method to adjust them, which is relatively simple and can yield good results.

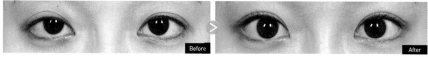

Blepharoplasty surgery

The patient had double eyelid surgery and medial epicanthoplasty, but there was a slight overexposure of medial canthus and uneven high fold. Epicanthus restoration was performed to create a softer appearance and double fold is lowered for more natural and refined look.

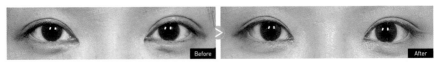

Epicanthus restoration surgery

TIP_Revision surgery, surgery information					
Surgery time	Anesthetizing method	Hospitalization	Stitch removal	Recovery time	Length of stay
1 hour	sleep, Local anesthesia	No hospitalization	7 days	7days	7days

| Middle age eyelid surgery

It is important to rejuvenate naturally, not artificially. Depending on your needs, upper blepharoplasty, upper lid lift, and lower eyelid surgery can be performed.

If the skin on the upper eyelid is thin and the sagging is not severe, we can create a more youthful appearance by simply removing the skin with upper blepharoplasty.

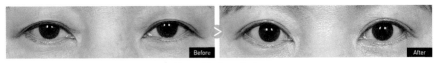

Upper blepharoplasty

If the lower eyelid is sagging and there is a lot of protruding fat, the first target for improvement will be the protruding under-eye fat and the deep hollows beneath the fat.

Rather than simply removing fat only, surgery that maintains the volume of the under-eye, while lifting the volume upward (elevation) will create a more youthful appearance. If you are unhappy with your under-eye fat and only remove it, it may be a successful surgery if the goal is to remove fat, but in this case, you may end up with a hollow appearance, which makes you look older. A younger-looking under-eye area can only be achieved with a lower blepharoplasty that maintains the volume with improvement of the protruded fat and the hollow beneath it. Also anchoring the soft tissues and orbicularis oculi muscles upward can created more youthful appearance.

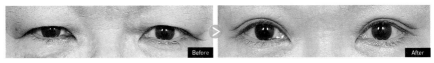

Lower blepharoplasty

There is sagging above and below the eyes, especially in the corners of the eyes, drooping of the upper eyelids. The amount of under-eye fat does not seem to be much, but the hollows underneath are visible. First of all, the upper eyelid hollowness can be improved by lowering the patient's original eye fat to create a more youthful appearance, and sagging skin at the corners will be removed. In the case of the lower eyelid, we performed lower blepharoplasty by relocating the fat rather than removing it, so that the volume of the lower eyelid is maintained and the hollowness is improved.

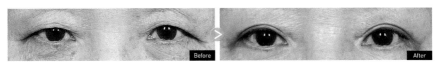

Upper and lower blepharoplasty

TIP_Middle age eyelid surgery, surgery information					
Surgery time	Anesthetizing method	Hospitalization	Stitch removal	Recovery time	Length of stay
1 hour	sleep, Local anesthesia	No hospitalization	7 days	7days	7days

| Low eyebrows

If the position of the eyebrows are low, forehead lift surgery may be an alternative.

In the case of low eyebrows, in the past, surgery was performed by making an incision horizontally across the scalp, but recently, in most cases, forehead lift surgery (=eyebrow lift surgery) using an endoscope is performed by making 3-5 small holes inside the hairline. We are using it to make improvements.

In the case of low eyebrows, if the cause is incorrectly identified and excessive eyelid skin is removed, there will be no need to create forehead wrinkles, and the position of the eyebrows will go down, creating an unnatural look.

In these cases, when you come for a consultation, even if you only plan to have surgery on the eye area, you often get much better results by expanding the scope of the surgery through sufficient consultation and performing forehead lift surgery and eye surgery together.

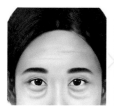 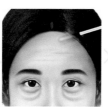 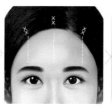 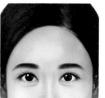

On the scalp above the hairline A small vertical incision of about 1 cm

Meticulous disection with full HD endoscope

After adjusting and fixing the muscles and fascia, adjust the shape of the eyebrows or forehead

After surgery

Not only middle-aged women, but also young women sometimes have low eyebrows. In the case of endoscopic forehead lift surgery, it is usually performed on middle-aged people, but in fact, many middle-aged women have low eyebrows, so middle-aged women are more likely to undergo surgery.

Even in young people, if the eyebrows are low, surgery is recommended. It becomes an indication.

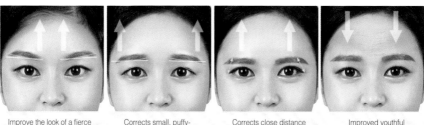

| Improve the look of a fierce or tired look by adjusting the position and angle of the eyebrows | Corrects small, puffy-looking eyes caused by sagging eyebrows and eyelids | Corrects close distance between the eyebrow and the eyes. | Improved youthful appearance by resolving wrinkles between the eyebrows and forehead |

In the case of young women, the eyebrows may look high in photos, but they are actually raised through the forehead muscles, and when the eyelid surgery is performed, the eyebrows may be lowered, creating a stuffy look. By performing double eyelid surgery and forehead lift together, you can observe the eyes that are bigger and larger than before the surgery.

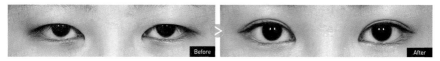

Forehead lift with blepharoplasty

In the case of endoscopic forehead elevation alone, the eyebrows are elevated, the horizontal wrinkles on the nasal bridge are stretched, and the hidden eyelids are exposed, giving a much younger and natural appearance.

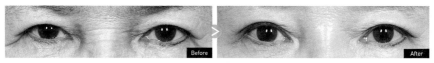

Forehead lift only

The eyebrows are much lower, the eyelids are thicker and drooping, and there is asymmetry, the eyebrows are lifted by the forehead muscles. Through endoscopic forehead lift, the eyebrows were raised and at the same time, the upper eyelid surgery was performed to remove the puffy eyelids and create a double eyelid line to create a younger-looking eye.

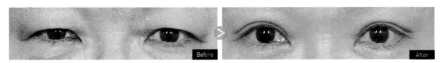
Upper blepharoplasty with forehead lift

In the case of endoscopic forehead lift alone, wrinkles on the nasal bridge and the eyes were improved, and the distance between the eyes and eyebrows was increased to reveal the hidden double eyelids, creating a natural and youthful appearance.

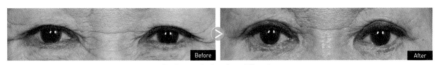
Endoscopic forehead lift only

As you can see, when it comes to eyelid and periocular surgery, the type of surgery you need will depend on your current eye condition.

TIP_Low eyebrows surgery information

Surgery time	Anesthetizing method	Hospitalization	Stitch removal	Recovery time	Length of stay
1 hour	sleep, Local anesthesia	No hospitalization	7~10 days	2 weeks	10~14 days

코성형(Rhinoplasty)
코의 유형에 따른 코수술 방법(Surgical techniques according to the pattern of nose)
코재수술(Revisional rhinoplasty)

얼굴이라는 숲 속에 자연스럽게 잘 어울리는 나무인 코

A naturally harmonious tree called nose in the forest called face

이목구비 등 얼굴 전체의 균형을 고려하지 않고 무리하게 진행하는 코수술의 결과는 불만족으로 이어지고, 코재수술로 이어지는 경우가 허다하다.

The results of rhinoplasty performed without considering the balance of the entire face, including other facial features, often lead to dissatisfaction and finally revisional rhinoplasty.

더플러스성형외과
THE PLUS Plastic Surgery

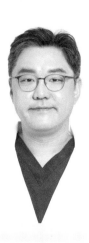

www.theplusnose.com

김택균(Taek-Kyun Kim)

• 성형외과 전문의 / 의학박사(Board certified Plastic Surgeon, MD, PhD)
• 현)더플러스성형외과 대표원장(Director of THE PLUS Plastic Surgery, Seoul, Korea)
대한성형외과학회 정회원(Active Member, Korean Society of Plastic and Reconstructive Surgeons(KPRS))
대한성형외과학회 코성형연구회 학술위원(Scientific Member, Korean Society of Rhinoplasty Surgeons)
• 미국성형외과학회 정회원(Active Member, American Society of Plastic Surgeons(ASPS))
• Exchange-clerkship at Mass. Eye&Ear Infirmary (MEEI), Harvard Medical School(Boston, USA)

02-1 코 성형의 메가 트렌드 코 재수술

코성형수술, 변화의 바람

한국의 성형수술은 2000년대에 전성기를 맞이하며, 아시아의 주변국에 큰 위상을 알렸다. 2020년대에는 K-pop의 활약에 힘입어 전 세계적으로 그 영향력을 뻗기에 이르렀다. 1980년대 미국 할리우드 영화의 인기에 힘입어 한국인들이 서양인의 코 모양에 열광했던 것과 같이 여러 나라의 환자들이 한국을 방문해서 한국 아이돌 가수의 코 모양을 갖고 싶어 하는 것도 어렵지 않게 볼 수 있다. 이와 더불어 일본과 태국을 비롯한 여러 동남아 국가의 성형외과 의사들도 한국의 코성형을 배우기 위해서 문의 및 방문하는 경우가 늘고 있다.

국내 환자들의 코 성형에 대한 취향과 트렌드도 십수 년간에 걸쳐 변화되어 가는 추세이다. 예를 들어 예전에는 콧대와 코끝을 높이는 데 치중했다면, 최근에는 조금은 더 자연스럽고 얼굴과 조화로운 코성형을 추구하는 추세이다. 또한 코성형수술에 사용되는 재료가 더욱 다양화되고, 코의 모양뿐만 아니라 기능적인 측면도 고려하는 환자가 늘고 있다. 이러한 변화는 코성형수술 이후 재수술이라는 영역을 확대해 가고 있다. 현재 코성형수술의 상당수는 코재수술이 차지하고 있다. 인구 구조의 변화 및 환자들의 취향 변화는 이러한 코재수술 시장을 키워가고 있으며, 차후에는 코성형수술의 주축이 될 것이라 믿어 의심치 않는다. 따라서 필자는 코재수술에 대한 내용에도 비중을 두고 독자들이 쉽게 이해할 수 있도록 기술하도록 하겠다.

수술 전 상담

코성형수술의 첫 번째 단계는 환자와 의사와의 만남이다. 상담이라고 불리는 이 단계는 환자가 의사를 믿고 수술하기로 선택하게 되는 가장 중요한 과정이며, 집도 의사는 단시간 내에 환자가 원하는 것을 알아내고, 그에 대해 설명하며, 설득하여 수술로 진행시키는 일련의 과정이다. 아무리 좋은 수술기술이 있더라도 환자가 수술하기로 동의하지 않는다면 무슨 소용이 있겠는가? 이때 중요한 것이 환자와 비슷한 유형의 케이스 전후 사진일 것이다. 하지만, 얼굴 전체의 이미지나 구조가 다른데 코만 예쁘다고 한들 아름다운 얼굴을 완성할 수는 없을 것이다.

| 코성형

얼굴에서 성형수술이 많이 이뤄지는 대표적인 부위가 눈과 코다. 이 중에서 코는 얼굴의 중앙부에 위치, 얼굴의 전체적인 인상에 큰 영향을 미치는 부위다.

1. 절개(Incision)

2. 연골채취(Harvest Cartilage)

귀연골(Ear)　비중격연골(Septum)　늑연골(Rip)

3. 코끝수술(Tip-plasty)

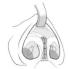

비주연골 이식
(Columellar strut graft)　비연골묶기
(Suture technique)

코끝연골이식
(Tip only graft)

4. 비골절골(Osteotomy)

5. 콧대수술(Dorsum)

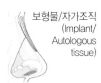

보형물/자가조직
(Implant/
Autologous
tissue)

6. 콧볼축소(Alar base reduction)

코성형수술을 먼저 부위별로 나눠본다면 미용적 측면을 담당하는 코끝, 콧대, 코뼈, 콧볼이 있으며, 기능적인 측면을 담당하는 비중격, 하비갑개, 상악동이 있다.

각 부위에 대한 수술방법을 간단히 살펴보면, 코끝은 비익(콧날개) 연골(물렁뼈)의 모양을 봉합사로 묶거나 귀연골, 비중격연골, 늑연골 등의 연골을 채취해서 필요한 모양으로 조각하여 이식해 주는 방법으로 모양을 개선하게 된다. 콧대는 우리가 익히 잘 알고 있는 실리콘 보형물이나, 고어텍스 보형물, 기증진피, 또는 늑연골, 진피지방, 두피근막 등의 자가(본인)조직을 콧대 피부아래 넣어서 콧대를 높여주게 된다. 코뼈는 절골(뼈를 자르는) 과정을 통해서 코뼈의 위치와 너비를 변화시키게 되고, 콧볼은 넓은 경우 피부를 절제하고 봉합사로 양측을 묶어서 좁히는 방식으로 진행된다.

다음으로 비중격이 심하게 휘어있는 비중격만곡증으로 비호흡(코로 숨쉬기)이 힘든 경우 휘어있는 연골과 뼈 부위를 제거하고 남아있는 부분을 강화시킨다. 하비갑개는 비중격과 함께 비호흡에 중요한 부위로 비중격만곡증과 동반되어 커지게 되면 비후성 하비갑개, 일반적으로 비염이라고 불리게 되어 수술이 필요하게 된다. 마지막으로 이러한 비염이 지속되면, 코 옆에 상악동이라고 불리는 공간에 염증이 발생하게 되며(축농증), 약물적 또는 수술적 치료가 필요하게 된다.

코의 유형에 따른 코수술 방법

부위별 코성형수술을 이해하였다면, 우리가 일반적으로 언급하는 유형별 코성형수술, 즉 낮은코, 매부리코, 휜코, 복코 등에 대한 코성형수술도 쉽게 이해할 수 있다.

01 낮은코

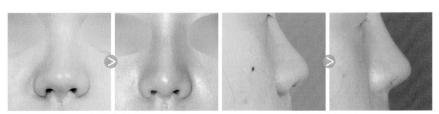

코성형 수술전후   코성형 수술전후

낮은코는 주로 콧대가 낮은 것을 이야기하지만, 대부분 코끝도 함께 낮고 작은 경우가 많다. 한국인을 포함한 동양인에서 가장 흔한 유형이다. 앞서 언급한 코끝과 콧대 수술이 필요하며, 코뼈나 콧볼이 넓다면 절골이나 콧볼축소를 함께 시행한다.

02 매부리코

매부리코는 코의 상부 1/3 지점의 코뼈와 연골이 만나는 부분이 튀어나와 코끝이 매의 부리를 닮았다고 해서 붙여진 이름이다. 이 경우에는 콧대가 발달하여 있는 경우 그냥 매부리 부분을 다듬거나 잘라내는 것만으로도 좋아질 수 있지만, 대부분의 경우에는 코끝을 함께 높여줘야 더 나은 모양을 얻을 수 있다. 또한 매부리 윗쪽 미간 부위가 낮다면 그 부위에 연골이나 기증진피 등을 넣어주거나, 실리콘 등으로 전체 콧대를 높여줄 수도 있다.

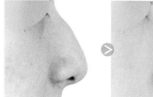
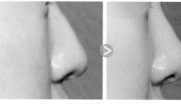

매부리코 수술전후   매부리코 수술전후

03 휜코

휜코는 선천적인 경우 또는 외상 등으로 인한 후천적 경우가 있다. 대부분의 경우에는 코뼈와 비중격이 함께 휘어있는 경우가 흔하므로 코뼈절골과 비중격만곡증 교정이 함께 이루어지는 경우가 많다. 코끝의 경우에도 콧대와 함께 휘어져 있어

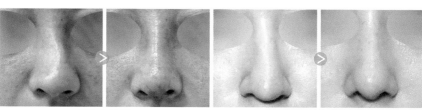

휜코 수술전후   휜코 수술전후

코끝 수술 또한 필요한 경우가 많다. 휜코의 경우에는 얼굴의 전체적 축과도 함께 생각해 봐야 하는데, 코만 너무 바르게 하면 오히려 턱이 휘어 보이는 경우도 있으니 전체적인 균형에 대한 고려도 필요하다.

최근에는 3D 프린팅 기술의 발전으로 의료기기에도 많은 성과를 보이면서 2020년부터는 환자의 CT 데이터를 기반으로 한 3D 프린팅 실리콘 보형물이 사용가능하게 되었다. 이로 인

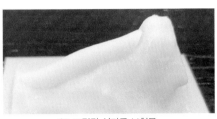
3D 프린팅 실리콘 보형물

해 수술 시간의 단축과 함께 개개인의 코에 맞춤형 보형물 사용으로 염증 가능성을 낮추고 경한 매부리코나 휜코의 경우에는 매부리 부분 절제나 코뼈 절골을 하지 않고도 교정이 가능하게 되어 회복 기간 또한 단축하는 효과 내고 있다.

04 복코

복코는 주로 코끝이 뭉툭한 경우를 일컫는 경우가 많으며, 서양인과는 달리 연골이 크기보다는 피부가 두꺼운 경우가 흔하다. 따라서 이에 대한 교정은 코끝 연골을 얇게 조작하는 것뿐만 아니라 코의 피부를 얇게 만드는 과정도 필요하다.

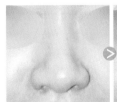
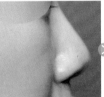
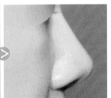

복코 수술전후   복코 수술전후

| **TIP**_코성형 수술정보 | | | | |
수술시간	마취방법	입원여부	회복기간	체류기간
1~1시간 30분	국소 및 수면마취	필요없음	2주일	10일

코재수술

코재수술의 경우는 크게 두 가지 원인으로 나눠진다. 단순히 미용적으로 또는 기능적으로 더 나은 개선을 원하는 경우와 여러 가지 복합적인 문제를 동반하는 경우이다.

미용적인 측면에서 재수술을 고려하는 경우에는 보형물이 휘어서 콧대가 휘었다든지, 코끝에 이식한 연골이 약해지면서 코끝이 아래로 떨어져 보인다든지, 비중격 연골 채취 이후에 비중격이 휘면서 하비갑개가 커져 한쪽 코로 숨쉬기가 힘들다든지 하는 케이스이다.

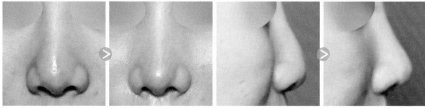

코 재수술 전후   코 재수술 전후

반면 기능 및 복합적인 문제로 인해 재수술을 고려하는 경우다. 이 경우에는 상당수의 경우 염증이 발생하여 만성적으로 피부의 구축을 일으켜 코끝이 들려 보이고 코가 전체적으로 변형되는 케이스이다. 그 이외에도 보형물이 피부나 점막을 뚫고 나오는 경우 등도 있다.

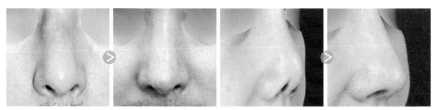

코 재수술 전후   코 재수술 전후

코재수술 시 고려해야 할 점들

코재수술의 경우에는 수술 자체도 첫 수술과 다르지만, 그 이전에 이루어지는 상담 및 검사도 더 신경을 써야 한다. 환자들이 이전수술의 결과로 인해 추가적인 수술에 대한 두려움이 많기에 질문 또한 더 많고 복잡한 경우가 많다. 충분한 상담

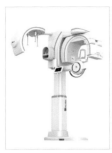 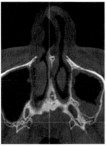 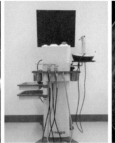 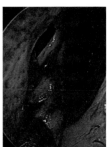

| CT | CT 소견 | 내시경 | 내시경 소견 |

으로 신체적인 부분뿐만 아니라 심리적인 부분까지 환자가 원하는 바를 확실하게 파악하는 것이 중요하다.

일반적으로 많이 사용하는 귀연골이나 비중격연골이 없는 경우도 흔하고, 피부 상태가 좋지 않아 실리콘 보형물 등을 사용할 수 없어 자가조직을 사용해야 하는 경우 또한 허다하다. 코재수술을 수회 내지 10회 정도 했던 환자들의 경우에는 더 더욱 그러하다. 따라서 수술 전에 시행해야 할 검사 또한 놓치지 않아야 한다. CT 와 비내시경 검사가 바로 그것이다. 코안의 상태를 100% 다 알려주지는 못하지만, 보형물의 크기, 위치와 상태, 비중격 천공이나 유착 여부, 비염이나 상악동염(축농 증) 등의 여부를 미리 알 수 있다. 불확실성의 측면에서 코재수술은 코성형수술과 는 또 다른 장르의 수술이라고 할 수 있다.

TIP_코재수술 정보

수술시간	마취방법	입원여부	회복기간	체류기간
2~3시간	국소 및 수면 또는 전신마취	필요없음	2주	10일

최후의 보루인 복합조직이식술과 이마피판술

코성형 수술과 코재수술이 보편화되면서 코수술의 횟수가 잦아져서 코의 상태가 최악으로 치닫게 되면, 코 연골의 문제뿐만 아니라 코 피부의 문제가 더욱 심각해 진다. 사실 코 연골이 약해지거나 염증으로 인해 흡수되더라도 늑연골 등을 채취

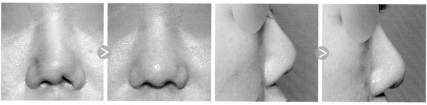

코성형수술전후   코성형수술전후

해서 그 역할을 대신할 수 있게 할 수 있지만, 피부의 경우, 특히 비주(콧기둥) 부위의 피부에 결손이 생기면 재건하는 것은 쉽지 않다. 피부와 연골을 함께 이식하는 복합조직이식술 또는 이마의 피부를 가져오는 이마피판술 등의 방법만이 최후의 보루가 된다. 복합조직이식술의 경우 성공률이 낮고 성공하더라도 흡수율이 높으며, 이마피판술의 경우 회복 과정이 오래 걸리고 이마에 커다란 흉터를 남기게 된다. 따라서 이러한 문제가 생기지 않도록 코 첫 수술이나 재수술에서 결과에 대해 너무 큰 욕심을 부리지 않는 것을 추천한다. 이러한 문제가 생기는 경우는 대부분의 경우 환자나 수술자의 과도한 욕심에서 기인하는 경우가 흔하기 때문이다.

코 수술 후 치료 및 관리

코 수술 후 관리 또한 코성형수술 및 코재수술에서 중요한 단계라고 할 수 있다. 먼저 수술 직후에 드레싱 과정에서 코피가 나는 것을 방지하기 위해 코를 솜으로 막고 하루 정도 후에 제거한다. 또한 피부 테이프와 부목을 하게 되는데, 이는 붓기를 최소화하고 외부로부터 코를 보호하는 역할을 하게 된다. 통상적으로 5일가량을 적용하게 되고, 비주의 실밥을 함께 제거한다. 수술 10일 후에는 코안과 연골이나 진피지방, 두피근막 등을 채취한 부위의 실밥을 제거하며 일단락된다. 수술 후 1, 3, 6개월 정도의 정기 경과를 관찰하며 필요시 흉터 주사나 레이저 관리 등을 시행한다. 일반적으로 코성형수술 후, 2주 정도라면 멍과 큰 붓기는 빠지게 되지만, 붓기는 오랜 기간에 걸쳐 빠지게 된다. 통상적으로 수술 후 1개월째 70%, 3개월째 90%, 6개월째 거의 100%의 붓기가 빠지게 된다고 설명하지만, 코재수술의 경우 이보다 2배 정도의 기간이 소요된다.

02-1 Megatrends in Rhinoplasty Revisional Rhinoplasty

Wind of Change in Rhinoplasty

Korea's plastic surgery industry boomed in the 2000s, positioning the country as a leading destination for cosmetic procedures in Asia. By the 2020s, the global popularity of K-pop further propelled its influence. Many international patients now flock to Korea, inspired by the facial features of Korean idols, reminiscent of the 1980s when Koreans admired Western nasal shapes popularized by Hollywood. Additionally, many plastic surgeons from Japan, Thailand, and other Southeast Asian nations seek to learn Korean rhinoplasty techniques.

Tastes and trends in rhinoplasty among domestic patients have evolved over the past decade. While past preferences leaned towards higher nose bridges and more pronounced tips, current trends favor natural-looking results that harmonize with facial features. The materials and techniques have diversified, with patients considering both aesthetics and functionality. This shift has also widened the scope for revisional surgery following rhinoplasty.

Currently, revisional rhinoplasty constitutes a significant portion of all rhinoplasty surgeries. Changes in demographic structures and evolving patient preferences are enlarging the market for revisional rhinoplasties. It's clear that revisional rhinoplasty will play a dominant role in the future, so this article aims to provide a comprehensive overview for readers.

Preoperative Consultation

The initial consultation between the patient and surgeon is crucial. It fosters trust and sets the stage for the upcoming surgery. During this meeting, the surgeon gauges the patient's desires, providing explanations and guidance. Surgical success is contingent on mutual understanding and agreement. Before-and-after photos can help, but individual facial structures differ, so achieving beauty isn't solely about a perfect nose.

| Rhinoplasty

This is a surgery to improve or change the tip of the nose and is performed when the shape, size, or asymmetry of the tip of the nose is to be corrected. Since each individual's facial structure and desired results are different, it must be customized and planned with this in mind.

Breaking down the procedure, rhinoplasty focuses on cosmetic aspects like the nasal tip, bridge, nasal bone and alar base, as well as functional areas like the nasal septum, inferior turbinate, and maxillary sinuses.

Various surgical techniques are used to reshape, augment, or improve functionality. Looking briefly at the surgical method for each part, for the nasal tip, the shape of the alar cartilage is tied with sutures, or cartilage such as ear cartilage, septal cartilage, and costal cartilage is harvested, sculpted into the necessary shape, and then grafted to improve the shape. The nasal bridge is raised by placing well-known Silicone implants (SOFTXIL), Gore-Tex implants, donated dermis, or autologous tissues such as costal cartilage, dermal fat, and temporal fascia under the skin of nasal bridge. The position and width of the nasal bone are changed through the osteotomy on the nasal bone, and if the alar base is wide, the alar skin is excised and then both sides are tied with cinching sutures to narrow it.

Next, if nasal breathing is difficult due to a severely bent septal septum, the deviated cartilage and bone are removed and the remaining parts are strengthened. The inferior turbinate, along with the nasal septum, is an important part of nasal respiration. When it enlarges accompanied by a deviated septum, it is called hypertrophic inferior turbinate,

1. 절개(Incision)

2. 연골채취(Harvest Cartilage)

귀연골(Ear) 비중격연골(Septum) 늑연골(Rip)

3. 코끝수술(Tip-plasty)

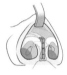

비주연골 이식 비연골묶기
(Columellar strut graft) (Suture technique)

4. 비골절골(Osteotomy) 5. 콧대수술(Dorsum)

보형물/자가조직
(Implant/
Autologous
tissue)

6. 콧볼축소(Alar base reduction)

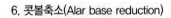

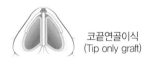

코끝연골이식
(Tip only graft)

commonly called rhinitis, and requires surgery as well. Finally, if this rhinitis persists, inflammation occurs in the space called the maxillary sinus next to the nose (sinusitis), and medical or surgical treatment is required.

If you understand the rhinoplasty by part, you can easily understand the rhinoplasty by type that we generally refer to, that is, rhinoplasty for a low nose, a hump nose, a deviated nose, and a bulbous nose.

Surgical techniques according to the pattern of nose

If you understand rhinoplasty surgery by region, you can understand the types of rhinoplasty surgery we commonly refer to, namely low nose, hooked nose, Rhinoplasty surgery for crooked nose, double nose, etc. is also easy to understand.

01 Low nose

A low nose mainly refers to a low nasal bridge, but in most cases, the tip of the nose is also low and small. It is the most common type among Asians, including Koreans. The nasal tip-plasty and bridge augmentation mentioned above are necessary, and if the nasal bone or alar base is wide, an osteotomy or alar reduction is performed together.

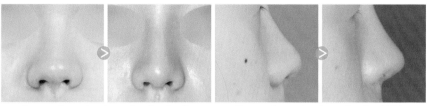

Preoperative and postoperative view (front),   Preoperative and postoperative view (side)

02 Hump nose

A hump nose is named because the part where the nasal bone and cartilage meet at the upper third of the nose protrudes, and it resembles the beak of a hawk. In this case, it can be improved by simply trimming or cutting the hump, but in most cases, a better shape can be obtained by raising the nasal tip together since it usually looks droopy. In addition, if the glabellar area above the hump is low, cartilage or donated dermis can be put in that area, or the entire nasal bridge including glabella can be raised with silicone implant.

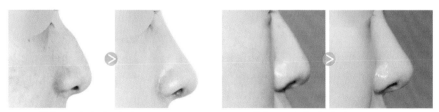

Before and after hooked nose surgery   Before and after hooked nose surgery

03 Crooked nose

A deviated nose may be congenital or acquired due to trauma. In most cases, the nasal bone and septum are bent together, so osteotomy and septoplasty are often performed together. In the case of the nasal tip, it is also curved along with the nasal bridge, so there are many cases where tip-plasty is also required. In the case of a deviated nose, it is necessary to consider the overall axis of the face as well, but if only the nose is set too straight, the chin may look even more deviated, so it is necessary to consider the overall balance.

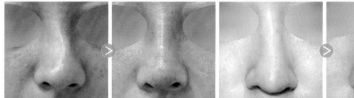

Preoperative and postoperative view (front)   Preoperative and postoperative view (front)

Recently, with the development of 3D printing technology, many achievements have been made in medical devices. Since 2020, 3D printing silicone implants based on patient CT data have become available. As a result, the surgery time is

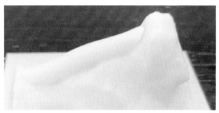

3D printed silicone implants

shortened, and the possibility of inflammation is reduced by using more precise fitting implant for each individual nose. In the case with a mild hump or deviation, it is possible to correct it without resection of the hump nose or osteotomy of the nasal bone, which has the effect of shortening the recovery period.

04 Bulbous Nose

A bulbous nose mainly refers to cases where the nasal tip is blunt and wide, and unlike Caucasians, it is commonly due to have thick skin rather than large cartilage among Asians. Therefore, correction of this requires not only narrowing the nasal tip cartilage, but also a process of thinning of the nasal skin.

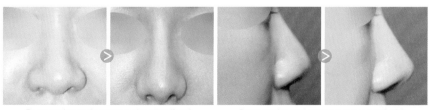

Preoperative and postoperative view (front)   Preoperative and postoperative view (side)

TIP_Rhinoplasty Information

Operation time	Anesthetizing	Hospitalization	Recovery period	Staying period
1-1.5 hours	Local & sedative anesthesia	No need	2 weeks	10 days

| Revisional rhinoplasty

In the case of revision rhinoplasty, there are two main reasons. It is a case of simply wanting better cosmetic or functional improvement, or a case accompanied by various complex problems.

In the case of revision rhinoplasty, there are two main reasons. It is a case of simply wanting better cosmetic or functional improvement, or a case accompanied by various complex problems.

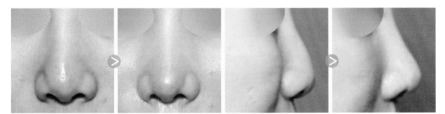

Preoperative and postoperative view (front)   Preoperative and postoperative view (side)

On the other hand, in the case of the latter, inflammation occurs in many cases and chronic contracture of the skin makes the nasal tip looking up-turned or the entire nose is deformed. In addition, there are cases in which the implant penetrates the skin or mucosa.

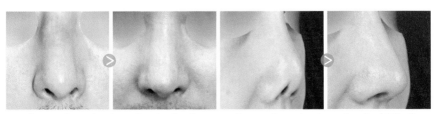

Preoperative and postoperative view (front)   Preoperative and postoperative view (oblique)

Considerations during revisional rhinoplasty

In the case of revisional rhinoplasty, the surgery itself is different from the first surgery, but more attention to the consultation and examination that take place before the revisional rhinoplasty is necessary. Since patients have a lot of fear of additional surgery due to the results of the previous surgery, the questions are often more and even complicated. It is important to have a clear understanding of what the patient wants not only physically but also psychologically through sufficient counseling. It is common for cases where there is no ear cartilage or septum cartilage, which are commonly used, and it is also common to use autologous tissue because silicone implants cannot be used due to poor skin conditions.

This is especially true for patients who have undergone several to ten rhinoplasty surgeries. Therefore, it is also important not to miss the examinations that should be performed before surgery including CT and nasal endoscopy. Although it cannot tell 100% of the condition inside the nose, the size, location and condition of the implant, perforation of the septum or adhesions, rhinitis or maxillary sinusitis (sinusitis) can be informed in advance. In terms of uncertainty, revisional rhinoplasty can be called as a different genre of surgery from rhinoplasty.

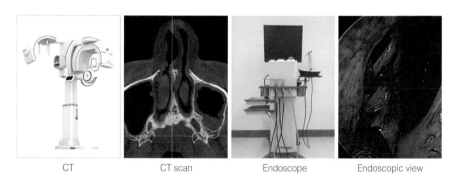

| CT | CT scan | Endoscope | Endoscopic view |

TIP_Revisional rhinoplasty Information				
Operation time	Anesthetizing	Hospitalization	Recovery period	Staying period
2-3 hours	Local & sedative or general	No need	2 weeks	10 days

Composite graft or forehead flap surgery as the last option

As rhinoplasty and revisional rhinoplasty become more common, the number of rhinoplasty increases, and when the condition of the nose reaches its worst, not only the problem of nasal cartilage but also the problem of the nasal skin becomes more serious. In fact, even if nasal cartilage is weakened or absorbed due to inflammation, costal cartilage can be harvested to replace its role. Only methods such as composite graft in which skin and cartilage are transplanted together or forehead flap surgery in which the skin of the forehead is taken are the last resort. In the case of composite graft, the success rate is low and even if successful, the absorption rate is quite high. In the case of forehead flap, the recovery process takes a long time and leaves a vertical long scar on the forehead. Therefore, it is recommended not to be too greedy about the results of the first rhinoplasty or revisional rhinoplasty to prevent such problems from occurring. This is because most of these problems are caused by excessive greed of the patient or the surgeon.

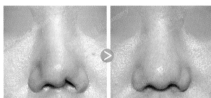
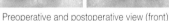
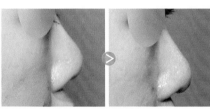

Preoperative and postoperative view (front)　　Preoperative and postoperative view (side)

Postoperative care and management

Problems may arise if left alone after the surgery, and it will take longer to obtain the final result. Therefore, postoperative management can also be considered as an important step in rhinoplasty and revisional rhinoplasty.

First, the dressing process immediately after surgery is in order to prevent nasal bleeding. The nose is blocked with cotton and removed about a day later. In addition, skin tape and splints are applied, which minimize swelling and protect the nose from the outside. Usually, it is applied for about 5 days, and the stitches of the nose are removed together. Ten days after the operation, the stitches are removed from the area where the nose itself and donor site for cartilage, dermal fat, and scalp fascia were collected.

After that, the regular follow-up is 1, 3, and 6 months after the surgery, and if necessary, injection or laser for scar management is performed. In general, after rhinoplasty, bruises and large swelling go away in about two weeks, but swelling goes away over a long period of time. Normally, it is explained that swelling is reduced by 70% at 1 month, 90% at 3 months, and almost 100% at 6 months after surgery, but in the case of revision rhinoplasty, it takes about twice as long.

Many people ask about bruise cream and swelling laser, but in reality, cold compresses are applied during the first two days after surgery to prevent more swelling, and warm massage for the next two weeks helps blood circulation to subside the swelling as quickly as possible. In addition, light walking is effective to reduce postoperative swelling. There are many inquiries about scar ointment and scar laser as well. After stitch removal, the ointment is available to apply for several months, and if it is still noticeable afterwards, laser is performed. A scar on columella is usually not prominent in 1 year after the rhinoplasty if it is not case with previous multiple rhinoplasties.

코끝 재수술(Revision Tip plasty)
다양한 코재수술(Various types of Revision Rhinoplasty)
맞춤보형물 코재수술(Revision Customized Implant Rhinoplasty)

어떠한 경우에도 진정한 마지막을 위해…
자연스럽게 살리는 코재수술

No matter how your nose condition is
Expect for a genuine final outcome

코 재수술은 1차 수술에 비해 난이도가 높기 때문에 코재수술 경험이 풍부하고 코의 해부학적 구조를 잘 알고 있는 병원에서 적합한 수술을 받아야 또 다시 수술에 실패하는 일을 막을 수 있다.

Revision rhinoplasty is more challenging than the primary surgery, so a suitable surgery must be performed at a hospital with extensive experience and well-acquainted with the anatomical structure of the nose in revision nose surgeries to prevent another surgical failure.

CDU 청담유성형외과
CDU Cheongdam U Plastic Surgery

www.cdups.co.kr

양동준(Dong-Jun Yang)

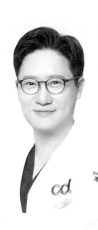

- CDU 청담유성형외과 대표원장(Director of CDU Cheongdam U Plastic Surgery)
- 대한성형외과학회 코성형연구회 정회원(Full member, Rhinoplasty Research Society at the Korean Society of Plastic and Reconstructive Surgeons)
- 대한성형외과학회의사회 정회원 (Full member, Korean Society of Plastic and Reconstructive Surgeons)
- 미국성형외과학회(ASPS) 정회원 (Full member, American Society of Plastic Surgeons (ASPS))

02-2 정확한 **실패 원인** 및 개인의 **니즈**까지 고려한 **코 재수술**

코 해부학에 대한 정확한 지식과 다양한 임상 경험이 필요

과거 코수술을 시행했으나 만족스럽지 못하였거나 보형물에 문제가 발생했을 경우 재수술을 고려하기 마련이다. 코는 얼굴의 중심에서 얼굴 전체의 조화를 맞추는 데 있어서 가장 중요한 구조물이다. 또한 미용적인 목적에서뿐만 아니라 숨을 쉬는 아주 중요한 구조물이기 때문에 수술적인 면에서 신중할 필요가 있다.

코 수술은 10년에 한 번씩 재수술을 해야 한다는 말이 있지만 이건 잘못된 정보이다. 한번 잘 된 코 수술은 평생 다시 하지 않아도 되기 때문에 첫 수술이 아주 중요하고, 혹여나 여러 가지 이유 때문에 재수술을 한다고 했을 때는 더는 수술을 하지 않도록 정확한 원인 파악과 함께 그 원인에 맞는 수술이 가능한 경험이 많은 성형외과 전문의에게 수술을 받는 것이 아주 중요하다.

코는 개개인이 다 다르다. 피부 두께와 탄력도, 모공의 크기, 연부 조직의 양, 연골의 크기와 탄력도 등이 다 다르기 때문에 수술 시 예쁘고 멋진 코를 만들기 위해서는 코 해부학에 대한 정확한 지식이 있어야 한다. 또한 각기 다른 케이스별로 수술했을 때 제대로 된 코 모양이 나오는 것에 대한 아주 다양한 임상 경험이 뒷받침되어야 한다.

코끝 재수술

코끝 재수술은 한번 건드린 조직을 다시 건드려야 하는 고도의 수술이다. 어떤 원인으로 코끝 재수술이 필요한지 환자의 상태와 원인을 면밀하게 분석 후 수술을 진행해야 한다.

코끝이 떨어진 경우

코끝이 떨어진 경우는 지지대인 비주가 약하거나, 코끝의 연골이 벌어지면서 코끝이 넓어지면서 떨어지는 경우가 많다. 재수술로 들어가서 비주를 체크하여 비주가 약한 경우에는 귀연골, 늑연골, 비중격연골 등으로 약한 기둥을 더 지지해 줘야하고, 코끝 연골이 벌어진 경우에는 비익 연골을 묶어주는 수술을 해야 한다.

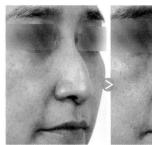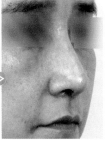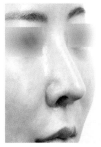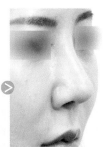

코끝이 떨어진 경우 수술전후   코끝이 떨어진 경우 수술전후

코끝이 들린 경우

염증이 생겼는데 오랫동안 방치하거나, L 타입 보형물을 쓴 경우에 흔하게 나타

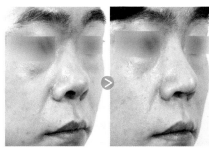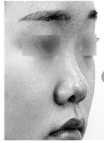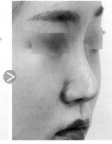

코끝이 들린 경우 수술전후   코끝이 들린 경우 수술전후

난다. 이런 경우에는 코끝을 내려주는 수술을 해야 한다. 코끝의 비익연골(lower lateral cartilage)을 지지하고 붙잡고 있는 여러 가지 인대조직(ligamentous structure)을 잘 박리해서 비익연골이 자유롭게 움직이도록 한 다음에, 비익연골을 아래로 내려주는 것이 가장 중요하다.

코끝이 뭉퉁해 보이는 경우

코끝이 뭉퉁해 보이는 이유는 다양하다.

코끝이 떨어졌거나, 코 끝에 있는 지방(fat), 연부조직(soft tissue), 근막층(SMAS), 연골(cartilage) 등이 덜 제거되었기 때문입니다. 이때는 코끝에 있는 여러 조직들을 제거해야 하고, 코끝 연골의 일부를 절제하거나, 코끝 연골을 묶어줘서 코끝이 날렵하게 보여주도록 해야 한다. 또 자가 연골 등을 이용하여 코끝을 더 높이 세워줘야 한다.

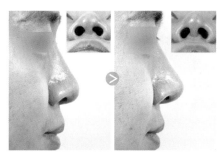

코끝이 뭉퉁해 보이는 경우 수술전후

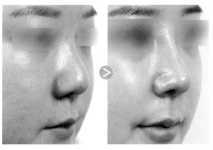

코끝이 뭉퉁해 보이는 경우 수술전후

코끝 피부가 얇아진 경우

피부가 얇아서 연골이 비치거나, 피부색이 빨갛게 된 경우는, 높이를 낮춰서 피부가 받는 텐션(tension)을 낮춰주거나, 진피를 덧대서 얇아진 피부의 두께를 보충해 줘야 한다.

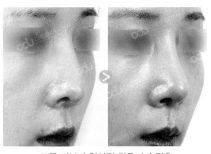
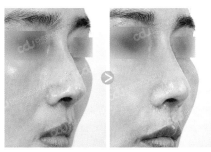

코끝 피부가 얇아진 경우 수술전후   코끝 피부가 얇아진 경우 수술전후

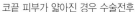

TIP_코끝재수술 정보				
수술시간	마취방법	입원여부	회복기간	체류기간
60분	수면	–	7일	3~5일

다양한 코재수술

코재수술을 필요로 하는 상황은 다양하다. 각기 다른 케이스별로 수술법이 모두 다르기 때문에 풍부한 임상 경험이 뒷받침되어 좀 더 신중하고 섬세하게 수술이 계획되어야 한다.

코가 낮은 경우

전체적으로 낮은 경우는 기존의 낮은 보형물을 빼고, 더 높은 보형물로 바꿔줘야 하고, 코끝에는 기증 진피(alloderm)이나 연골(cartilage)을 보충해 줘야 한다.

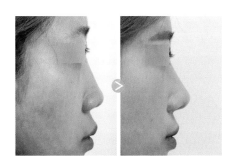
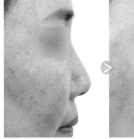
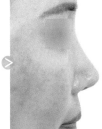

낮은코 수술전후   낮은코 수술전후

기존에 제품화되어 있는 보형물보다 더 높게 원하는 경우에는 맞춤 보형물로 최대한 높게 수술을 할 수도 있다.

코가 길어 보이는 경우

일반적으로 코의 길이는 얼굴 길이를 3등분했을 때 1/3 정도가 이상적인 코의 길이라고 알고 있지만, 실제로는 꼭 그렇지는 않다. 예를 들어 얼굴이 긴 사람의 경우 코의 길이를 얼굴의 길이에 맞춰서 1/3로 한다면 코가 길어 보여서 오히려 전체적인 얼굴의 길이가 더욱 길어 보일 수 있다.

이처럼 코의 길이는 수학 공식처럼 1/3이 아니라 전체적인 얼굴을 파악하고 거기에 맞추는 것이 가장 정확하다고 보인다. 코가 길어 보이는 이유는 두 가지이다. 첫째는 미간이 높을 때이며, 두 번째는 코끝이 화살코처럼 내려온 경우이다. 그래서 코를 짧아 보이게 하기 위해서는 미간의 높이를 낮추거나, 화살코 교정을 해야 한다. 또한 선택하는 보형물에 있어서 일반적으로 미간을 높이는 보형물이 아니라 코끝을 위주로 높이는 보형물인 비스툴의 NB 타입을 선택해야 한다.

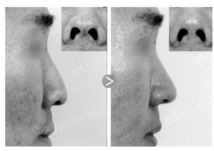
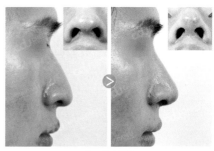

긴코 수술전후   긴코 수술전후

콧구멍이 들린 경우

콧구멍이 들린 것을 교정하는 방법은 콧구멍에 귀연골 등을 덧대주거나, 콧날개를 올려줌으로써 콧구멍이 덜 들려 보이게 할 수도 있고, 코끝 길이 연장을 해줌으

로써 콧구멍이 들린 것을 좋아지게 할 수 있다.

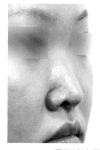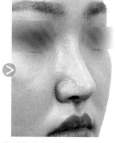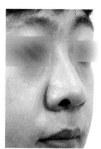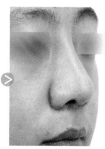

콧구멍이 들린 경우 수술전후   콧구멍이 들린 경우 수술전후

매부리가 남은 경우

기존에 있던 매부리(hump)를 덜 제거한 경우에는 수술로 매부리를 더 깎아주고, 매부리와 맞닿는 부분의 보형물의 바닥도 깎아줘야 한다(carving). 또한 필요시 미간이나 코끝을 더 올려줌으로써 매부리는 해결될 수 있다.

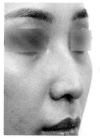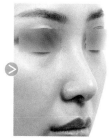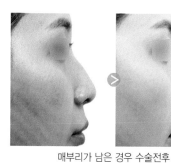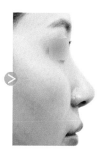
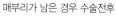

매부리가 남은 경우 수술전후   매부리가 남은 경우 수술전후

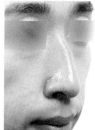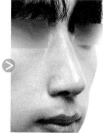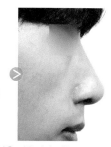

매부리가 남은 경우 수술전후   매부리가 남은 경우 수술전후

코가 휜 경우

보형물이 휜 경우에는 기존 보형물을 감쌌던 피막(capsule)을 제거하고, 다시 새로운 공간을 만든 후에 다시 보형물을 넣어주는 수술을 해야 한다.

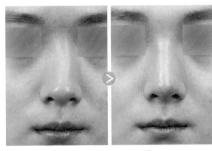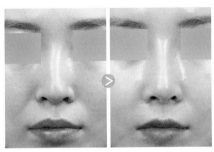

코가 휜 경우 수술전후   코가 휜 경우 수술전후

콧볼축소술

콧볼을 줄였음에도 불구하고 아직도 콧볼이 크다고 느끼는 경우에는 두 가지 수술 방법이 있다. 조금만 줄어들고 콧날개가 약간 위쪽으로 올라가 콧구멍이 덜 보이기를 원하는 경우에는 비절개 콧볼 축소를 시행하고, 콧날개 크기를 확실히 줄이고자 하는 경우에는 피부를 제거하는 절개법으로 하는 것이 맞다.

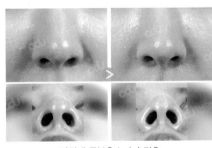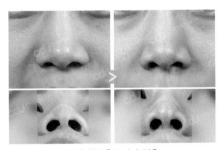

비절개 콧볼축소 수술전후   절개 콧볼축소 수술전후

TIP_다양한 코재수술 정보				
수술시간	마취방법	입원여부	회복기간	체류기간
60분	수면	–	7일	2~8일

맞춤보형물 코재수술

환자의 CT 데이터를 기반으로 제작되는 개인별 맞춤형 보형물은 보다 정확한 수술 결과 예측이 가능하며, 재수술의 위험 요소를 현저하게 감소시켜준다.

맞춤 보형물 수술

CT 촬영을 해서 현재 코의 형태를 면밀히 파악하고, 환자의 현재 상태와 원하시는 모양에 맞게 보형물을 맞춤 제작하게 된다. 맞춤 보형물의 장점은 아주 많다. 빈 공간 없이 바로 뼈에 딱 맞게 밀착이 되기 때문에 회복이 빠르고, 코뼈나 코 연골이 휘어진 경우에 절골 없이 맞춤 보형물로 꺼진 부위를 채워줌으로써 휘어 보이는 것을 교정해 줄 수 있다. 또한 매부리를 깎을 필요 없이 교정할 수 있고, 환자마다 원하는 미간, 코끝의 높이가 각각 다르기 때문에 환자가 원하는 형태로 만들 수 있다. 그래서 재수술 시 일반 보형물이 아닌 맞춤 보형물로 수술하는 경우에 보다 더 정확한 수술을 할 수 있다.

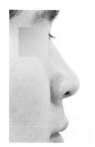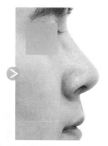

맞춤 보형물 수술전후

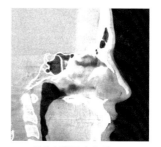

맞춤 보형물 수술 후 3D CT

TIP_맞춤보형물 코재수술 정보				
수술시간	마취방법	입원여부	회복기간	체류기간
60분	수면	–	7일	2~8일

02-2

Revision Rhinoplasty: Identify the exact cause of failure and individual needs

Need accurate knowledge of nose anatomy and diverse clinical experience

The surgery for those who already had previous rhinoplasty but haven't satisfied with the result or issues arose with implant, revision is likely to be considered. The surgery for those who already had previous rhinoplasty but haven't satisfied with the result or issues arose with implant, revision is likely to be considered.

The nose is the most important structure in achieving overall facial harmony, located at the center of the face. Furthermore, not only for aesthetic purposes but also as a vital structure for breathing, one needs to be cautious when considering surgery.

There's a misconception that nose surgery needs to be redone every 10 years, but this information is incorrect. Once a nose surgery is done well, it can last a lifetime, which is why the initial surgery is crucial. If, for various reasons, a revision surgery becomes necessary, it's vital to accurately identify the cause and undergo the procedure with a plastic surgeon who has enriched experience in addressing such issues to ensure no further surgeries are needed. Every individual's nose is unique. Due to differences in skin thickness, elasticity, pore size, the amount of soft tissue, cartilage size, and cartilage elasticity, creating a beautiful and attractive nose during surgery requires precise knowledge of nasal anatomy. Additionally, a wide range of clinical experience is essential to understand how to achieve the right nasal shape for various individual cases. I will explain the surgery with various cases along with photos.

| Revision Tip plasty

Revision Tip plasty involves a high degree of complexity as it requires reworking tissues that have already been operated on. It's crucial to thoroughly analyze the patient's condition and the reasons for the revision before proceeding with the surgery.

Nose with droopy tip

When the nasal tip droops, it often occurs due to weakened supporting structures, or the nasal cartilage spreading, causing it to widen and droop.

In revision surgery, the case of the support structure is weak, additional support has to be provided using ear cartilage, septal cartilage or columellar strut.

If the nasal tip cartilage has spread apart, a surgical procedure that ties the alar cartilage together is necessary.

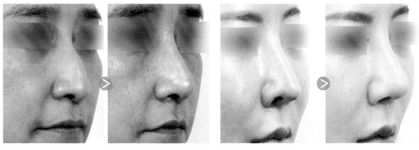

Droopy tip surgery Before & Affter

Nose with upturned nasal tip

If inflammation has been neglected for a long time or if an L-type implant has been used, it can commonly occur. In such cases, surgery is needed to lower the tip of the nose. It's essential to carefully dissect the various ligamentous structures that support and hold the lower lateral cartilage of the nasal tip to allow the cartilage to move freely. After that, lowering the lower lateral cartilage. These are the most important procedures.

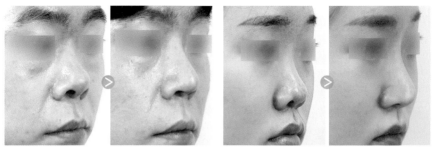

Upturned nasal tip surgery Before & Affter

Nose with bulbous nasal tip

The reason for a bulbous or rounded-looking nasal tip can vary. It can be due to the nasal tip drooping or fat, soft tissue, SMAS layer, or cartilage in the nasal tip were not adequately removed. In such cases, various tissues in the nasal tip need to be removed. It may also be necessary to excise a part of the nasal tip cartilage or tie the nasal tip cartilage to give a more refined appearance. Additionally, autologous cartilage or other materials may be used to elevate the nasal tip higher.

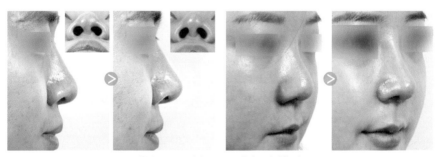

Bulbous nasal tip surgery Before & Affter)

Nose with thin skinned nasal tip

If the skin is getting thinner, causing cartilage to show through or the skin to appear red, lowering the height to reduce the tension on the skin or adding dermis to supplement the thickness of the thin skin.

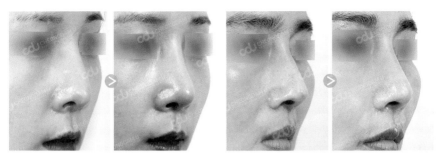

Thin skinned nasal tip surgery Before & Affter

TIP_Revision Tip plasty Information

Operation time	Anesthetizing method	Hospitalization	Convalescent period	The length of one's visit
60 min	Sedation	-	7 days	3~5 days

Various types of Revision Rhinoplasty

There are various situations that require revision rhinoplasty. Since the surgical methods vary for each case, it is essential to plan the surgery with careful consideration and precision, supported by extensive clinical experience.

Nose with low nasal bridge

In cases where the entire nose is low, it's necessary to replace the existing low implant with a higher one, and the nose tip needs to be supplemented with allograft dermis (alloderm) or cartilage.

If you want a higher profile than what's available with standard implants, customized implants can be used to achieve the desired height as closely as possible.

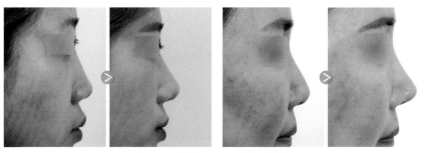

Low nasal bridge surgery Before & Affter

Long nose

It's commonly believed that the ideal nose length should be about one third of the total face length when the face is divided into three equal parts, this isn't always the case in reality.

For instance, for someone with a long face, adjusting the nose length precisel to one third of the facial length, it might make the nose appear disproportionately long and further accentuate the length of the face.

Thus, determining the length of the nose is not as simple as a mathematical formula of 1/3, but rather, it is most accurate when considering the overall facial proportions and adjusting accordingly.

There are two main reasons why a nose might appear long. Firstly, it can be due to a high nasal bridge, And secondly, it might be because the tip of the nose droops down, resembling an arrowhead. To make the nose appear shorter, it's essential to either reduce the height of the

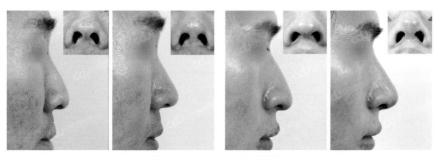

Long nose surgery Before & Affter

nasal bridge or correct the arrowhead-shaped tip.

Furthermore, when choosing the implant material, it's generally advisable to select the NB Type of implant from Bistool, which primarily focuses on raising the tip of the nose, rather than a common implant that raises the bridge.

Nose with raised nostrils

Correcting visible nostrils can be done by adding ear cartilage(or other materials) or by lifting the nostril wings. Also by extending the length of the nasal tip, the appearance of raised nostrils can be less visible.

Additionally, it's possible to correct raised nostrils that appear triangular from the front by filling them with filler.

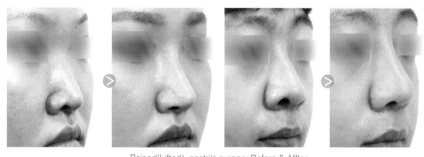

Raised(Lifted) nostrils surgery Before & Affter

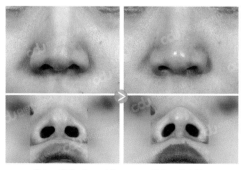

Raised(Lifted) nostrils surgery Before & Affter

Nose with deviated implant

When the implant is deviated, the existing capsule that enveloped the existing implant must be removed. After creating a new space, a new implant is then inserted.

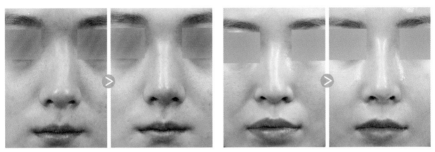

Deviated nose surgery Before & Affter

Nose with remained hump

In cases where the existing hump has not been sufficiently removed, it is necessary to further

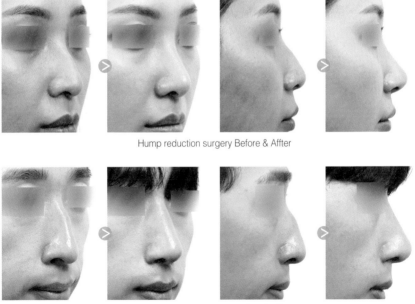

Hump reduction surgery Before & Affter

Hump reduction surgery Before & Affter

reduce the hump and also carve the base of the implant that touches the hump. Additionally, if necessary, elevating the glabella or the tip of the nose can help to address the hump.

Alar reduction

If the alar base is still look big even after reduction, there are two surgical methods.

For those who want only a slight reduction and prefer the nostril wings to rise slightly so that the nostrils are less visible, a non-incisional alar reduction is performed.

On the other hand, if someone want to significantly reduce the size of the alar bases, it is appropriate to remove some skin through an incisional method.

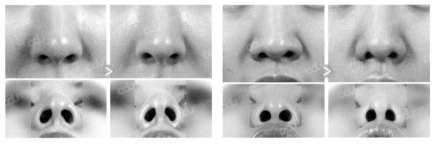

Non incisional alar reduction surgery Before & Affter

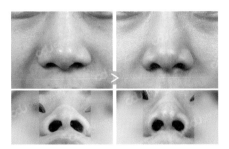

Incisioanl alar reduction surgery Before & Affter

TIP_Various types of Revision Rhinoplasty Information				
Operation time	Anesthetizing method	Hospitalization	Convalescent period	The length of one's visit
60 min	Sedation	-	7 days	2~8 days

Revision Customized Implant Rhinoplasty

Customized implants based on the patient's CT data allow for more accurate predictions of surgical outcomes and significantly reduce the risk factors for revision surgery.

Customized implant surgery

Through CT imaging, meticulously analyze the current shape of the nose, and then custom manufacture the implant based on the patient's current condition and desired shape.

There are many advantages to customized implants.

It fits perfectly onto the bone without any gaps, leading to faster recovery. Additionally, in cases where the nasal bone or cartilage is bent, a customized implant can fill in the recessed areas without the need for osteotomy, correcting the appearance of bending.

Therefore, when undergoing revision surgery, using a customized implant rather than a standard one allows for a more precise operation.

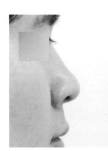 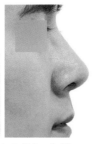

Customized Rhinoplasty Before & Affter

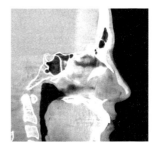

CT scan after customized implant surgery

TIP_Revision Customized Implant Rhinoplasty Information

Operation time	Anesthetizing method	Hospitalization	Convalescent period	The length of one's visit
60 min	Sedation	-	7 days	2~8 days

입꼬리 올림술(Mouth corner lifting surgery)
인중 축소술(Phil trum reduction)
입술 성형술(Lip augmentation)
입매 비대칭의 교정(Correction of mouth asymmetry)

얼굴의 전체적인 조화와 아름다움을 입매가 완성한다

Lip Reshaping Can Enhance the Beauty of the Entire Face

입매는 안면부의 다른 부위보다 전체적인 인상과 표정에 강한 영향을 준다. 아름다운 입매란 입매를 구성하는 각 부위별 아름다움 뿐 아니라 밝은 인상과 좋은 이미지를 다른 사람에게 각인시킬 수 있도록 얼굴 형태에 맞게 조화가 이뤄져야 한다.

The mouth has a stronger influence on the overall impression and expression than other parts of the face. A beautiful mouth should not only be beautiful in each part of the mouth, but should also harmonize with the shape of the face so that a bright impression and good image can be imprinted on others.

V&MJ 골든뷰 피부과 · 성형외과
V&MJ Golden View Dermatology·Plastic Surgery

www.mjpsclinic.com

송상훈(Sang-Hoon Song)

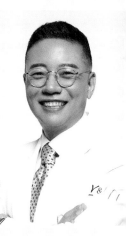

• 성형외과 전문의(Board certified plastic surgeon)
• V&MJ 골든뷰 성형외과 센터장(Director of V&MJ Golden View Plastic Surgery Center)
• 대한성형외과학회 정회원(Active member, Korean Society of Plastic and Reconstructive Surgeons)
• 대한미용성형외과학회 정회원(Active member, Korean Society for Aesthetic Plastic Surgery)
• 전) 고려대학교 성형외과 임상교수
(Former) Professor, Dept. of Plastic and Reconstructive Surgery, Korea University)

03 매력적인 미소와 조화로운 입매로 완성되는 아름다움

어떠한 얼굴도 호감이 가는 좋은 이미지로 아름다워 보일 수 있다

최근 성형의 트랜드는 이미지 성형이다. 기존 성형이 특정 부위를 예쁘게 만들려는 목적이 강했다면 이미지 성형은 전체적인 조화를 추구하는 점이 특징인데 그중 무뚝뚝해 보이는 인상을 개선하여 미소 짓는 부드러운 인상으로 만들어 주는 입매성형이 이미지 성형의 중심에 있다.

입매성형은 입술의 크기와 모양을 개선하는 입술성형뿐 아니라 입꼬리의 형태나 위치의 교정, 인중길이의 교정, 부비부(팔자주름 부위)의 함몰교정, 앞턱의 돌출 정도에 따른 교정, 잘못된 입매성형의 후유증이나 이물질 등을 제거하고 복원하는 등 입을 중심으로 주위조직과의 자연스러운 조화를 이루는 것이 목적이며 이로 인한 좋은 이미지와 기억에 오래 남는 개성의 표출이 덤으로 따라오는 수술을 뜻한다.

하지만, 이러한 입매수술에서 가장 중요한 것은 "절대로 과하지 않게 하는 것"(Don't to do it too much)이다. 수술이 과하게 되면 복원이 매우 어려우며 때로는 복원이 불가능할 수도 있으므로 지나치게 욕심을 내지 않도록 하는 것이 중요하다.

입꼬리 올림술

입꼬리 올림술은 처진 입꼬리로 인해 우울하게 보이거나 화나 보이는 표정을 밝고 부드럽고 환한 인상을 갖도록 해준다.

입꼬리가 올라가면 밝고 부드러운 이미지로 바뀐다

선천적으로 입의 길이가 짧고 입꼬리가 처져있거나, 나이가 들면서 볼살과 함께 입꼬리도 처져 내려와 입가주름이 있는 생긴 경우, 입술의 두께나 길이가 작은 사람이 양악수술을 시행한 후에 생긴 부작용으로 입술이 말려 들어가게 되고 입꼬리가 처지게 되는 경우는 다른 사람들에게 무뚝뚝하게 보이거나 화난 사람처럼 보여 차가운 인상을 주게 된다. 입꼬리 올림술은 이처럼 처진 입꼬리로 인해 우울하거나 화난 사람처럼 느껴지는 것을 밝고 부드러운 이미지로 바뀌게 한다.

따라서 노화로 인한 입꼬리 처짐이나 처진 입매로 고민 중인 결혼을 앞둔 신부, 안면윤곽수술이나 치아교정 후 입매 관련 후유증이 있는 사람, 미소가 중요한 항공기 승무원, 기타 서비스 관련 종사자에게 필요한 수술이다.

입꼬리수술의 수술방법

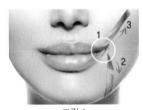

그림 1

입꼬리수술은 ① 입꼬리 주변으로 작은 삼각형 모양의 피부를 절제하고, ② 입꼬리를 내리는 근육을 약화시키고, ③ 입꼬리를 올리는 근육의 힘을 강화하여 새로운 입꼬리의 모양과 위치를 만드는 것이다.

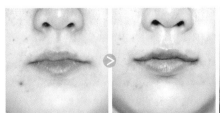

입꼬리 수술전후

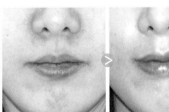

입꼬리 수술전후

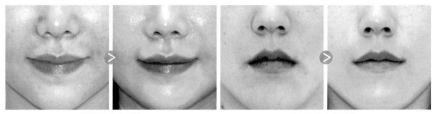

입꼬리 수술전후   입꼬리 수술전후

TIP_입꼬리수술 정보

수술시간	마취방법	입원여부	회복기간	실밥제거	체류기간
2시간	국소, 수면마취	입원없음	7일	5~7일 후	6~10일

※ 부작용 : 흉터, 함몰, 입가주름, 착색, 저교정, 과교정 등

│ 인중 축소술

이상적인 인중은 보통 아랫입술부터 턱까지 거리의 절반 정도이다. 인중축소술은 얼굴형에 맞지 않는 긴 인중의 길이를 적당히 맞춰서 얼굴의 균형을 잡는 수술이다.

자신에게 맞는 균형 잡힌 인중

인중이 길고 윗입술이 얇고 가지런하면 인자하고 근엄하게 보일 수 있으나, 대부분의 긴 인중을 가진 이들은 얼굴 전체가 길어 보이고 나이 들어 보이며 약간 무기력하게 비춰지는 경우가 많다.

선천적인 원인 이외의 인중 길이가 변화되는 요인으로는 다음과 같다.

1. 입술 주위 조직의 노화로 인해 인중 피부의 탄력이 감소하여 인중이 길어지고 윗입술이 말려 얇아지며 입꼬리가 처지는 현상이 발생한다.

2. 양악수술이나 치과적인 교정 후 인중이 길어지며 윗입술이 말려 들어가고 볼이 처지는 등의 부작용이 발생한다.

인중축소술 후 줄어든 인중의 길이 변화로 자신의 나이보다 적어 보이게 되며 얼굴의 크기가 작아 보이고 인상이 활기차고 자신감 있는 모습으로 변화된다.

또한 윗입술의 볼륨이 커져 말려 있는 입술라인이 되살아나 생동감 있는 모습이 된다.

인중축소 수술방법

인중축소수술은 코밑경계 주름 부위의 피부절개를 하는 방법(Bull Horn Lift)과 빨간 입술(홍순)과 피부의 경계면인 윗입술라인 절개를 통한 수술방법(Gull Wing Lift), 코밑절개와 입술라인 절개의 장단점을 융합한 하이브리드 인중축소법(Goldenview hybrid Lift)이 있다.

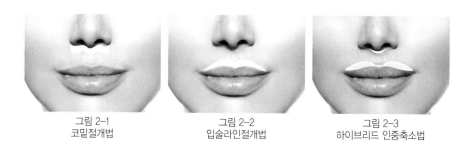

그림 2-1	그림 2-2	그림 2-3
코밑절개법	입술라인절개법	하이브리드 인중축소법

코밑절개 인중축소는 입술두께에 큰 변화를 주지 않으면서 인중길이를 줄이고자 할 경우, 입술라인을 통한 절개는 입술이 얇으면서 입술경계선이 불분명하고 평평할 때 적용된다.

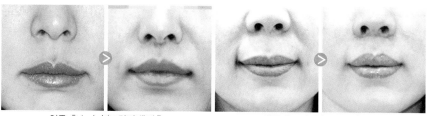

인중 축소 수술(코밑절개)전후   인중 축소 수술(코밑절개)전후

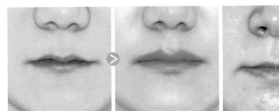

인중 축소 수술(입술라인절개)전후

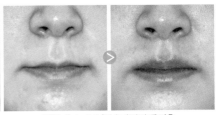

인중 축소 수술(입술라인절개)전후

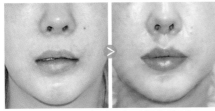

인중 축소 수술(하이브리드 인중축소)전후

이중에서 골든뷰 하이브리드 인중 축소는 기존의 코밑절개와 입술라인 절개 방법의 장점을 살리고 단점을 최소화한 융합수술방법으로 최근에 가장 많이 이용되는 수술법이다.

TIP_인중 축소수술 정보

수술시간	마취방법	입원여부	회복기간	실밥제거	체류기간
2시간	국소, 수면마취	입원없음	7일	7일 후	6~10일

※ 부작용 : 흉터, 착색, 콧구멍 변형(코밑절개), 부종, 저교정, 과교정

| 입술 성형술

입술의 형태와 두께로 고민하고 걱정하는 사람들이 의외로 많다. 각자의 얼굴 형태에 적합하면서도 본인이 선호하는 입술을 찾는 게 필요하다.

입술 축소술

입술이 크고 두꺼운 경우에는 입술을 얇게 하는 입술축소술(Lip Reduction)을 이용하여 원하는 두께와 모양으로 줄일 수 있다. 입술의 경우 1~2mm의 두께 차이에도 큰 이미지 변화를 느낄 수 있다.

입술 축소수술 방법

입술축소술은 입술 내측 구강점막에 절개를 넣고 미리 정한 절제량만큼 점막이나 근육을 절제한 후 다시 재봉합하는 과정으로 봉합할 때는 녹는 실을 사용하기 때문에 나중에 실밥을 제거할 필요는 없다.

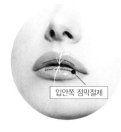

1 Step
입술내측 절제
원하는 입술크기와 얼굴 비율과 어울리는 입술크기를 정한 후 입술내측 구강점막에 절개를 넣고 미리 정한 절재량만큼 점막을 절제

입안쪽 점막절제

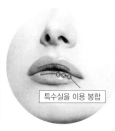

2 Step
특수실 미세봉합
인체에 무해한 녹는 실을 이용하여 섬세하고 꼼꼼하게 봉합. 녹는 실은 자연스럽게 녹아 없어지기에 실밥 제거로 따로 방문할 필요성이 없음

특수실을 이용 봉합

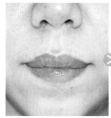
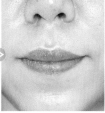

입술 축소 수술전후

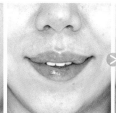
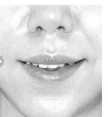

입술 축 소수술전후

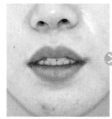
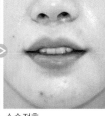

입술 축소 수술전후

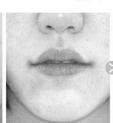
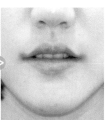

입술 축소 수술전후

입술 확대술

입술이 얇고 입술외형이 빈약한 경우에 도톰하면서 볼륨 있는 입술을 만들 수 있는 다양한 시술법과 수술법이 있다. 이중 가장 효과적이며 반영구적인 수술법은 입술 확대술(Lip Augmentation)이다.

입술확대 수술방법

수술방법은 점막전진술(Mucosal advancement)과 입술라인확대술(Lip line augmentation)이 있다. 점막전진술은 주로 아랫입술의 확대 시에 사용되는데, 입술 내측 점막을 전외측으로 외번(Rolling Out)시켜 앞으로 이동시키는 방법이다. 입술라인확대술은 주로 윗입술의 확대 시에 사용되며 홍순과 인중피부의 경계라인을 절제 봉합하는 수술법이다. 입술라인인중축소술(Bull horn lift)과 동일한 수술이며 입술 경계선이 불분명하고 얇으면서 볼륨감이 없고 편평한 경우에 효과적이다.

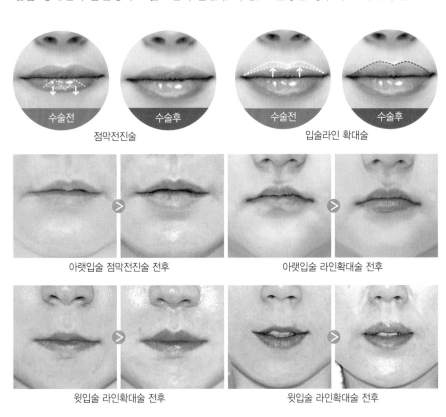

점막전진술

입술라인 확대술

아랫입술 점막전진술 전후

아랫입술 라인확대술 전후

윗입술 라인확대술 전후

윗입술 라인확대술 전후

TIP_입술성형 수술정보

수술시간	마취방법	입원여부	회복기간	실밥제거	체류기간
1~2시간	국소, 수면마취	입원없음	7일	필요없음	6~10일

※ 부작용 : 부종, 감각저하, 수술부 조직의 연화지연(delay of the softening), 함몰, 착색, 저교정, 과교정 등

입매성형수술 시의 주의사항

　입매수술 후 첫 3~4일간은 냉찜질을 하는 것이 초기 부종의 예방 및 감소에 도움이 된다. 실밥을 제거하기 전에도 거품세안과 샤워는 가능하다.

　수술 후 무엇보다도 중요한 것은 최소 2개월 정도는 말을 많이 하지 말고, 치과치료와 같이 입을 크게 벌리지 않도록 주의하는 것이다. 또한 지속적인 흉터 연고나 보습제, 자외선 차단제의 사용이 중요하다.

입매 비대칭의 교정

입매비대칭의 원인은 선천적, 후천적 안면신경마비, 얼굴골격의 비대칭, 입술이나 입꼬리의 비대칭, 치조골과 치아의 비대칭, 입술주위 근육의 활성도의 차이 등 다양하다.

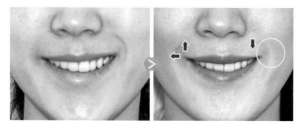

입매비대칭교정 전후

입매비대칭 교정법

　입매비대칭의 교정은 양악수술 등 골격수술이 반드시 필요한 경우도 있겠지만, 일반적으로는 적절하게 볼륨을 맞추고(지방이식, 윤곽 필러 등) 근육의 활성도를 조절하면(보톡스 시술) 생각보다 좋은 결과를 얻을 수 있다.

TIP_입매비대칭 교정 시술정보

시술시간	마취방법	입원여부	회복기간	실밥제거	체류기간
30분 내외	국소, 연고마취	입원없음	즉시	필요없음	1일

※ 부작용 : 멍, 부종, 염증, (말하기, 씹기, 삼키기 등의 일시적인 가벼운) 운동장애, 저교정

03 Beauty completed by charming smile and harmonious

Any face can look beautiful with a good, likable image

I have performed over a thousand lip reshaping procedures. The shape of the mouth is a major factor that determines the overall balance of the facial features. Beautifully shaped lips can drastically enhance your smile and the beauty of the face.

Beautiful faces have certain aspects in common. They may have strong, pronounced features, soft, small features, a narrow bone structure or even angular bone structure, etc. but all have a certain type of harmony among the features.

The shape of the lip, in particular, contributes to the overall balance of the facial features. A tiny difference in the shape of the lips can drastically change one's smile and create a uniquely attractive face.

The shapes of the eyes and lips are the most important factors that determine the overall impression of the face. Plastic surgery and other procedures of the eyes have been commonly performed, however, undesirable shapes of the lips, wrinkles around the mouth, and drooping mouth corners have been dismissed as less important or could not be corrected due to lack of effective procedures.

The shape of the mouth greatly influences facial expressions and the general impression others get from your face. Lip volume, shape of the mouth corner, nasolabial lines, shape of the chin and jaw lines(bimaxillary) can be corrected to improve one's smile and create a more youthful appearance. Aesthetic surgery of the lips can be performed to create a balance between lips and surrounding tissues, as well as more unique, individualized beauty.

Types of lip reshaping surgery.

01 Mouth corner lift for descending mouth corners

02 Lateral upper lip lift for very thin or non-existent lateral upper lip

03 Philtrum reduction(Lip lift) for rejuvenation

04 Cupid's bow surgery for volumizing the middle of the upper lip

05 Aesthetic reconstruction of the philtral ridge

06 Lip reduction for unattractively large lips

07 Lip augmentation for very thin or non-existent lips

08 Nasolabial fold, mariotte line and chin correction

09 Lip reshaping procedures for correcting asymmetry of the lips and reconstruction/removal of previously injected foreign body or filler materials, etc.

| Mouth corner lift

Descended corners of the mouth give the face a grumpy look. They can be caused by congenitally drooping corners of the mouth with a shorter and protruding mouth or aging and reduced elasticity of the skin.

When the corners of the mouth rise, the image changes to a bright and soft image

Patients with thin lips or shorter horizontal length of the mouth often suffer from a smaller mouth, drooping mouth corners or thinned lips after bimaxillary surgery. Mouth corner lift can create a happier and friendlier appearance by elevating the drooping corners of the mouth.

Procedures of the mouth corner lift

Mouth corner lift will be conducted as follows :

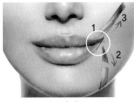

1 painting

① cuts triangle-shaped skins around the corners of the mouth, ② weakens the depressor anguli oris muscles, and ③ makes new shapes and locations of the corners of the mouth by strengthening the power of the muscles lifting the lips.

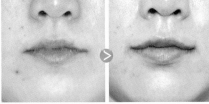
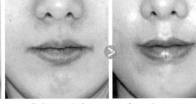

Before and after corner of mouth surgery   Before and after corner of mouth surgery

The surgery is carried out under local anesthesia alone or with simultaneous sedation anesthesia if necessary. The surgery takes about 1-2 hours. The Incision is carefully sutured with a thin thread which is removed in 5 days.

If mouth corners have descended due to age, the corrective surgery can bring a more rejuvenated and softer appearance. Patients will be particularly pleased with a drastically improved look when they smile.

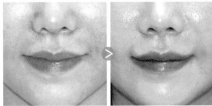
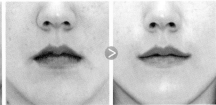

Before and after corner of mouth surgery   Before and after corner of mouth surgery

TIP_Mouth corner surgery information

Treatment time	Anesthetizing method	Hospitalization	Recovery time	Stitch removal	Stay time
2 hours	Local and sedative anesthesia	No hospitalization	7 days	5~7 days later	6~10 days

Side effects : scars, depressions, wrinkles around the mouth, pigmentation, under-correction, over-correction, etc.

| Phil trum reduction

An ideal length of the philtrum is about half of the distance between the lower lip to the bottom of the chin. Philtrum reduction surgery helps create better balance of the face by adjusting the overly long philtrum.

A balanced philtrum that suits you

Asians tend to have a flatter top part of philtrum compared to caucasians, which makes the mouth appear to protrude. This creates a rather stubborn and aggressive appearance. Aging of the perioral tissues reduces the elasticity of the philtrum skin, thins the upper lip and pushes down the corners of the mouth, resulting in a longer philtrum. The philtrum length can also change from the retreating upper jaw and protruding lower jaw after bimaxillary surgery. This increases the nasolabial angle, lengthens the philtrum, thins the upper lip and even lowers the isthmus. Protrusion of the alveolar bone or upper teeth, dental correction of snaggle tooth, etc. can also result in a longer philtrum and thinner upper lip.

Outcome and surgical method of philtrum reduction

A shorter philtrum makes the face appear younger, smaller, more confident and energetic. The added benefit of this procedure is the thickened upper lip, giving the face a more animated appearance with a fuller mouth.

There are two surgical methods to philtrum reduction;

01 Bull's horn incision under the nose

02 Gull wing incision.vermilion border of lip

03 Goldenview hybrid lip ift that combines the advantages of the two surgeries above mentioned

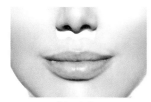
2-1 painting
Subnasal incision method

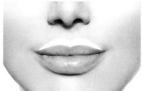
2-2 painting
Lip line incision method

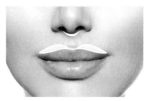
2-3 painting
Hybrid philtrum reduction method

The under nose incision can be carried out to reduce the philtrum while leaving the upper lip unchanged. The vermilion border incision can be applied when the upper lip is thin with unclear or flat border. Among them, goldenview hybrid lip lift is a surgery that has mostly been used nowadays as it combines the advantages of the two other surgeries and minimizes the advantages, if it fits the surgical indications.

1St Bleeding, edema, infection, asymmetry, relapse, and scarring can occur in rare cases. Side effects also include under-correction, over-correction, and skin bumps. Under nose incision can result in a wider nose or larger nasolabial angle depending on the extent of incision.

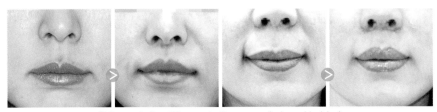

Before and after philtrum reduction surgery (subnasal incision)

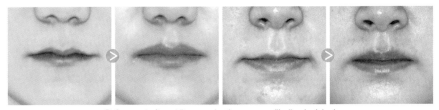

Before and after philtrum reduction surgery (lip line incision)

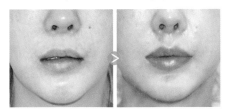

Before and after philtrum reduction surgery (hybrid philtrum reduction)

TIP_Philtrum reduction surgery information

Treatment time	Anesthetizing method	Hospitalization	Recovery time	Stitch removal	Stay time
2 hours	Local and sedative anesthesia	No hospitalization	7 days	7 days later	6~10 days

Lip reshaping

Ideal thickness and shape of lips depend on subjective standards. Many people fret that their lips are too thick or thin. Undesirably thick lips give an unsophisticated appearance. Recent trends favor plump lips with healthy gloss. It is important to accurately assess the need for the lip shaping procedure. If there are problems with teeth or alveolar bone, orthodontic, mouth protrusion correction, chin augmentation, or mid-facial contouring can be combined for better outcome.

LIP REDUCTION

A slight difference of 1-2mm in lip thickness can drastically change the entire facial image. The ideal ratio of lower lip to upper lip thickness in women is 7 to 10, with the lower lip being slightly thicker. Men are expected to have a thicker lower lip. This ratio should be considered in lip reduction surgery.

Surgical method of lip reduction

In lip reduction surgery, a medial lip incision is made in the mucous membrane of the oral cavity and a predetermined amount of mucous membrane or muscle is resected

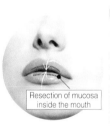

1 Step

medial lip resection

desired lip size and face
After determining the size
of the lips that matches the
proportions, an incision is
made in the oral mucosa
inside the lip and the
mucosa is excised for a
predetermined amount of
incision.

Resection of mucosa inside the mouth

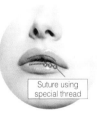

2 Step

Special thread microsuture

Sutured delicately and
meticulously using soluble
thread that is harmless to the
human body. There is no need
for a separate visit to remove
the thread as the meltable
thread naturally dissolves and
disappears.

Suture using special thread

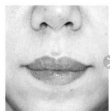
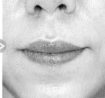

Before and after lip reduction surgery

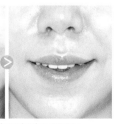

Before and after lip reduction surgery

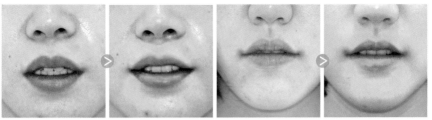

Before and after lip reduction surgery   Before and after lip reduction surgery

before suture. As absorbable thread is used in suture, there is no need to remove stitches. The surgery is performed under local anesthesia or intravenous sedation anesthesia as needed. The surgery takes about 30-40 minutes for one lip.

Cautions to be taken after surgery

Food ingestion is possible immediately after surgery, however, spicy or hard food should be avoided. Severe swelling lasts about 2-3 days after surgery but gradually disappears. In about a week, the patient can comfortably go outdoors as normal. The incision area of the medial lip feels hardened in the beginning but returns to normal texture in 2-3 months. Temporary sensory paralysis or mild numbness could follow lip reduction but sensation returns to normal in 2-3 month

LIP AUGMENTATION

Various treatments and surgical procedures are available to volumize and plump up thin and flat lips.

Surgical method of lip augmentation

Surgical methods of lip augmentation include lip mucosal advancement and lip line enhancement. The lip mucosal advancement is a flap surgery of lip mucosa. This method brings eversion and appropriate level of volume enhancement without excessive thickening. It is mainly used for lower lip augmentation along with lip line augmentation of the upper lip.

Mucosal advancement is the anterior adjustment of the medial lip mucosa and increases the lip volume by anterior- lateral eversion. Patients with a clear boundary of the lip and without excessively long philtrum or chin, scar-prone skin or keloids can experience natural-looking fuller lips. Lip augmentation using the upper lip line is the same procedure as the vermilion border of the lip incision of philtrum reduction(Gull wing lip lift). This method makes an incision along the vermilion border of the lip and is beneficial for patients with thin, flat lips and unclear borders of the mouth.

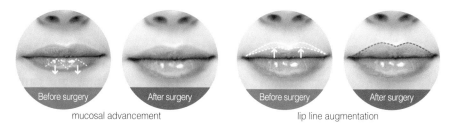

mucosal advancement · lip line augmentation

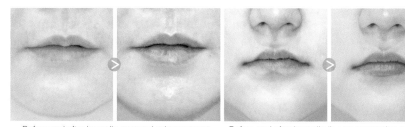

Before and after lower lip mucosal advancement · Before and after lower lip line augmentation surgery

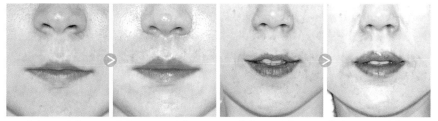

Before and after upper lip line augmentation · Before and after upper lip line augmentation

TIP_Lip reshaping surgery information

Treatment time	Anesthetizing method	Hospitalization	Recovery time	Stitch removal	Stay time
1~2 hours	Local and sedative anesthesia	No hospitalization	7 days	Not needed	6~10 days

Side effects : Edema. Decreased sensation, delay of the softening of surgical tissue. Denting, pigmentation, undercorrection

Cautions to be taken after surgery

The lip mucosa is very sensitive and can experience severe edema during the first 2-3 days after surgery. The swelling subsides gradually to only about 20-30% remaining in about a week and the patient can return to normal daily activities. As with lip reduction surgery, the mucosal sensation is numbed immediately following surgery but returns in about 2-3 months. Spicy or hard food should be avoided for a while after surgery.

Corrective procedure on the asymmetric shape of the lip

Reasons for an asymmetric shape of the mouth vary; natural and acquired facial paralysis, skeletal asymmetry of the face, asymmetry of the lip shape or the corners of the lips, asymmetry of the alveolar bone and teeth, and the differences in the activities of the muscles aroundthe lips.

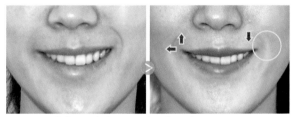

Before and after correction of mouth asymmetry

To correct these, there may be cases that need skeletal surgeries, though there are ways to yield a better result than expected such as making a balanced volume (through fat transplantation, fillers, etc.) and adjusting the activities of the muscles (through Botulinum toxin)

TIP_Lip reshaping surgery information

Treatment time	Anesthetizing method	Hospitalization	Recovery time	Stitch removal	Stay time
approximately 30 minutes	Local and sedative anesthesia	No hospitalization	immediately	not needed	1 day

Side effects : Bruising, swelling, inflammation, temporary and mild motor problems such as speaking, chewing, and swallowing. undercorrection

아트볼륨이마성형(Art Volume Forehead Surgery)
눈썹뼈 절삭술(Brow Bone Reduction Surgery)
이마재수술(Revisional Forehead-plasty)
아트내시경이마거상술(Endoscopic Forehead Surgery)
이마여성화수술(Forehead Feminization Surgery)

"

이마가 아름다움을 완성한다

The forehead completes the beauty

"

굴곡 없이 매끄럽고 얼굴과 조화를 이루는 이마는 모두의 바람이다. 이마에 관한 모든 문제에 대해 획기적이고 종합적인 해법을 제시한다.

A smooth, even forehead that harmonizes the face is something everyone wants. We offer groundbreaking and comprehensive solutions to all your forehead problems.

K아트성형외과의원
K-Art Plastic Surgery

www.k-artps.com

김남복(Nam-Bok Kim)

- 성형외과 전문의, 의학박사(Plastic Surgeon, MD.Ph.D)
- 충남대학교 의과대학 외래교수
(Outpatient Professor, Chungnam National University School of Medicine)
- 대한성형외과학회 정회원(Member of the Korean Society of Plastic Surgeons)
- 대한미용성형외과 학회 정회원(Member of the Korean Society of Aesthetic Plastic Surgery)
- 대한두개안면성형학회 정회원(Member of the Korean Society of Craniofacial Plastic Surgery)

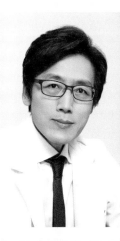

04 내시경을 이용한 신개념의 이마 수술

흠 없는 예쁜 이마 만들기. 이마성형의 모든 것!

동글고 환한 이마는 예로부터 고귀함의 상징으로 인식되어 왔다. 반듯하고 자연스러운 라인을 그리는 이마는 기품이 있고, 밝고 건강한 매력을 느끼게 한다. 예나 지금이나 예쁜 이마는 불변의 미의 기준이다.

볼륨 있고 매끄러운 이마를 얻기 위해서 다양한 방법들이 사용되어 왔다. 이마에 자가지방을 이식하는 지방이식, 필러로 이마의 부족한 부분을 채우는 시술, 보형물을 사용하여 적당한 이마 볼륨을 만드는 방법 등이 있었다. 하지만 모두 한계와 부작용들이 너무 많이 생겨, 더 이상 사용해서는 안 되는 것이 증명되고 있다. 또한 이러한 잘못된 여러 가지 이마성형 때문에 이마재수술이 필요한 경우도 크게 늘고 있는 실정이다. 또, 나이가 들면서 생기는 이마와 눈가의 주름과 눈썹과 눈꺼풀 처짐으로 인한 여러 가지 문제도 이마 수술로 함께 개선해 주어야 한다. 그에 따라, 안전하고 영구적인 새로운 방법이 요구되고 있다. 나아가 환자가 필요한 각각의 상태에 따라, 이마의 볼륨과 눈썹 뼈 절삭 등 모양에 관한 문제뿐 아니라, 처진 눈썹과 주름에 대한 이마거상, 이마의 확대 및 축소, 재수술 등 모든 요구에 따라, 이를 총체적으로 해결할 수 있는 종합적 이마성형이 실현될 수 있어야 한다. 이제 내시경 수술의 발전으로, 그러한 요구에 부응할 수 있게 되었다.

아트볼륨이마성형

기존의 지방이식이나 보형물은 문제점이 많아 지양되어야 한다. 안전하고 리프팅까지 가능한 신개념의 내시경 수술법 아트볼륨이마수술을 소개한다.

보형물 없이 완성하는 자연스럽고 볼륨 있는 이마 만들기

많은 사람이 동글고 예쁜 이마를 연예인의 외모의 조건으로 꼽는다. 그런 이마를 갖기 위해 여러 가지 방법들이 동원되어 왔다. 하지만 지방이식은 흡수가 일어나 여러 차례 반복 시술을 해야 하며, 생착과 흡수가 고르지 않아 아래로 흐르며 요철을 일으킨다. 보형물은 수년 후 물이나 피가 차고, 뼈가 함몰되는 문제가 심각하다. 모두 마땅한 방법이 아니다.

이에 필자는 내시경의 발달과 함께 획기적인 이마 융기법을 개발하게 되었다. 핵심은 아무런 삽입물을 넣지 않고, 자신의 살로 채워 올라오도록 하는 것이다.

필자의 아트볼륨이마수술은 두피에 작은 절개를 통하여 내시경으로 수술하는 방법으로, 돌출된 눈썹부의 조직을 이마의 고랑으로 재배치함으로써, 높은 가장자리는 낮추고, 낮은 이마의 중심부는 옮긴 살로 채워 높게 만드는 완전히 새로운 이마 융기법이다. 이 수술은 매우 간단하며 안전하고, 효과 또한 탁월하며 영구적인 것이 장점이다. 보형물이 전혀 들어가지 않는 만큼 그에 따른 부작용을 모두 피할 수 있고, 지방이식처럼 흡수나 울퉁불퉁한 요철의 염려도 없다. 한 번의 수술로 충분한 효과를 얻을 수 있고, 처진 이마와 눈썹도 함께 리프팅 가능하며, 눈썹뼈가 돌출된 경우에는 이도 깎아서 낮출 수 있다. 많은 효과를 한 번에 얻을 수 있다. 아트볼륨이마수술은 기존 이마성형의 문제점들을 종합적으로 보완한 신개념의 획

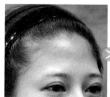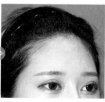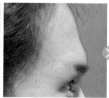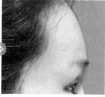

아트볼륨이마성형 수술전후   아트볼륨이마성형 수술전후

기적 수술 방법이라 할 수 있다.

TIP_아트볼륨이마성형 수술정보

수술시간	마취방법	입원여부	회복기간	실밥제거	체류기간
1시간	국소, 수면마취	입원없음	약 2주	12일	1~2주

눈썹뼈 절삭술

이마에 볼륨뿐 아니라 기존에는 불가능했던 눈썹뼈 설삭까시 본원에서 세계 최초로 니시경으로 기능케 하였다.

미남의 조건, 멋진 이마를 만드는 남자이마수술

매끈하고 훤한 이마는 세련된 도시의 남성 이미지로, 모두가 갖고 싶어 하는 모습일 것이다. 시원하게 뒤로 올린 머리로 드러낸 훤한 이마는 남자의 자신감을 보여준다. 남자의 경우에는 눈썹뼈가 튀어나온 경우가 흔하다. 이러한 경우 돌출된 눈썹뼈에 맞추어 보형물이나 지방이식 등으로 윗이마를 채우게 되면, 이마는 더욱 튀어나오고, 눈은 더욱 깊어지게 되어, 속칭 앞짱구와 같이 어색하고 강한 인상이 되어 낭패를 보기 쉽다.

눈썹뼈가 돌출된 경우에는 이를 깎아서 낮춰야 비로소 자연스러운 이마를 얻을 수 있다. 하지만 눈썹뼈를 깎으려면, 과거에는 두피 내에 긴 절개를 가해야만 가능하여서, 머리가 짧은 남성들은 사실상 시행이 불가능하였던 것이 사실이다. 게다가 전신 마취도 요하였다.

하지만 이제 가능해졌다. 필자가 세계 최초로 간단한 내시경만으로 이를 가능케 하였다. 두피에 아주 작은 절개를 통하여, 안전하게 눈썹뼈의 절삭이 가능하다. 돌출이 심한 경우에는 절골하여 안으로 밀어 넣으면 더욱 큰 효과를 볼 수 있다. 흉은 문제가 되지 않고, 입원도 필요 없으며, 수면마취와 부분마취만으로 모두 시행

가능하다. 또, 동시에 이마에 볼륨과 리프팅 효과도 얻을 수 있다. 가히 획기적인 수술이라 할 수 있다.

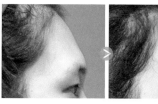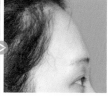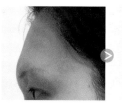

눈썹뼈 절삭술 및 내절골술 수술전후   눈썹뼈 절삭술 및 내절골술 수술전후

TIP_눈썹뼈 절삭술 수술정보					
수술시간	마취방법	입원여부	회복기간	실밥제거	체류기간
2시간 30분	국소, 수면마취	입원없음	약 2주	12일	1~2주

| 이마재수술

이마수술 부작용의 완전한 해결책! 지방이식과 보형물로 인한 부작용을 제거와 동시에 재융기를 시켜주는 신개념의 방법이다.

두 번의 실패는 없다. 내 인생의 마지막 이마성형! 이마재수술

  이마에 지방이식이나 보형물 삽입이 증가하면서, 그에 따른 부작용도 크게 증가하고 있다. 지방이식은 흡수로 인하여, 여러 차례 반복 시행하여야 하는 문제도 있지만, 흡수되고 나면 아래로 흐르기도 하고 울퉁불퉁한 요철을 남기게 되어, 흡인으로 다시 제거해야 하는 경우가 많이 늘고 있다. 또, 보형물은 전위나 신경자극 등의 문제를 일으키기도 하지만, 시간이 지남에 따라 피나 물이 차게 되는 경우가 허다하다. 보통 삽입 후 5년에서 10년 정도 지나 갑자기 발생하는 경우가 대부분이다. 그러한 이유는 일종의 지연성 거부반응이기 때문이다. 한 번 피나 물이 차기 시작하면, 점차 그 주기가 짧아지고, 결국은 제거를 해야만 한다.

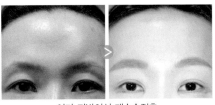
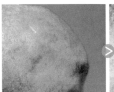
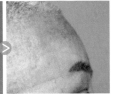

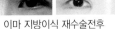
이마 지방이식 재수술전후

이마보형물 재수술전후

보다 문제는, 그 사이 뼈가 함몰되고 있었다는 것이다. 시간이 지남에 따라 보형물에 의하여 이마뼈가 계속 침식되어 가라앉게 되는 것인데, 이는 매우 심각한 문제라 할 수 있다. 보형물을 제거하고 나면, 그대로 지낼 수는 없고 거부반응이 있는 보형물을 다시 넣을 수도 없어서 고민이 된다.

아트볼륨이마재수술은 이런 고민을 근본적으로 해결할 수 있는 방법이다. 보형물을 제거함과 동시에 침식으로 인해 낮아진 이마를 자가조직 재배치로 재융기할 수 있다. 동시에 이마의 거상도 가능하고, 눈썹뼈가 돌출된 경우에는, 이를 깎는 것까지도 가능하다.

TIP_이마재수술 수술정보

수술시간	마취방법	입원여부	회복기간	실밥제거	체류기간
2시간	국소, 수면마취	입원없음	약 2주	12일	1~2주

아트내시경이마거상술

내시경수술로 흉터 걱정 없이 처진 눈꺼풀과 눈썹을 자연스럽게 되돌려주는 눈썹이마거상술. 또한, 볼륨까지 만들어주는 다중 효과의 최신 수술법이다.

이마에 대한 총체적 해법! 일거다득 이마거상술

젊어서 예뻤던 쌍꺼풀이 나이가 들면서 점차 처지고 덮게 된다. 이때 보통은 눈꺼풀이 내려왔다고 생각하고, 쌍꺼풀 위의 눈꺼풀을 잘라내고 쌍꺼풀 수술을 시행하는 경우가 흔하다. 하지만 실제 처진 것의 대부분은 눈꺼풀이 아니라 눈썹 즉, 이마가 처지며 그에 매달려 있는 눈꺼풀이 따라서 처지게 되는 것이다. 이 경우 처진 윗눈썹을 그대로 두고, 눈꺼풀 피부를 잘라 쌍꺼풀 수술을 하게 되면, 윗눈썹과 쌍꺼풀 사이가 더 좁아지게 되고 인상이 아주 강하게 변하게 된다.

또, 눈썹 밑에서 피부를 잘라 거상하는 즉, 눈썹밑 거상술을 시행하는 경우도 있는데, 이는 흉만 남기고 유지가 되지 않을 뿐 아니라, 나중에 제대로 된 이마거상술을 시행하려하면, 피부가 모자라 문제가 되는 경우가 많다.

이와 같이 나이가 들며 눈꺼풀이 처진 경우에는, 눈이 아니라 처진 원인이 되는 눈썹 즉, 이마를 당겨 올려주어야 자연스럽고 제대로 된 원인 교정이 되는 것이다.

과거에는 이마를 당겨 올릴 때 머리 속에서 긴 가로 절개를 해야 하고, 그에 따라 수술도 커지고 긴 흉터와 두피의 감각저하 등 여러 가지로 수반되는 문제점들이 많아 쉽게 시행하기 어려웠다. 하지만 내시경이 나온 지금은 그러한 절개에 따른 문제점들을 모두 극복하고, 두피 속의 작은 절개만을 통하여 매우 간단하게, 이마와 눈썹 그리고 눈꺼풀까지 되돌려 올려놓을 수 있게 되었다.

또, 두피에서 당겨 올리게 되면 이마의 주름도 펴지고, 눈가와 콧등 주름도 펼 수 있다. 처진 눈썹이 당겨 올라가면 인상이 젊고 밝아지며 처진 눈꺼풀이 걷어져, 젊어서 예뻤던 시원한 눈으로 되돌릴 수 있다. 또, 미간에 찌푸린 주름도 원인이 되는 추미근을 잘라내어 영구적으로 없앨 수 있다. 또한, 이마가 좁거나 고랑진 경우 이마 거상과 동시에 좁은 이마를 넓힐 수도 있고, 고랑진 이마를 융기시켜 젊고 예쁜 이마를 만들 수 있다. 나이가 들면서 발생하는 눈과 이마의 모든 문제점을 근원적으로 교정하는, 일거다득의 총체적 해결법이라 할 수 있다.

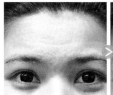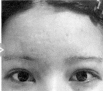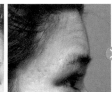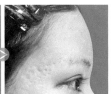

아트내시경이마거상술 전후　　아트내시경이마거상술 전후

수술시간	마취방법	입원여부	회복기간	실밥제거	체류기간
1시간 30분	국소, 수면마취	입원없음	약 2주	12일	1~2주

이마여성화수술

안면 여성화는 예쁜 이마로 완성된다. 내시경 수술로 가능해진 이마 여성화 수술!

안전하고 볼륨까지 얻는 내시경이마확대술

남성과 여성의 이마는 매우 많이 다른 점을 가지고 있다. 전체적으로 남성의 이마는 판판하고 각이 져 있으며, 눈썹뼈나 아이홀뼈가 많이 돌출되어 굴곡이 심하다. 이마 중앙부는 흔히 꺼져 있고 깊게 위치한 눈을 가지고 있으며, 눈썹의 위치는 낮은 반면 눈썹의 바깥쪽은 높아 기운이 뻗친 모양을 보이고, 미간을 찌푸리는 근육의 힘은 세어 미간 주름이 생기기 십상이다. 헤어라인은 높고 흔히 M-자형 탈모를 보인다.

이에 반해, 여성의 이마는 전체적으로 동그란 느낌을 주며, 이마가 둥글고 볼륨감이 있다. 또한 눈썹뼈나 아이홀뼈 등의 돌출이 없어서 매끄러운 이마의 윤곽선을 가지고 있으며 이마 중앙부가 동글게 튀어나와 있다. 눈의 위치도 남자보다 옅게 위치하고, 눈썹의 위치는 높으면서 눈썹은 비교적 수평에 가까운 모양을 띤다. 미간을 찌푸리는 근육의 힘은 세지 않아 미간 주름이 생기는 경우가 적고, 헤어라인은 낮고 둥근 모양의 헤어라인을 보인다.

트랜스젠더로서 안면 여성화를 하려는 경우 이마의 여성화도 매우 중요하며 최근 그 중요성에 대한 인식도 증가하고 있다. 과거에는 이러한 이마 여성화 수술을 하려면 헤어라인을 따라 길게 절개하거나, 두피 내에 귀에서 반대쪽 귀까지에 이르는 긴 절개선을 가하여야만 가능했다. 현재도 본원을 제외한 나머지 모든 병원에서 그렇게 절개하고 수술을 하고 있는 실정이다. 하지만, 그러한 긴 절개선은 헤어라인이나 두피 내에 크게 눈에 띄는 탈모를 동반한 긴 흉터를 남기고, 또 절개선 후방에 감각저하 같은 신경 증상을 흔히 발생시켜, 얻는 것보다 잃는 것이 더 많다는 말이 나오는 것도 사실이다.

더욱이 그러한 수술 방법으로는 여성화에 꼭 필요한 이마 중앙의 볼륨을 만들지 못하고, 아이홀뼈도 절삭해 낮추지 못한다. 잃는 것은 많으나, 얻는 것은 매우 제한적인 것이다.

이에 본원에서는 긴 절개선 흉터를 남기지 않고 이마 볼륨까지 만들 수 있는 내시경 이마 여성화 수술을 개발해 시행하고 있다. 앞서 소개한 내시경 볼륨이마 수술과 거상술 그리고 눈썹뼈 절삭술 및 내절골술 또 아이홀뼈 절삭술이 그것이다. 이 모두를 조합하여 시행하면 이마의 여러 남성적 특징들을 없애고 동글고 볼륨있는 예쁜 여성의 이마를 만들 수 있다. 나아가 두피 절개와 같이 전신 마취나 입원도 필요 없고, 수면마취와 국소마취 하에서 시행이 가능하고, 입원도 필요하지 않다. 또 내시경 수술이어서 절개선이 매우 작으므로 흉터도 문제가 되지 않지만 회복도 매우 빨라서 약 2주 정도면 거의 표가 나지 않을 정도로 회복이 빠르다.

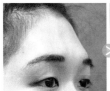 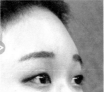 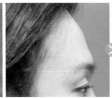 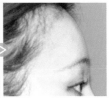

이마 여성화 수술전후   이마 여성화 수술전후

TIP_이마 여성화 수술 정보

수술시간	마취방법	입원여부	회복기간	실밥제거	체류기간
3~3시간 30분	국소. 수면마취	입원없음	약 2주	12일	1~2주

04 Groundbreaking New Concepts of Forehead Surgery Using Endoscope

A Novel Approach to Forehead Surgery Using Endoscopy Creating a Flawless, Pretty Forehead. All About Forehead Surgery!

A round, bright forehead has long been recognized as a symbol of nobility. A well-defined and naturally shaped forehead exudes elegance, cheerfulness, and a sense of radiant well-being. A beautiful forehead has always been a timeless standard of beauty.

To achieve a voluminous and smooth forehead, various methods have been commonly used. Fat grafting, in which an individual's own fat is transplanted to the forehead, fillers to fill in gaps in the forehead, and implants to enhance forehead volume. However, they all have limitations and a host of side effects that are now being shown to be avoidable.

In addition, the number of patients needing revision forehead surgery is increasing due to these various botched procedures. There are many other problems that can be addressed with forehead surgery, such as wrinkles on the forehead and around the eyes, sagging eyebrows and eyelids that can occur with age. As a result, there is a need for new methods that are safe and permanent.

Depending on the individual needs of the patient, a comprehensive forehead surgery system is now available that can address not only shape issues such as forehead volume and brow bone reduction, but all needs such as forehead lifting for sagging brows and wrinkles, forehead augmentation and reduction, and revision surgery. With advances in endoscopic surgery, this is now a feasible option.

| Art Volume Forehead Surgery

Conventional fat grafting and implants have many problems but are no longer the only option. Introducing Art Volume Forehead Surgery, a new concept in endoscopic surgery which is safe and allows for simultaneous lifting

Create a natural, voluminous forehead without implants!

Many people consider a rounded, beautiful forehead to be a prerequisite for celebrity appeal. Various methods have previously been used to achieve such a forehead. However, fat grafting can be counterproductive and risky, with multiple repeat procedures needed due to absorption, uneven placement, and downward movement that causes unevenness in the face.

Implants are prone to induce seroma or hematoma and bone depression after a few years. None of these are acceptable. With the development of endoscopy, I've developed a revolutionary forehead ridge method. The key is to use the patient's own tissue to fill in the gaps, without any inserts.

Introducing Art Volume Forehead Surgery, a novel method of forehead elevation that is performed endoscopically through a small incision in the scalp and relocates tissue from the protruding brow into the furrow of the forehead, lowering the higher bumps while raising the center of the lower forehead with transferred soft tissue.

The procedure is simple, safe, effective, and permanent. Since there are no implants involved, you can avoid the side effects that come with them, and you don't have to worry about absorption or unevenness like with fat grafting.

In just one surgery, you can lift your sagging forehead and eyebrows, and if you have a

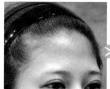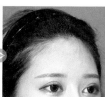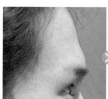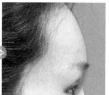

Before and After Art Volume Forehead Surgery

protruding brow bone, you can shave it down at the same time.

Many effects can be achieved at once. Art Volume Forehead Surgery is a novel concept and groundbreaking surgical method that comprehensively complements the problems of existing forehead surgery.

TIP_Art Volume Forehead Surgery information					
Operation time	Anesthetizing method	Hospitalization	Recovery time	Stitch removal	Stay time
1 hour	Local + Sleep anesthesia	No hospitalization	Approx. 2weeks	12 days	1~2 weeks

| Brow Bone Reduction Surgery

We are the first in the world to perform endoscopic forehead surgery that not only enhances forehead volume, but cuts down excessively protruding brow bone, which was previously impossible to do while also providing natural volume.

Men's Forehead Surgery : What Makes a Good-looking Forehead

A smooth and defined forehead is the signature of a sophisticated urban man, and it's a look that everyone aspires to have. A well-defined forehead with a cool slicked-back hairstyle shows a man's confidence. It's common for men to have a protruding brow bone, but if the upper forehead is filled with implants or fat grafting to match the protruding brow bone, the forehead will protrude even more and the eyes will appear even deeper.

If you have a protruding brow bone, you can shave it down to achieve a natural-looking forehead. In the past this procedure used general anesthesia and was made with a long incision across the scalp. For men with short hair, an obvious scar would be left across the head, making it hard to disguise.

For the first time, I've made it possible to avoid these issues by using a simple endoscope. The brow bone can be safely shaved through small incisions on the scalp.

Even with a severe protrusion, the brow bone can be rasped and in-fractured to achieve a greater effect. Scarring is not an issue, no hospitalization is required, and the procedure can be performed under sleep and local anesthesia. With this procedure, the forehead can be volumized and lifted, making it truly a breakthrough surgery.

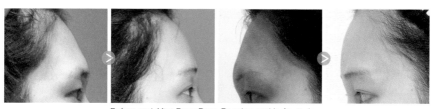

Before and After Brow Bone Rasping and In-fracturing

TIP_Brow Bone Reduction Surgery Information					
Operation time	Anesthetizing method	Hospitalization	Recovery time	Stitch removal	Stay time
2 hours 30 minutes	Local + Sleep anesthesia	No hospitalization	Approx. 2weeks	12 days	1~2 weeks

| Forehead Revision Surgery

The perfect solution to forehead surgery side effects! This novel method treats side effects caused by fat grafting and implants while simultaneously rejuvenating the forehead.

The last forehead surgery you'll ever need! Forehead Revision Surgery

As the number of people getting fat grafts and implants in the forehead has increased, resulting in the number of people suffering the side effects as well. Fat grafting has the problem of resorption, which requires repetition to keep the effect. Additionally, the grafted fat may flow down and leave a bumpy irregularity, which needs to be removed again. Implants can also cause problems such as dislocation and nerve irritation, they can even fill with blood or seroma over time. This usually happens suddenly, about five to ten years after implantation. This is because it's a type of delayed rejection. Once it starts to bleed or ooze, it will gradually become more frequent, and eventually need to be removed. The effect of using implants is even more dangerous, as severe bony erosion can occur over time.

As implants erode the bone in the forehead, the forehead sinks lower. These are serious problems for patients seeking to improve their foreheads in a sustainable manner. Once the implant is removed, the results of bony erosion remain, and implants should not be used again once they've been rejected.

Art Volume Forehead Revision Surgery is a radical solution to this problem. In addition to removing the implants, foreheads damaged due to erosion can be resurfaced using the patient's own soft tissue from the surrounding area, repositioning it to the depressions left by bone erosion. At the same time, the forehead can be lifted, and where the brow bone may be protruding, it can be shaved.

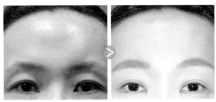

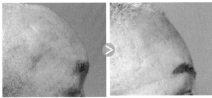

Fat Injection Removal : Before and After   Forehead Implant Revision : Before, Introperation and After

TIP_Forehead Revision Surgery Information

Operation time	Anesthetizing method	Hospitalization	Recovery time	Stitch removal	Stay time
2 hours	Local + Sleep anesthesia	No hospitalization	Approx. 2weeks	12 days	1~2 weeks

| Endoscopic Forehead Lift Surgery

Art forehead lift is an endoscopic surgery that naturally rejuvenates drooping eyelids and eyebrows without the risk of scarring. It is the latest surgical method with multi-effects combined together to safely create volume.

A comprehensive solution for your forehead! All-in-one forehead lift surgery

With aging, the eyelids that were once stunning in our youth gradually droop, concealing the eyes. With drooping eyelids, it's common to get corrective eyelid surgery which cuts away the upper eyelid.

However, most of the time, it's not the eyelids that are drooping, but the eyebrows or forehead that droops; the eyelids then hang from them covering the eye. In this case, if you leave the drooping upper eyebrows in place and perform a double eyelid surgery by cutting the eyelid skin, a narrower gap between the upper eyebrows and the eyelids is created, resulting in an uncanny expression.

In addition, there are cases where skin is cut from under the eyebrows to perform a brow lift, which is called a sub-brow lift. This is not only an impermanent solution, but also leaves a scar, and these patients cannot perform a proper forehead lift later on because of insufficient skin.

Therefore, if the eyelids are drooping due to age, then the cause of the drooping is not the eyes, but the eyebrows, which should be lifted to correct the problem naturally.

In the past, it has been difficult to perform forehead lifting because it required a long horizontal incision on the scalp or along the hairline. This was accompanied by various problems due to being a major surgery such as long scars and decreased sensation in the scalp.

However, with the introduction of the endoscope, it's possible to overcome all the problems associated with long incisions and simply lift the forehead, eyebrows, and eyelids, using only a few small incisions made on the scalp.

By lifting the skin up from the scalp, wrinkles on the forehead are smoothed out, in addition to the wrinkles around the eyes and on the bridge of the nose. Drooping

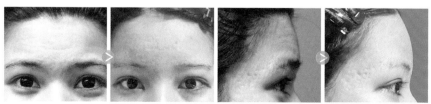

Before and After Art Endoscopic Forehead Lift

eyebrows can be pulled up to make the face look younger and brighter, and drooping eyelids can be lifted to restore the freshness of youthful eyes. Frown lines on the brow can also be permanently eliminated by removing the furrowing muscles that cause them.

If you have a narrow or furrowed forehead, you can widen the narrow forehead at the same time as a forehead lift, or you can increase the volume on the furrowed forehead to create a youthful and beautiful forehead.

It's a holistic solution to correct all the problems of the eyes and forehead that occur with age.

TIP_Endoscopic Forehead Lift Surgery Information

Operation time	Anesthetizing method	Hospitalization	Recovery time	Stitch removal	Stay time
1 hour 30 minutes	Local + Sleep anesthesia	No hospitalization	Approx. 2weeks	12 days	1~2 weeks

| Forehead Feminization Surgery

Facial Feminization is Complete with a Pretty Forehead!
Endoscopic Forehead Feminization Surgery is now possible!

Developing endoscopic forehead feminization surgery to support transgender people

The foreheads of men and women are generally very different. Men have characteristically flat and angular foreheads, irregular surface protruding eyebrow and eyehole bones overshadowing the eyes.

The middle of the forehead is low and recessed, and the eyes are deeply set. The eyebrows are generally positioned low and the peak at the corners and canted end high, giving a strong masculine appearance.

Muscles used for frowning are well developed and lead to frown lines between the eyebrows. The typical male hairline is higher than for women, and often has an M-shape. In contrast, a woman's forehead is rounder and full of volume. With a smooth forehead contour yet without brow bone or eyehole bone protrusions or deep eye sockets. The middle of the forehead is round and not recessed. Her eyebrows sit higher up and are more horizontal. Her frowning muscles are naturally less developed and will not be as strong, so frown lines are less likely to develop. And her hairline is low and rounded.

For transgender people who want to facial feminization, the feminization of the forehead is also very important. Awareness of the impact of a feminine forehead is increasing and becoming more and more popular with our method.

In the past, forehead feminization surgery was only possible by making a long incision along the hairline or by making a long incision on the scalp from one ear to the other. These are still the default methods in all hospitals except ours. However, long incision lines leave long scars, leading to noticeable hair loss along the hairline or scalp. Often times, neurological symptoms such as numbness occur behind the incision line, so the risks can often outweigh the benefits.

Moreover, such surgical methods do not create the volume in the center of the forehead, which is essential for feminization, and the eyehole bone cannot be rasped and lowered. There is much to lose, but very limited to gain.

Therefore, our hospital has developed and performed endoscopic forehead feminization surgery that can create forehead volume without leaving long incision scars.

These include the endoscopic volume forehead surgery, brow lift, brow and eyehole bone rasping, and frontal sinus in-fracturing. By combining all of these, you can get rid of many of the masculine features of the forehead and create a round, voluminous,

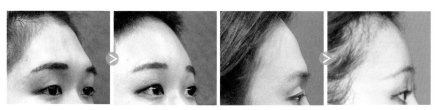

Before and After Forehead Feminization Surgery

beautiful feminine forehead.

Furthermore, it does not require general anesthesia or hospitalization like the incision method, and it can be performed under sleep anesthesia plus local anesthesia, which does not require hospitalization. Also, since it is a completely endoscopic surgery, the incision lines are very small, recovery is so fast hardly noticeable after two weeks, and scars usually will be fine.

An exciting new development in forehead feminization surgery is now available for transgender people!

TIP_Forehead Feminization Surgery Information					
Operation time	Anesthetizing method	Hospitalization	Recovery time	Stitch removal	Stay time
3~3 hours 30 minutes	Local + Sleep anesthesia	No hospitalization	Approx. 2weeks	12 days	1~2 weeks

이중턱 지방흡입술(Double chin liposuction)
이중턱 근육 묶기(Platysma muscle surgery)
아래 얼굴거상술(Lower face lift)

효과적인 이중턱 개선을 위한 다양한 이중턱 성형술

Various double chin cosmetic procedures for effective double chin improvement

얼굴의 두 겹으로 자리 잡은 이중턱을 개선할 수 있는 이중턱 지방흡입부터 늘어진 이중턱 근육묶기 수술까지 알아보도록 한다.

Let's explore the range of procedures available to improve double chins that have settled in the two layers of the face, from double chin liposuction to muscle tightening surgery for sagging double chins.

정우성형외과
Jung Woo Plastic Surgery

www.jwps.co.kr

이정우(Jung-Woo Lee)

• 성형외과 전문의 (Plastic Surgeon)
• 대한성형외과 학회 정회원(Full Member of Korean Society of Plastic Surgery)
• 대한미용성형외과 학회 정회원(Full Member of the Korean Society for Aesthetic Plastic Surgery)
대한두개안면성형외과 학회 정회원(Full member of the Korean Society of Craniofacial Plastic Surgery)
• 대한 성형외과 학회 안면윤곽 연구회 총무이사
(Managing Director of Facial Contour Research Group, Korean Society of Plastic Surgery)
• 現) 정우성형외과 대표원장(Current Director of Jungwoo Plastic Surgery)

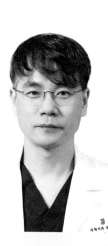

05 피하지방과 **턱뼈** 크기, 그리고 **근육**을 고려한 맞춤형 이중턱 성형술

이중턱 성형술의 목적

미의 기준은 시대에 따라 변화한다. 과거에는 전반적으로 동그란 형태의 얼굴이 '귀티 나고 복스럽다' 여겨졌다면, 오늘날에는 작고 갸름한 V라인의 얼굴형이 남녀노소를 불문하고 미의 기준으로 자리 잡았다. 조금 더 작고 갸름한 얼굴형을 원하는 트렌드 속에서 턱 아래에 두 겹으로 자리 잡고 있는 '이중턱'은 불청객이 아닐 수 없다.

이중턱이 있으면 얼굴과 목의 경계가 모호하게 보이기 때문에 인상이 둔해 보일 뿐 아니라 입체감이 사라지기 때문에 실제 보다 더 평면적으로 보이고 살쪄 보이게까지 한다. 사람은 전반적인 실루엣을 통해 사물을 인지하기 때문에 얼굴형은 이목구비를 담고 있는 밑바탕이자 이미지의 전반적인 분위기를 좌우하고 첫인상을 결정짓는데 중요한 역할을 하고 있어 많은 사람들이 이중턱을 개선할 수 있는 솔루션을 찾고 있다. 많은 사람들이 다이어트 또는 식단 관리를 통해 이중턱을 해결하려 노력하고 있지만 이중턱과 같이 국소 부위에 살 만을 빼는 것은 쉽지 않을뿐더러 많은 시간과 노력이 필요한 부분이다. 이러한 니즈에 발맞추어 미용성형 분야에서는 발 빠르게 '이중턱 성형술'을 내놓았다. 이중턱이 생기는 원인을 단순하게 불필요한 피하지방이 많은 경우로만 생각할 수 있다. 하지만 이중턱 부위는 다른 부위와 다르게 지방뿐 아니라 턱뼈의 크기와 모양 그리고 이중턱 아랫부분의 근육의 영향으로 발생하는 경우도 있다.

따라서 '이중턱 성형술'은 단순히 지방의 양만 줄일 것이 아니라 이중턱이 발생하는 원인에 따른 적합한 솔루션으로 근본적인 개선을 통해 이중턱의 부피를 줄이고 매끄럽고 갸름한 얼굴라인을 만드는 것을 목적으로 한다.

이중턱 지방흡입술

이중턱 부위에 불필요한 피하지방이 이중턱 부위에 쌓이게 되면서 두 겹으로 접히는 경우, 아큐스컬프 레이저를 조사하여 미세 캐뉼라(Micro Cannula)로 융해된 지방을 흡입해 개선할 수 있다.

원래 불필요한 지방을 제거해 주는 '지방흡입술'은 복부나 허벅지같이 지방층이 두꺼운 곳에서 주로 많이 시행되었다. 하지만 우리의 얼굴도 다른 신체 부위처럼 피부밑에 피하지방이 존재하고 많은 환자들의 얼굴지방을 국소적으로 제거하려는 니즈를 수용해 많은 성형외과 전문의들의 연구로 얼굴 지방 흡입을 시행하게 되었다. 얼굴 부위와 더불어 이중턱 부위의 불필요한 지방을 효과적으로 개선할 수 있는 방법으로는 아큐스컬프 레이저를 이용한 이중턱 지방 흡입이 개선책이 될 수 있다.

수술 방법

아큐스컬프 레이저는 지방을 타깃으로 하는 1,444nm의 파장을 가지고 있는 레이저기기로 지방을 태우는 목적으로 사용되는 레이저 기기이다. 하지만, 임상을 통해 확인한 결과 아큐스컬프 레이저를 통해 지방을 태우고 환자가 눈에 띌 만큼 효과를 보기에는 한계점이 있다. 따라서 이중턱 지방을 흡입하기 전 아큐스컬프 레이저를 피하지방에 조사하여 조직을 느슨하게 만든 다음 지방을 미세캐뉼라를 통해 핸드메이드 방식으로 흡입하는 방법으로 이중턱 지방을 개선한다.

이 수술 방법은 이중턱 부위에 피하지방층이 두터운 경우에 더욱 효과적이기 때문에 수술 전 상담 단계에서 초음파 검사를 통해서 지방의 양을 확인하는 것이 중요하다. 수술은 국소 또는 수면마취로 진행이 가능하며, 턱 끝 밑과 턱 양옆 쪽에 작은 절개창을 이용해 투메센트 용액을 주입한 후 아큐스컬프 레이저를 조사한 후 같은 절개 부위를 통해 미세캐뉼라를 이용해 핸드메이드 방식으로 흡입을 하여 진행한다.

이중턱 부위의 지방을 흡입하기 위해서는 얼굴 부위인 만큼 부작용과 조직 손상을 낮추기 위해 기존의 지방 흡입의 방법보다 조금 더 섬세한 방법을 필요로 한다. 따라서 기존의 흡입관이 아닌 얇은 미세캐뉼라를 이용해 높은 압력으로 지방을 흡입하는 것이 아니라 1cc 또는 3cc 정도의 주사기를 이용하여 낮은 압력으로 반복하여 섬세하게 지방을 흡입해야 한다.

수술 후 관리 및 효과

이중턱 지방 흡입 수술 후에는 1~2일 정도 급성 부기가 발생할 수 있다. 이 기간에는 차가운 찜질팩을 수건이나 거즈에 감싸 냉찜질을 해주고 3일차부터는 온찜질을 통해 혈액순환을 증진시켜 부기에 도움이 된다.

수술 후 지방이 빠져나간 부위의 조직이 잘 달라붙을 수 있도록 가멘트(압박용 땡김이)를 착용 후 퇴원을 하게 된다. 가멘트 착용 여부는 최종 수술 결과에는 영향을 주지 않지만, 빠른 회복과 부기를 빨리 빼는 데 도움을 준다. 따라서 가멘트의 경우 이중턱 부위에 잘 밀착될 수 있도록 보정속옷을 입는 정도의 강도로 착용하되 너무 오랜 시간 착용하기보다는 착용 후 휴식을 반복해 주는 것이 회복에 도움이 된다.

이중턱 지방 흡입의 효과는 환자의 개인마다 차이가 있지만, 수술 후 한 달 정도 경과한 후 림프에 부종이 빠지고 지방을 흡입한 공간이 달라 붓는 느낌이 나면서 라인이 나오게 되며 잔 부기가 서서히 빠지면서 최종적인 결과는 6개월 정도의 시간이 소요된다.

수술 후 유지 기간

우리 몸의 지방세포는 유아기와 청소년기에는 지방의 세포가 지속적으로 늘어나지만, 성인이 되면 지방세포의 숫자는 고정이 된다. 이렇게 고정된 지방세포의 수는 변동이 없게 된다. 지방 흡입 수술은 우리의 몸에서 지방을 빼내는 수술이기 때문에 한번 빠지게 된 지방세포는 다시 생성되지 않게 된다. 따라서 이중턱 지방 흡입을 받은 결과는 시간이 지나 노화 현상으로 자연스럽게 처짐이 올 수 있지만, 살이 찌지 않는 이상은 효과가 계속 유지된다.

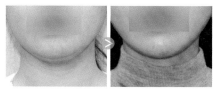

이중턱 지방흡입 수술 정면   이중턱 지방흡입 수술 측면

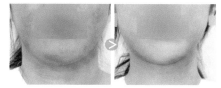

이중턱 지방흡입 수술 정면

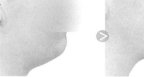

이중턱 지방흡입 수술 측면

TIP_이중턱 지방흡입 시술정보				
시술시간	마취방법	입원여부	회복기간	체류기간
30분 ~1시간	수면, 국소마취	입원없음	5~7일	7일

이중턱 근육 묶기

아래턱뼈의 크기가 작거나 후방으로 들어가 있는 무턱, 턱 끝을 줄이는 안면윤곽 또는 양악 수술을 받은 사람의 경우에 효과적인 수술 방법이다.

이중턱이 발생하는 이유는 앞서 언급한 피하지방의 축적이 원인이기도 하지만 턱뼈의 크기나 모양도 이중턱이 발생하는 요인 중 하나이다. 아래턱뼈가 작은 경우 또는 턱 끝이 후방으로 들어가 있는 무턱의 경우에는 턱밑에 라인을 잡아주고 있는 근육들이 팽팽하게 잡아주지 못하고 아래 방향으로 늘어지게 되면서 이중턱이 발생할 수 있다. 또한 턱 끝의 길이나 폭을 줄이는 안면윤곽 수술이나 상악과 하악을 함께 수술하는 양악 수술을 이전에 시행했던 환자에게도 후천적으로 이중턱이 발생할 수 있다.

그 이유는 안면윤곽 또는 양악 수술의 과정에서 턱 라인 밑쪽에 위치한 근육을 박리하게 되고 이로 인해 근육이 떨어지면서 늘어나 이중턱이 발생하게 된다.

이렇게 지방뿐 아니라 턱뼈의 크기와 근육의 처짐으로 인한 이중턱이 발생한 경우에는 '이중턱 근육 묶기'가 효과적인 대안이 될 수 있다.

수술 방법

'이중턱 근육 묶기' 수술 전에는 피하지방을 흡입하는 지방 흡입 과정을 선 진행 후 근육 묶기를 진행한다. 수술은 이중턱의 정도와 지방량에 따라 한 시간 반에서 두 시간 정도 시간이 소요되며, 구레나룻 쪽이나 턱 아래쪽에 지방 흡입을 위한 1~2mm의 작은 절개창을 통해 지방 흡입이 시행되고 턱 끝 아래쪽 밑부분에 약 2~3cm 정도의 절개를 통해 이중턱 근육 묶기 수술이 진행된다.

'넓은 목근(Platysma)'과 피부 사이를 박리하고 넓은 목근 안쪽에 지방 흡입 방법으로는 흡입되지 않는 지방과 근육 사이에 위치해 있는 지방주머니를 충분히 수술적으로 절제하여 제거하고 양쪽 넓은 목근 사이의 공간을 확보한 후 목 근육을 신발 끈 묶듯이 꼼꼼하게 봉합을 하게 되면 근육이 타이트하게 당겨 올라가면서 이중턱이 개선된다.

흉터 및 회복 기간

이중턱 근육 묶기는 턱 아래 2~3cm 정도의 절개를 통해 시행되는 수술인 만큼 환자가 흉터에 대한 걱정과 부담이 있는 수술 방법이다. 하지만 대부분 턱뼈와 목의 경계 부위의 주름을 이용하여 수술을 진행하기 때문에 정면에서는 절개 흉터가 보이지 않으며, 수술 시 숙련된 전문의가 꼼꼼하게 봉합을 한다면 흉터는 잘 보이지 않는다. 수술 후에도 흉터연고를 꾸준히 발라서 관리해 주면, 개인마다 기간이나 정도의 차이는 있겠지만, 1~2개월 정도는 흉터가 붉은 기를 보이다 6개월 정도 시간이 경과하면 흐려져서 잘 안 보이게 된다.

이 수술은 이중턱 부위의 지방 흡입과 지방절제, 근육 묶기가 복합적으로 병행되는 수술인 만큼 앞서 말한 이중턱 지방 흡입만 시행 한 경우보다는 출혈이 발생할 가능성이 조금 더 높은 편이다.

수술 중 집도의가 꼼꼼하게 지혈을 해도 수술 후 개인에 따라 수술 후 멍이나 부기가 발생할 수 있다. 특히 멍의 경우 여성 환자보다는 남성 환자들에게 확률적으로 더 나타날 수 있는데, 그 이유는 여성에 비해 남성의 혈관이나 근육이 크기 때문이다. 대부분의 멍은 일주일 정도 경과하면 목 아래쪽으로 퍼지면서 빠지게 되고 경우에 따라 진하게 멍이 든 경우에는 2주 이상 소요될 수 있다.

수술 후 부착해 주는 압박테이프를 제거 한 후에는 마스크 착용이나 메이크업 등으로 가린 후 가벼운 일상생활은 가능하다.

효과 및 수술 후 주의사항

이 수술은 수술 후 3일째 붙여 놓았던 압박테이프를 제거한 후부터 즉각적인 효과를 볼 수 있다. 직접적으로 지방을 절제하고 근육 자체도 봉합을 통해 성형을 해주었기 때문에 수술 후 부기가 있는 것을 감안해도 육안으로 즉각적인 효과를 환자가 느낄 수 있다.

하지만 수술 과정에서 근육과 피부를 분리하는 과정이 있어 피부가 다시 잘 밀착될 수 있도록 압박해 주는 것이 중요하다. 박리했던 근육과 피부가 달라붙기 전까지는 수술 부위 쪽으로 출혈과 혈종이 발생할 가능성이 있어 수술 후 부착해 주는 압박테이프는 2~3일 정도 유지해 주는 게 도움이 되며, 가멘트는 수술 부위에 일주일 정도는 착용해 주는 것이 빠른 회복에 도움이 된다.

수술 후 일주일 경과 후에는 절개했던 부위의 실밥을 제거하게 되는데 가벼운 대화, 노래, 운동은 할 수 있지만, 무거운 중량을 들어야 하는 운동이나 고개를 많이 숙이거나 목을 움직이는 강도 높은 운동은 수술 후 한 달까지는 조심해 주어야 한다.

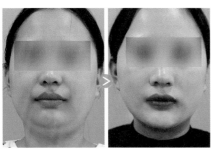

이중턱 근육묶기 정면

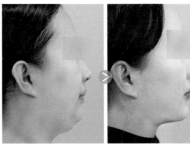

이중턱 근육묶기 측면

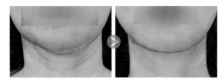

이중턱 근육묶기 정면

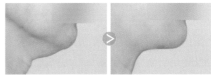

이중턱 근육묶기 측면

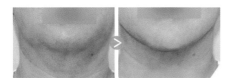

이중턱 근육묶기 정면

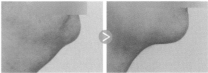

이중턱 근육묶기 측면

TIP_이중턱 근육묶기 시술정보

시술시간	마취방법	입원여부	회복기간	체류기간
1시간30분~2시간	수면 마취	입원없음	7~10일	14일

아래 얼굴거상술

노화로 인해 피부의 탄력이 저하되어 아래 방향으로 늘어지고 처지는 경우에는 '아래 얼굴거상술'을 통해서 개선할 수 있다.

노화는 우리의 신체의 자연스러운 현상이기도 하지만 동안이 하나의 자기관리의 척도가 되면서 중년층에서도 미용성형에 대한 관심이 높아지고 있다. 이중턱 성형술은 젊은 층에서도 니즈가 있는 수술이지만 노화로 인해서 탄력이 저하된 중년층에서도 관심을 가지는 수술이다. 하지만 앞서 말한 이중턱 성형술들은 목 부분보다는 턱 아래쪽과 목의 경계를 개선하는 수술 방법이기 때문에 아래턱의 중앙 부위의 개선은 충분히 될 수 있으나 나이가 들어 옆 턱선 피부의 탄력이 현저하게 저하되고 피부가 남아 처진 경우에는 이중턱 근육 묶기만으로는 한계가 있고 개선되기 어렵다.

이런 경우에는 귀 앞으로 절개를 통해 탄력이 떨어져 늘어진 피부를 탄력 있게 당겨주고 남는 피부를 절제하여 고정해 주는 '아래 얼굴 거상술'의 병행이 필요할 수 있다.

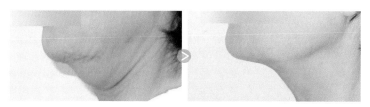

아래얼굴거상술 측면

TIP_아래 얼굴거상술 시술정보

시술시간	마취방법	입원여부	회복기간	체류기간
3~4시간	수면 마취	입원없음	7~10일	14일

05 Customized Double Chin Cosmetic Surgery Considering Subcutaneous Fat, Jawbone Size, and Muscles

The Objective of Double Chin Cosmetic Surgery

Beauty standards vary with the passage of time. In the past, a generally round facial shape was often considered elegant and charming. However, in today's world, a small and slender V-line facial shape has become the prevailing beauty ideal for people of all ages and genders. Within the trend of desiring a smaller and more slender facial shape, the 'double chin', residing beneath the chin in two layers, can be perceived as an unwelcome guest.

Having a double chin not only makes the boundary between the face and neck appear ambiguous but also eliminates the sense of dimension, making one's appearance flatter and even seemingly heavier than in reality. As humans perceive objects through overall silhouettes, facial shape serves as the foundation that holds facial features, influencing the general ambiance of an image and significantly impacting initial impressions. For this reason, many individuals are seeking solutions to improve the appearance of a double chin.

Many people make efforts to address a double chin through dieting or dietary management. However, specifically targeting localized fat such as a double chin is not easy and requires a significant amount of time and effort. In response to this need, the field of cosmetic surgery has rapidly introduced 'double chin plastic surgery'.

The cause of a double chin can be thought of as simply having too much unnecessary subcutaneous fat. However, unlike other areas, the double chin area may be caused not only by fat, but also by the size and shape of the jaw bone and the muscles under the double chin.

Therefore, 'Double Chin Surgery' aims not only to reduce the quantity of fat but also to provide a tailored solution based on the causes of double chin formation. Its primary goal is to achieve a fundamental improvement by reducing the volume of the double chin and creating a smoother and more slender facial contour.

| Double Chin Liposuction

When excess subcutaneous fat accumulates in the double chin area, causing it to fold into two layers, Accusculpt laser is employed to target and liquefy the fat, which is then aspirated using a microcannula to achieve improvement.

Just like other parts of our bodies, the face also has subcutaneous fat beneath the skin, and many patients desire localized fat reduction in their facial areas. In addition to other facial regions, a promising solution for effectively improving excess fat in the double chin area is double chin liposuction using the Accusculpt laser.

Surgical Method

The Accusculpt laser is a laser device with a wavelength of 1,444nm designed to target fat. In the process of double chin liposuction, the Accusculpt laser is applied to subcutaneous fat before aspirating the fat using a microcannula, allowing the tissue to become more pliable. This manual aspiration method helps improve double chin fat.

The effectiveness of this surgical method is notably enhanced when the subcutaneous fat layer in the double chin area is thicker. Therefore, it's crucial during the pre-surgical consultation phase to confirm the amount of fat through ultrasonic testing.

The surgery can be performed using local or sleep anesthesia. Small incisions are made beneath the chin and on either side of the chin tip. A tumescent solution is injected into these incisions. Following this, the Accusculpt laser is applied, and then a microcannula is used through the same incisions for manual aspiration, effectively improving the double chin fat.

To aspirate fat in the double chin area, a delicate approach is necessary, given the facial region, to minimize side effects and tissue damage. Therefore, instead of using the traditional suction cannula, a thin microcannula is employed. The fat is not suctioned at high pressure but rather extracted meticulously using a low-pressure, repetitive technique with 1cc or 3cc syringes for precision.

Aftercare and Effects Following Surgery

After undergoing double chin liposuction, acute swelling may occur for about 1~2 days. During this period, applying a cold compress wrapped in a towel or gauze can help with the swelling. Starting from the third day, using warm compresses can promote blood circulation and aid in reducing the swelling.

After the surgery, you will be discharged while wearing a garment (compression wear) to help the tissues adhere properly in the areas where the fat has been removed. Wearing this garment does not directly impact the final surgical results, but it aids in a faster recovery and reduces swelling.

Therefore, it is advisable to wear the garment with an intensity similar to that of shapewear to ensure good adherence to the double chin area. Instead of wearing it for extended periods, taking breaks intermittently after wearing the garment will aid in the recovery process.

The effects of double chin liposuction vary for each individual. However, approximately one month after the surgery, lymphatic swelling diminishes, and the area where fat was removed begins to show a more defined contour, although there might initially be a sensation of unevenness. Gradually, any residual swelling subsides, and the final results typically manifest over a period of about six months.

The duration of maintenance after surgery

During childhood and adolescence, fat cells in our body continuously increase in number, but once a person reaches adulthood, the quantity of fat cells remains relatively constant. The fixed number of fat cells does not significantly fluctuate.

Liposuction is a surgical procedure that removes fat from the body, and once these fat cells are removed, they typically do not regenerate. As a result, the outcome of double chin liposuction may naturally experience some sagging over time due to the aging process, but as long as weight is maintained, the effects generally persist without further gain in fat.

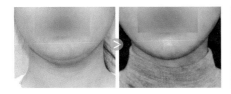 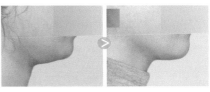

Double chin liposuction surgery case

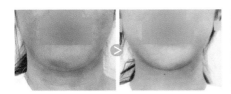 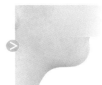

Double chin liposuction surgery case

| Platysma muscle surgery

The surgical method described is effective for individuals with a small or retrusive lower jaw, who have undergone chin reduction, or double jaw surgery to enhance facial contours.

The size and shape of the jawbone are indeed contributing factors to the development of a double chin. In cases where the lower jawbone is small or the chin tip is retruded, it can affect the muscles under the chin, preventing them from adequately supporting the jawline. This can lead to the development of a double chin as these muscles may loosen and sag downward.

Furthermore, patients who have previously undergone facial contouring surgery to reduce the length or width of the chin tip or double jaw surgery involving both the upper and lower jaws may develop a double chin as a secondary issue. This occurs because during the process of facial contouring or double jaw surgery, the muscles located beneath the jawline may become detached. As a result, the muscles sag and elongate, leading to the development of a double chin.

In cases where a double chin is caused by factors other than just excess fat, such as jawbone size and muscle sagging, 'Platysma muscle surgery' can be an effective alternative.

Surgical Method

Before the 'Platysma muscle surgery' procedure, liposuction to remove subcutaneous fat is performed as a preliminary step. Small incisions of 1~2mm are made under the chin or on the jawline for fat removal. Additionally, a 2~3cm incision is made beneath the chin tip to perform the Platysma muscle surgery.

The procedure involves dissecting between the Platysma muscle and the skin, thoroughly excising and removing the fat pockets located between the Platysma muscle and the underlying muscle. After creating a spacious area between the wide neck muscles on both sides, the neck muscles are meticulously sutured, much like tying shoelaces. This tightens the muscles, resulting in an improvement in the double chin.

Scars and Recovery Period

Platysma muscle surgery is a surgical procedure that involves an incision of about 2-3 cm below the chin, which can raise concerns and apprehension among patients due to worries about scarring.

However, since most of the surgery is performed using the natural creases at the border between the jawbone and the neck, the incision scars are not very visible when viewed from the front. Moreover, if a skilled surgeon carefully sutures the incision, the scars tend to be inconspicuous. Post-surgery, consistent use of scar cream can aid in managing the scarring.

While the duration and intensity may vary for each individual, scars typically appear red for 1~2 months after surgery and gradually become less noticeable over time, usually fading significantly by around 6 months.

As this procedure involves a combination of fat removal and excision in the double chin area, alongside muscle tightening, there is a slightly higher likelihood of bleeding compared to cases where only double chin liposuction is performed.

Even with meticulous care and attention to hemostasis by the surgeon during the operation, bruising or swelling can still occur after surgery, varying from person to person. Particularly, bruising might be more prevalent in male patients compared to female patients, likely due to larger blood vessels or muscles in males than in females. Most bruises tend to dissipate and spread downwards beneath the neck within about a week, while in some cases, more pronounced bruising might take more than two weeks to subside.

After removing the compression tape applied after surgery, patients can wear masks or use makeup to conceal the area. Light daily activities are generally feasible.

Surgical Effects and Post-Operative Precautions

This surgery yields immediate results starting from the third day after removing the compression tape that was applied during the surgery.

Since it involves direct removal of fat and reshaping of muscles through sutures, patients can experience visible results immediately after the surgery, even considering post-operative swelling.

However, it's crucial to support the skin to ensure it re adheres correctly after the muscle and skin separation during surgery. Until the separated muscle and skin properly reattach, there is a possibility of bleeding and hematoma formation at the surgical site. Therefore, keeping pressure on the area with adhesive tape for about 2~3 days post-surgery can be helpful. Wearing a compression garment for around a week following the procedure aids in a quicker recovery.

A week after the surgery, the stitches at the incision site are removed. Light conversation, singing, and light exercise are permissible, but it's essential to avoid heavy lifting and strenuous neck movements for up to a month following the surgery.

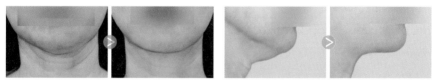

Platysma muscle surgery case

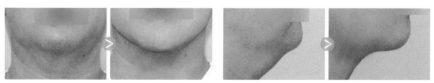

Platysma muscle surgery case

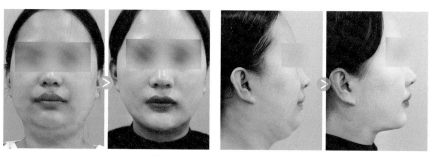

Platysma muscle surgery case

TIP_Platysma muscle surgery Procedure Information				
The surgical time	The anesthesia method	Hospitalization	The recovery period	The duration of stay
1 hour 30 minutes to 2 hours	Sleep anesthesia	No hospitalization	7~10 days	14 days

| Lower face lift

When skin elasticity is diminished due to aging, causing it to sag and droop downwards, 'Lower face lift' can be used to address and improve this condition.

Aging is a natural process in our bodies, but as time becomes a measure of self-care, interest in cosmetic procedures has increased among middle-aged individuals, becoming a gauge of self-management and personal enhancement.

Double chin plastic surgery is a procedure that appeals to both younger individuals and those in their middle years due to the effects of aging. However, the aforementioned double chin plastic surgeries primarily focus on improving the area below the chin and the boundary between the neck and the jawline.

As a result, these surgeries can effectively address the central area below the chin, but when skin elasticity significantly diminishes and the skin sags with age, especially along the sides of the jawline, Platysma muscle surgery alone may have limitations and prove challenging for improvement.

In such cases, a 'Lower face lift' may be necessary, which involves making an incision in front of the ear to lift and tighten the sagging skin, and then removing any excess skin to secure it, thereby restoring elasticity

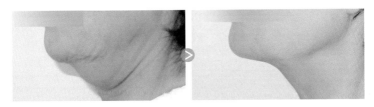

Lower face lift surgery case

TIP_Lower face lift Procedure Information				
The surgical time	The anesthesia method	Hospitalization	The recovery period	The duration of stay
3~4 hours	Sleep anesthesia	No hospitalization	7~10 days	14 days

가슴 확대술(Breast augmentation)
가슴 축소술(Breast reduction)

사랑을 부르는 가슴,
탄력과 볼륨감이 넘치는 매력적인 가슴은…
여성 그 자체!

Woman's breast that calls for love,

A sensual breast full of elasticity and
volume is the source of a woman's charm!

아름답고 건강한 가슴은 강력한 매력을 느끼게 하기에 여성 스스로의 자존감을 위해서도 중요하며
이성을 사로잡는 매력 포인트가 된다.

A beautiful and healthy breast not only evokes a powerful allure, but also crucial for a
woman's own self-esteem.

봉봉성형외과
The Bongbong Plastic Surgery

www.bongbongclinic.com

박성수(Seong-Su Park)

- 성형외과 전문의(Plastic Surgery Specialist)
- 대한 미용성형외과 정회원(Regular member of Korean Aesthetic Plastic Surgery)
- 국제 미용성형외과 정회원(International cosmetic surgery regular member)
- 국제줄기세포치료학회 정회원(Member of International Society of Stem Cell Therapeutics)
- 한국 유방성형 연구회 정회원(Member of Korean breast surgery Committee)

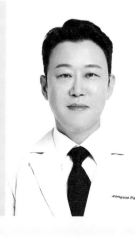

06 가슴성형, 여성이 원하고 만족도가 높은 성형수술

가슴성형 전문의가 생각하는 아름답고 매력적인 가슴의 조건

　과거와 달리 성형수술을 한 것에 대해서 굳이 숨기지 않는 분위기가 되면서 성형수술을 하는 여성들이 꾸준히 이어지고 있다. 그 중 가슴성형이야 말로 단연, 여성들이 가장 많이 원하는 부위로 만족도 또한 매우 높은 성형수술이다.

　저자는 20여 년 가까이 가슴성형만을 집도해오면서 2차, 3차 … 최고 8번째 가슴 재수술을 받는 여성을 만난 적도 있다. 물론 첫 수술로 단박에 원하는 가슴을 얻게 된다면 금상첨화겠지만 때로는 예기치 않은 부작용이 생기거나 만족스럽지 못한 사이즈, 모양, 단단한 촉감 때문에 재수술을 받게 되는 경우도 흔하다.

　봉봉 성형외과에는 보다 자연스러운 결과로 환자의 만족도를 업그레이드시키기 위해 하이브리드 가슴성형술을 세계 최초로 연구 개발하여 가슴성형에 사용해오고 있다. 무엇보다도 환자가 원하는 방향과 컨셉트, 즉 니즈(Needs)을 정확하게 캐치하고 이러한 희망사항을 부족함 없이 수술에 반영될 수 있도록 최선의 술기(Best surgical technique)를 구사해오고 있다. 그 결과 가슴성형 수술의 만족을 높이고 불필요한 추가 수술을 예방하는데 앞장서오고 있다.

만족스런 가슴성형을 위한 5가지 요소

가슴성형은 얼굴 못지않게 자신감에 큰 영향을 미치는 요소다. 가슴성형을 고려하고 있는 경우 만족스러운 결과를 얻기 위해 고려해야 할 몇 가지 중요한 요소가 있다. 사이즈, 위치, 밸런스, 좌우대칭 등이다.

1. 사이즈

B, C, D, E …. 각자마다 원하는 가슴 크기가 있다. 하지만 원하는 가슴 크기가 실제로도 잘 어울리고 몸에 무리가 되지 않아야 할 것이다. 지나치게 큰 보형물의 삽입은 자칫 머지않은 미래에 부작용과 후유증을 야기할 수 있다. 특히 흉곽 뼈의 함몰(꺼짐)이나 피부의 심각한 처짐과 얇아지는 문제를 일으키기도 한다.

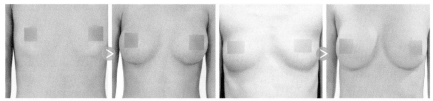

보형물 가슴확대, 유방밑 주름선 절개, 240cc, 라운드 스무스   보형물 가슴확대, 겨드랑이 절개, 260cc, 라운드, 스무스

2. 밸런스

유방은 여성 신체에서 일정한 비율을 이루면서 조화를 이루어야 한다. 가슴의 둘레와 허리의 둘레, 힙의 둘레비는 1.2 : 1 : 1.3~4 정도가 되는 것이 좋다. 슬림한 몸매의 여성에서 가슴 볼륨을 지나치게 강조하다 보면 자칫 이러한 비율이 깨지기 십상이다. 가슴의 크기가 적절하고 허리, 엉덩이와 적당한 비율을 이루었을 때 바디라인 전체가 매력적으로 보인다.

3. 대칭성

유방은 좌우에 하나씩 있다. 우측과 좌측의 가슴이 밸런스를 이룰 수 있어야 한다. 크기는 물론 유두와 유륜의 밸런스, 가슴 밑선의 좌우 대칭성이 유방의 미적 완성도에 매우 중요하다.

4. 가슴골

실제로 수술한 가슴이 인위적으로 보여지는 원인 중 가장 흔한 것은 부자연스러운 가슴골이다. 보형물을 삽입하더라도 가슴골은 충분한 연부조직의 유무에 따라 자연스러운 정도가 다르다. 넓게 분리된 가슴골은 수술한 느낌을 주게 되는데, 보다 자연스러운 결과를 내기 위해 보형물과 다른 재료를 같이 사용하는 하리브리드 가슴성형을 진행한다.

5. 다이내믹한 움직임

마시멜로, 모찌띡, 인절미처럼 가슴은 부드러운 촉감을 가져야 한다. 봉봉성형외과에서 하이브리드 가슴성형술을 창안하여, 체위 변동에 따라 자연스럽게 움직이며 달릴 때는 역동적인 출렁임을 보여준다. 특히 유방보형물만으로는 부족한 "Super-Naturalism(궁극의 자연미)"의 추구를 위해 줄기세포 자가지방 이식술과 바디필러의 사용 그리고 비수술적인 리프팅을 사용하기도 한다.

| 가슴 확대술

여성의 가슴은 크기만 크다고 하여 아름다워 보이지 않는다. 가슴성형에서 가장 중요한 부분은 가슴의 크기를 확대시키는 것보다 균형이 잡혀있고 개인의 신체의 조건과 조화를 이루는 자연스러운 라인을 만들어 주는 것이다.

사라진 희망을 찾는 여정, 유방 재건술

여성의 가슴은 크기만 크다고 해서 아름다워 보이지 않는다. 가슴성형에서 가장 중요한 부분은 가슴의 크기를 확대시키는 것보다 균형이 잡혀있고 개인의 신체의 조건과 조화를 이루는 자연스러운 라인을 만들어주는 것이다.

가슴에 삽입되는 보형물이 자리 잡을 공간을 임플란트 포켓(Implant Pocket)이라고 한다. 보형물이 머물게 되는 공간이다. 접근하는 경로에 따라서 겨드랑이 접근법, 유륜을 통한 접근법, 유방밑주름 접근법이 있다. 보형물이 삽입되는 깊이에 따라 근막하삽입법, 근육하삽입법, 이중평면법(변형된 근육하삽입법)이 있다.

가슴수술 시 중요 사항은 임플란트 포켓을 만들 때 출혈이 없이 깨끗하게 만듦으로써 얇고 신축성 있는 피막을 형성되도록 하고 조직 손상을 최소화하는 것이다. 이를 통해 빠른 회복과 적은 통증으로 하루 만에 일상 복귀를 가능하게 하는 "원데이가슴성형"을 고안하여 진료 중이다.

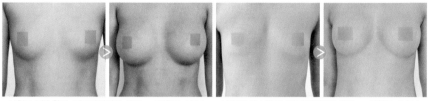

보형물 가슴확대, 겨드랑이절개, 260cc, 라운드 스무스　　보형물 가슴확대, 겨드랑이절개, 300cc, 라운드 스무스

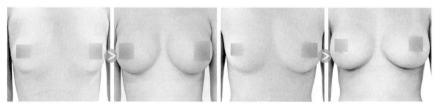

보형물 가슴확대, 유방밑 주름선 절개, 350cc, 라운드, 스무스　　보형물 가슴확대, 유방밑 주름선 절개, 380cc, 라운드, 스무스
[하이브리드 가슴성형]

가슴성형, 얼마나 크게 할 것인가?

여성들이 선망하는 가슴의 크기는 시대나 유행에 따라서도 조금씩 변해왔다. 아름다운 가슴의 기준은 단순히 가슴의 볼륨만을 나타내기보다는 전체적인 바디라인 안에서 가슴이 갖는 이상적 비율을 갖도록 해야 한다.

- **신체 비율** : 환자의 전체 신체 비율과 조화를 이루는 가슴의 크기가 중요하다. 어깨 넓이, 허리 크기, 힙 라인 등을 고려하여 가슴의 크기를 결정하며, 이를 통해 자연스러운 신체 라인을 만들 수 있다.
- **건강과 편안함** : 가슴의 크기가 너무 크면 척추에 부담을 줄 수 있으므로, 환자의 건강 상태와 생활 습관을 고려하여 적절한 크기를 선택한다.
- **환자의 의도와 취향** : 성형외과의 목표는 환자가 원하는 결과를 만족시키는 것이므로, 환자의 취향과 기대치를 충분히 듣고 이해하는 것이 중요하다.

- **자연스러운 모양과 느낌** : 인공적으로 보이지 않고 자연스러운 모양과 느낌을 중요시하는 환자들이 많으므로 신체와 잘 어울리는 크기와 형태를 선택한다.
- **전문 의사와의 상담** : 가슴 성형 수술은 전문 성형외과 의사와의 상담을 통해 개인별로 맞춤화된 계획을 세우는 것이 좋다. 환자의 신체 구조와 건강 상태, 기대치 등을 종합적으로 평가하여 이상적인 가슴의 크기와 형태를 제안해 드리고 있다.

성형외과적으로 이상적인 가슴의 크기는 표준화된 것이 아니라 환자의 개별 상황과 원하는 결과를 기반으로 결정되어야 하며, 전문의와의 충분한 상담과 검토를 거쳐 결정되는 것이 바람직하다.

한국 여성들은 대개 가슴이 빈약한 탓에 유방확대수술을 가장 많이 하고 있다. 가슴확대 수술법에는 유방조직 내에 인공 유방 보형물을 넣는 방법과 빈약한 가슴의 피부 아래에 적정량의 지방 세포를 주입하는 지방이식 가슴확대법이 있다.

가슴 수술은 크기뿐 아니라 몸매와의 조화와 균형을 이루는 것이 매우 중요하다. 환자의 키와 체격, 허리와 엉덩이 라인에 어울리는 가슴을 만들려면 가슴의 폭이나 넓이, 돌출의 정도, 경사도 등 3차원적인 형태를 고려하면서 수술을 해야 한다. 여기에 수술자의 예술적인 안목이 더해졌을 때 비로소 아름다운 가슴이 완성될 수 있게 된다.

지방이식 가슴확대술

가슴을 겉부터 속까지 살펴보면 가장 바깥 족이 피부, 피부아래지방층, 유선조직을 감싸는 쿠퍼씨인대, 유선조직, 대흉근을 둘러싼 근막, 대흉근, 얇은 섬유조직과 적은 양의 지방층, 소흉근, 늑골과 늑연골, 이렇게 되어있다. 이 중에서 부족한 피부 아래 지방층을 보강해 주는 방법이 바로 지방이식 가슴 확대술이다.

지방세포는 이식 후에 생착률, 즉 이식한 지방세포가 얼마나 많이 살아남는지에 따라 확대 효과와 만족도가 결정된다. 지방의 생착률을 높여주기 위해 성장인자와 줄기세포를 함께 사용한다.

지방이식을 통해 좋은 결과를 보기 위한 필요조건!

1. 우선 본인의 체내에 이식에 필요한 충분한 양의 지방이 있어야 한다.
2. 이식된 지방이 잘 생착 되도록 금연, 충분한 수면, 영양섭취
3. 두달간 마사지 금지

　지방이식을 통해 키울 수 있는 가슴의 크기는 대략 한컵 정도이다. 보형물 삽입 후에 적정량의 지방을 가슴골에 이식하여 "I"자형 클리비지(가슴사이 골)를 만들어주고 리플링(피부가 얇아져 보형물이 비쳐보이는 현상)이 있을 경우 피부아래 지방층에 주입하고 좌우 가슴크기의 비대칭이 있을 경우에는 볼륨업이 필요한 부위에 선택적으로 주입해줌으로써 더욱 자연스러운 가슴을 만들 수 있다.

필러를 이용한 가슴확대

　온전히 필러만으로 가슴을 확대하는 데에는 몇 가지 한계점이 있다.

1. 우선 안전한 바디필러의 선정이다. 일반적으로 히알루론산 필러가 보편적이나 다량의 히알루론산 필러의 사용은 때에 따라 가교제에 대한 예민한 면역반응이나 환자의 면역력이 나빠진 상태에서 지연 염증반응과 체액의 저류 등으로 필러의 이동 혹은 염증을 유발하여 부작용이 나타나는 경우도 적지 않다.

2. 무세포 동종진피 필러(Micronized Acellular Dermal Matrix)를 이용할 수 있으나 재료 자체의 비용이 상당히 고가이기에 단독으로 사용하기에는 비용적 부담이 있다.

3. PLA (Poly-lactic acid) 스킨 부스터는 콜라겐, 엘라스틴, 줄기세포 생성 등 다양한 조직 재생에 도움을 준다.

　봉봉성형외과에서는 다양한 필러의 대용량 사용 임상 경험을 바탕으로 "환자 맞춤형 바디 필러 시술"로 안전성을 높이고 있다.

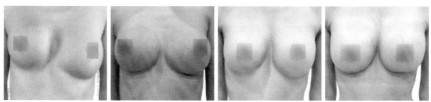

유방비대칭과 촉감 모양 불만족에 대한 가슴재수술　　더블라인 변형과 밑 빠짐 교정을 위한 가슴재수술
[하이브리드 가슴성형]

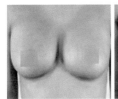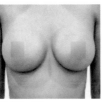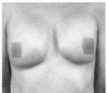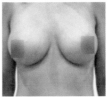

가슴재수술, 윗볼록 교정   가슴재수술, 구형구축 교정, 가슴골 교정 [하이브리드 가슴성형]

TIP_보형물 가슴 확대술 수술정보				
수술시간	마취방법	입원여부	회복기간	체류기간
1~2시간	수면, 전신마취	입원없음	5일~1주일	1주일

| 가슴 축소술

가슴이 본인의 체형에 비해 지나치게 크다면 이 역시 외모 콤플렉스가 될 수 있다. 함몰유도와 거대유도 또한 마찬가지다. 절개 방법도 다양하므로 각자에게 맞는 방법을 찾아야 한다.

유방 축소

유방이 지나치게 큰 경우 그로 인한 골격계의 무리와 피부염을 일으키게 되므로 축소 수술이 필요하다. 피부 디자인은 유방 처짐 교정수술과 크게 다르지 않으나 유선조직과 지방조직을 절제하는 양을 충분히 하여 축소를 원하는 만큼 해주는 것이 환자의 불편을 줄이는 데 중요하다.

함몰유두

선천적 혹은 후천적으로 유두가 함몰되는 경우, 피부 안으로 함입된 유두는 위생적인 문제와 미용적 불편을 야기한다. 많은 경우 함몰유두는 유관발달의 장애를 동반하기도 한다. 저자는 "흉터 걱정 없는 함몰유두 교정법"을 개발하여 국제 성형 논문에 보고한 바 있으며 유관의 기능을 보존하면서 유두의 함몰을 교정하고 있다.

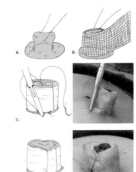

저자가 미국 미용성형외과 학회에 발표한
흉터를 만들지 않는 함몰유두 교정법

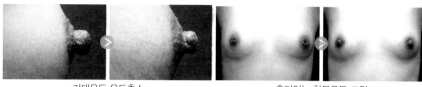

거대유두 유두축소   흉터없는 함몰유두 교정

거대유두

　이상적인 유두의 크기를 절대적인 수치화할 수는 없으나 기본적으로 유두 : 유륜 : 유방의 가로 폭 비율이 1 : 3 : 9인 것을 이상적인 비율로 본다. 유두의 직경은 1~1.5㎝ 돌출은 1㎝ 안팎인 것이 좋다. 지나치게 유두가 크거나 오랜 수유를 거치면서 늘어나고 처진 경우라면 적절한 크기로 줄이는 유두 축소 수술이 필요하다. 유방의 크기와 모양만큼이나 유두의 크기와 모양 역시 전체적인 유방의 미적 완성도를 결정하는 중요한 부분이다.

유륜 미백과 몽고메리 결절 축소

　유륜의 색조가 너무 짙거나 좁쌀 알갱이처럼 도드라진 몽고메리 결절이 지나치게 많거나 큰 경우 미용적인 문제를 일으키게 된다. 유륜의 색소 침착은 몇 차례의 미백 약물 주입과 레이저 치료를 통해 색조가 점차 연해지게 되며 유륜의 크기 및 몽고메리 결절은 특수하게 고안된 전문 장비를 이용하여 치료될 수 있다.

부유방 축소

　사람 몸에 있는 한 쌍의 유방 외에 기형적으로 더 달린 유방을 부유방이라 한다. 겨드랑이 앞쪽의 유두 혹은 유선 조직이 남아서 호르몬의 영향으로 커지게 되는 경우 옷맵시가 나지 않고 상반신의 미적 완성도를 떨어뜨리기 때문에 시술이 필요하다.

수술시간	마취방법	입원여부	회복기간	체류기간
2~3시간	수면, 진정, 전신마취	입원없음	5일	7~10일

TIP_가슴축소술 수술정보

06 Breast augmentation is by far the most desired by women and has a very high satisfaction rate

Conditions of beautiful and attractive breasts :

The author has been a plastic surgeon specializing in breast surgeries for 20 years.

Over the years, I experienced many women's breast surgeries. There are cases where it's the first breast surgery, but there are also times when a 2nd, 3rd... or even an 8th revision surgery is performed. While there are best-case scenarios where the patient gets the desired result from the first surgery, there are often cases where unexpected side effects occur, or they undergo a revision surgery due to dissatisfaction with the size, shape, or hardness of the implant.

As a plastic surgeon handling female patients, applying the best surgical techniques is undeniably crucial. However, it's even more important to accurately grasp the patient's desires and concepts, that is, their needs, and ensure that these needs are fully reflected in the surgery. This helps increase surgical satisfaction and prevent unnecessary additional surgeries.

At Bongbong Plastic Surgery, they have pioneered the use of hybrid breast augmentation surgery to achieve more natural results and maximize patient satisfaction, being the first in the world to develop and use this technique for breast augmentation.

Five key elements for satisfactory breast augmentation

Chest plastic surgery is a factor that has a great influence on confidence as much as the face. If breast implants are being considered, there are several important factors to consider in order to achieve satisfactory results. Size, location, Balance, left-right symmetry, etc.

1. Size

Women who visit the clinic each have their preferred breast size. B, C, D, E... Surgery should make it possible to achieve the desired size. The desired breast size should also be realistically suitable and not strain the body. If a patient wants an unrealistically large size, it's essential to explain the potential problems. Too large implants use can cause complications and sequelae in the not-too-distant future. They can also cause the chest bones to sink or the skin to sag and thin significantly.

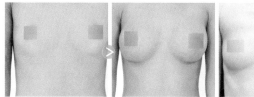
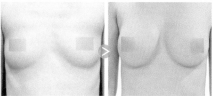

Breast augmentation by implant, inframammary incision, 240cc, round, smooth

Breast augmentation by implant, axillary incision, 260cc, round, smooth

2. Balance

Breasts should harmonize with a certain proportion of the female body. The ideal ratio between the circumference of the chest, waist, and hips is approximately 1.2 : 1 : 1.3~4. Emphasizing too much breast volume in a slim-bodied woman can disrupt this balance. When the breast size is appropriate, and it forms a proportionate balance with the waist and buttocks, the entire body line looks attractive.

3. Symmetry

There are two breasts, one on the left and one on the right. The right and left breasts should balance each other. The balance of size, the balance between the nipple and areola, and the symmetry of the breast folds are very important for the aesthetic completion of the breasts.

4. Breast cleavage

One of the most common reasons breast surgeries look artificial is due to an unnatural sternum. Even with the insertion of implants, the naturalness of the cleavage varies depending on the presence of enough soft tissue. A widely separated breast cleavage gives a post-operative look, a look that clearly shows surgery was done and this is why there's an increasing need for hybrid breast augmentation.

5. Dynamic Movement

- The breast should have a soft touch feel.
- Achieving an extreme softness, often compared to marshmallow, mochi, injeolmi (Korean rice cake), or cotton candy.
- I can be an ultimate goal of breast surgery.
- For the surgically augmented breast to be soft, first and foremost, there should be no capsular contracture. A thin and elastic membrane should form around the implant.
- Enough soft tissue, including subcutaneous fat, should cover the implant.
- When all these conditions are met, the breast can naturally move according to posture changes and can dynamically bounce when running.

"The reason the author devised the hybrid breast augmentation technique was to achieve such natural-looking and soft breasts. The realization of "Super-Naturalism", which is insufficient with just breast implants, is possible through stem cell autologous fat transplantation, the use of safe body fillers, and non- surgical lifting."

| Breast augmentation

A woman's chest doesn't look beautiful just because it's big. The most important part of breast implants is to create a natural line that is balanced and harmonizes with the conditions of an individual's body rather than expanding the size of the chest.

Women's breasts often appear as a regular topic on television programs. That's why the breasts symbolize femininity, can also be a source of complex for some women. The breast size that women desire has changed slightly over time and trends. The standard for beautiful breasts is not just about the volume of the breasts but should also ensure that they maintain an ideal proportion within the overall body line. The size and shape of the breasts should harmonize with the entire body and maintaining the health of the breasts can also be considered a standard for beautiful breasts. Defining the ideal breast size in plastic surgery is a complex issue. It takes into account the patient's body structure, health condition, personal preferences, and lifestyle habits."

- **Body Proportion** : The size of the breasts that harmonize with a patient's overall body proportion is essential. Considering factors such as shoulder width, waist size, and hip line, the breast size is determined, allowing for a natural body line.

- **Health and Comfort** : If the breast size is too large, it can put a strain on the spine. Therefore, the right size is selected, considering the patient's health status and lifestyle.

- **Patient's Intent and Preference** : The goal in plastic surgery is to satisfy the results the patient desires. Hence, it is crucial to listen to and understand the patient's preferences and expectations.

- **Natural Shape and Feel** : Many patients prioritize having a natural shape and feel that doesn't look artificial. The size and form that fit well with the body are chosen.

- **Consultation with a Specialist** : It's advisable to formulate a personalized plan for breast augmentation surgery through a consultation with a specialist in plastic surgery. The author evaluates the patient's body structure, health status, and expectations comprehensively and suggests the ideal size and shape of the breasts. In conclusion, the ideal breast size in plastic surgery isn't standardized but should be determined based on the individual patient's circumstances and desired outcome. An ideal decision comes after ample consultation and consideration with a specialist.

Asian women mostly opt for breast enlargement surgeries due to having small breasts. Breast enlargement methods include inserting artificial breast implants within the breast tissue or injecting a suitable amount of fat cells under the skin.

Breast surgery isn't just about size; it's vital to harmonize and balance with the body. Considering the patient's height, physique, waist, and hip line, the surgery should account for the breast's width, protrusion, slope, and other three-dimensional aspects.

Only when combined with the surgeon's artistic insight can one achieve truly beautiful breasts.

Breast Implant Augmentation :

The space where the implant settles in the breast is called the "implant pocket." It is the area where the implant stays.

Depending on the approach, there are axillary, through the areola, and inframammary fold methods. Depending on the depth of the implant insertion, there are subfascial, submuscular, and dual-plane (modified submuscular) methods.

With the advancement in biomedical engineering, the material and composition of implants are evolving. The properties of silicone materials have been changing to emulate the inherent softness of the breast. Different manufacturers offer varying viscosities and elasticity of the gel, and the shell's surface microstructure differs.

In the not-so-distant future, custom-made implants will be produced and used. With the advancement of tissue engineering, the era of "bio-implant breast augmentation" that can add volume using biological materials is anticipated.

BongBong Plastic Surgery Clinic

At BongBong Plastic Surgery Clinic, we have devised and implemented a "One-Day Breast Surgery" that enables a swift return to daily life in just one day with minimal pain. This is achieved by creating a pocket for the implant during breast surgery without bleeding and ensuring a clean procedure. This approach forms a thin and elastic membrane(implant capsule), minimizes tissue damage, and promotes faster recovery.

Fat Grafting Breast Augmentation

Looking at the breast from the outside to the inside, it consists of the skin, subcutaneous fat layer, Cooper's ligaments that encase the mammary tissue, mammary tissue, fascia surrounding the pectoralis major muscle, the muscle itself, thin fibrous tissue with a small fat layer, pectoralis minor muscle, rib, and

costal cartilage. The fat grafting breast augmentation technique is used to enhance the insufficient subcutaneous fat layer. The enlargement effect and satisfaction depend on the survival rate of the transferred fat cells after transplantation. To increase the survival rate of the fat, growth factors and stem cells are used together.

Essential Conditions for Successful Fat Grafting

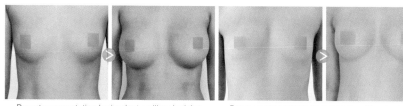

Breast augmentation by implant, axillary incision, 260cc, round, smooth

Breast augmentation by implant, axillary incision, 300cc, round, smooth

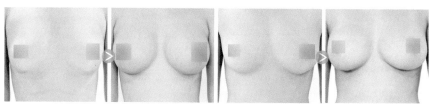

Breast augmentation by implant, inframammary incision, 350cc, round, smooth [Hybrid Case]

Breast augmentation by implant, inframammary incision, 380cc, round, smooth

- The patient should have a sufficient amount of fat for transplantation.
- To ensure the transferred fat survives well: avoid smoking, get enough sleep, and have proper nutrition.
- Massage is prohibited for two months.
- The size of the breasts that can be enhanced through fat grafting is roughly one cup.
- After inserting the implant, a moderate amount of fat is grafted to the sternum to create an "I" shaped cleavage.
- If there's rippling (a phenomenon where the implant is visible due to thin skin), fat is injected under the skin.
- If there's an asymmetry in the size of the breasts, the volume is selectively injected where needed to create more natural-looking breasts.

Breast Augmentation Using Fillers

Using fillers alone for breast augmentation has limitations. The main concern is the safe selection of body fillers. Hyaluronic acid fillers are common, but using them in large quantities can sometimes trigger sensitive immune reactions to the cross-linking agent. This can lead to inflammation or the migration of the filler, causing side effects.

Micronized Acellular Dermal Matrix filler can be used, it can be integrated with soft

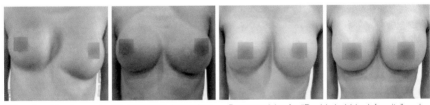

Breast revision for asymmetry correction, improving touch feel and shape [Hybrid Case]

Breast revision for "Double bubble deformity" and "Buttoming out deformity"

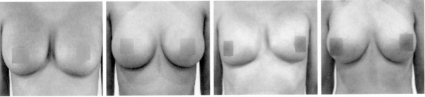

Breast revision for "Upper pole Fullness"

Breast revision for "Capsular contracture", "intermammary cleavage" [Hybrid Case]

tissue but it's price is quite expensive. The PLA (Poly-lactic acid) skin booster aids in the regeneration of various tissues like collagen, elastin, and stem cells.

The author enhances safety by customizing filler compositions based on extensive clinical experience with a diverse range of patients.

TIP_Breast Augmentation by Implant, Surgery Information				
Operation Time	Anesthesia method	Hospital Admission	Recovery time	Stay time
1~2 hours	IV sedation or General Anesthesia	Not needed	5~7 days	1 week

| Breast Reduction

If the breasts are too large, it can cause strain on the skeletal system and induce skin irritations, necessitating a reduction surgery. The surgical design is similar to breast lift procedure, and it's crucial to remove an ample amount of mammary and fatty tissue to alleviate the patient's discomfort.

Inverted Nipple

There are congenital or acquired cases of inverted nipples. Inverted nipples can cause hygienic and aesthetic concerns. In many cases, inverted nipples are accompanied by a developmental disorder of the milk ducts. The author has developed a "Scar-Free Inverted Nipple Correction Method", which has been reported in international plastic surgery journals. This corrects the inversion while preserving the function of the milk ducts.

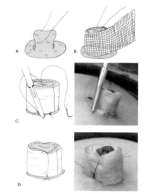

The author's presentation at the American Society of Plastic Surgery on a "Scarless Technique for inverted nipples correction."

Prominent Nipples

There's no absolute measure for the ideal nipple size, but typically the width ratio of nipple:areola:breast is considered ideal at 1:3:9. The diameter of the nipple should be

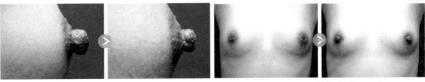

Giant Nipple, Nipple Correction   Scar-free Inverted Nipple Correction

between 1-1.5 cm, and the projection about 1 cm. If the nipple is excessively large or has stretched and sagged due to prolonged breastfeeding, a nipple reduction surgery is required.

Areola Whitening and Montgomery Tubercle Reduction

A very dark areola or overly prominent Montgomery tubercles can pose aesthetic problems. Pigmentation of the areola can be gradually lightened through several injections of whitening drugs and laser treatments. The size of the areola and the Montgomery tubercles can be treated with specially designed equipment. Accessory

Breast Reduction

Humans are mammals and, embryologically, multiple nipples and mammary tissues align on both sides of the chest. Typically, except for one pair, the rest regress. However, when the nipple or mammary tissue remains in the front of the armpit and enlarges due to hormonal influence, it's called an accessory breast. If it's large, it ruins the silhouette

TIP_Breast Reduction surgery information				
Operation Time	Anesthesia method	Hospital Admission	Recovery time	Stay time
2~3 hours	IV sedation or General Anesthesia	Not needed	5 days	7~10 weeks

페이스리프팅(Face lifting)
템플리프팅(Temple lifting)
실리프팅(Thread lifting)

잃어버린 10년의 세월을 되찾다

The time of 10 years that were lost is found back

사람의 얼굴은 세월의 흐름에 따라 주름이 생기고 깊어지며 피부가 처지기 시작한다. 시간은 되돌릴 수 없지만 젊음은 되돌릴 수 있다. 나이를 거스르는 동안 비법, 정답은 '리프팅'이다.

Regarding the face of a person, the wrinkles are generated and get deep, and the skin begins to sag according to the flow of the time. Although time cannot be reverted, youth can be reverted. While opposing the age, lifting is the secret and the right answer.

디엠성형외과
DM Plastic Surgery

www.dm-prs.com
www.dmps-en.com

유원민(Yoo-Won Min)

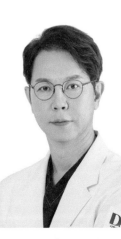

• 성형외과 전문의, 의학박사(Plastic surgery specialist/Doctor Of Medicine (MD))
• 연세대학교 의과대학 졸업(Graduate of Yonsei University Medical School/Doctor of Medicine)
• 대한성형외과학회 종신회원(KSPRS)
(Permanent member at The Korean Society of Plastic and Reconstructive Surgeons(KSPRS))
• 연세대학교 의과대학 세브란스병원 성형외과 교수/성형외과 과장
(Specialist/Professor at Yonsei University Severance Hospital Plastic Surgery Department)

07 나이를 거스르는 **동안 해법,** 정답은 '리프팅'

젊어지고 싶은 것이 사람의 기본적인 욕구

클레오파트라는 피부를 위해 우유, 장미수, 심지어 뱀의 독까지 사용했다는 이야기가 있으며, 중국의 미녀 양귀비는 제비집, 석류 등 피부 미용에 좋다는 것을 가리지 않았다고 전해진다. 이렇게 전해져 내려오는 이야기가 전부 진짜인지는 확인하기 어렵지만 동서고금을 막론하고 사람들이 얼마나 '젊음'을 추구했는지는 알 수 있는 부분임은 분명하다.

나이를 먹지 않는 사람은 없고, 나이를 먹게 되면 주름이 생기는 것은 당연한 결과이기 때문에 안티에이징은 어떤 시대건 간에 다양한 방법으로 존재해 왔으며 점차 새로운 방법으로 진화해 왔다.

특히, 현대의 의학 분야가 발전하면서 이러한 '안티에이징'은 다시 태어났다. '안티에이징(Anti-aging)은 나이가 들어가는 것을 막는다는 뜻으로 노화방지, 항노화의 의미를 가지고 있다. 근래에는 '안티에이징'과 관련해 노화를 늦추고 세포를 재생시키는 화장품이나 식품 등 다양한 기능성 제품이 있다. 하지만 이러한 것들이 주름살이 생기는 것을 어느 정도 예방시켜도 이미 얼굴에 생긴 주름살이나 중력에 의해 피부가 지속적으로 처지는 것까지 완벽하게 막을 수는 없다. 이러한 노화로 발생한 피부의 처짐과 노화현상을 개선시키기 위한 시술이 바로 '리프팅'이다.

페이스리프팅

팔자주름, 볼처짐, 입가주름, 목주름 등 안면의 전반적인 노화현상을 근본적인 원인부터 개선하여 피부의 탄력을 찾는 가장 확실한 수술법이다.

다시 한번 젊음을 되돌리는 마법의 '페이스리프팅'

    일반적으로 생활습관이나 얼굴표정으로 생긴 잔주름은 보톡스나 필러 등 간단하고 빠르게 해결할 수 있는 여러 방법이 있다. 하지만 세월이 흘러 나이가 들면서 생기는 깊은 팔자주름, 볼 처짐, 눈밑주름, 이마주름, 꺼진 볼살 등은 근본적인 원인을 해결하지 않으면 주름을 개선하기 어렵다. 노화로 인한 깊은 주름은 얼굴의 지방과 근육, 피부 등이 중력에 의해 인대가 늘어나 처지게 되면서 발생하게 되는데 이런 근본적인 원인을 해결하고 자연스럽게 주름을 개선하는 시술법이 바로 '페이스리프팅'이다.

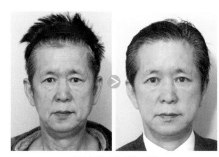
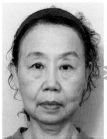
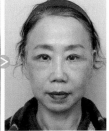

페이스리프팅 시술 전후   페이스리프팅 시술 전후

    페이스리프팅은 리프팅 시술 중 가장 확실한 효과를 얻을 수 있는 시술로써, 단순히 피부층만 당기는 시술이 아닌, 피부층과 함께 근막층(SMAS)을 당겨주는 근본적인 원인을 직접적으로 개선해주는 대표적인 리프팅 시술이다. 노화로 인해 처진 살과 주름에 대한 개선 효과가 가장 뚜렷하며 자연스러운 리프팅 효과를 볼 수 있다.

    단순히 피부만 당겨주는 일반적인 리프팅은 일시적으로 주름을 개선할 순 있지만, 자연스러운 결과를 얻을 수 없으며 시간이 지나면 피부가 다시 처지게 된다. 반면 '페이스리프팅'은 피부 아래쪽의 처진 지방과 근육을 함께 당겨주는 페임 (FAME) 테크닉을 통해 처진 지방패드를 분리 이동시킴으로써 자연스럽고 오랜 기간 유지되는 것이 큰 특징이며 어느 한 부위가 아닌 얼굴 전체적인 주름을 개선하는데 가장 효과가 좋다.

'페이스리프팅'은 근본적으로 주름개선을 위해 하는 수술이다. 환자마다 나이, 주름, 피부 노화 상태 등이 다르기 때문에 이를 면밀하고 정확하게 파악하여 개개인에게 맞는 진단을 하는 것이 선행된다. 이후 흉터가 가장 보이지 않는 귀의 윤곽선에 최소절개를 통해 주름의 원인 중 가장 큰 요소로 지목되는 근막층(SMAS) 조식을 일부 분리 후 세서하어 봉합해준다.

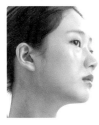 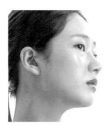 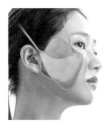 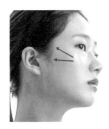

Step 1
고객 상태에 맞는 얼굴 라인을 진단한다.

Step 2
미리 디자인한 귀 앞쪽 1~2㎝가량을 절개한다.

Step 3
표시된 부위의 범위 내 스마스 조직을 분리 후 제거하고 봉합한다.

Step 4
스마스 조직을 분리 제거하고 봉합 후 피부를 덮는다.

수술 시간은 짧게, 젊음은 오래

주름의 원인을 파악하고 확실하게 개선하여 탄력을 더해주는 수술이기 때문에 주름 재발 걱정이 적으며 반영구적인 주름개선 효과를 볼 수 있다. 또한, 가장 보이지 않는 부위에 최소절개를 하기 때문에 흉터가 거의 눈에 보이지 않아 수술 티가 나지 않으며 시술시간과 회복시간이 짧아 일생생활 복귀가 매우 빠르다.

젊은 세대가 더 많이 하는 '리프팅'

갸름한 얼굴형을 원하는 20대부터 주름 개선과 어려 보이는 얼굴을 원하는 중년층까지 광범위한 연령대에서 리프팅 시술로 동안을 완성하고 있는 추세이다.

TIP_페이스리프팅 시술정보				
시술시간	마취방법	입원여부	회복기간	체류기간
3~4시간	수면마취	출혈여부에 따라	7~10일	7~10일

템플리프팅

처진 눈매로 인한 기능적인 부분부터 처진 눈가주름, 팔자주름, 볼살리프팅까지 미용적인 콤플렉스까지 한 번에 개선하는 수술법이다.

눈가 주름개선은 물론, 볼살리프팅 효과까지

　상안검, 하안검이 처지는 현상은 주로 노화가 진행되면서 나타나기도 하지만 선천적으로 눈꺼풀이 처진 경우도 있다. 눈꺼풀이 처진 것은 미용적인 부분뿐만 아니라 기능적인 부분에서도 큰 불편함을 초래하게 된다. 눈꺼풀이 시야를 가리게 되면서 시력이 저하되거나 눈을 뜨기 위해 이마의 근육을 사용하여 이마 주름이 생기는 등 기능적인 불편함 뿐 아니라 졸려 보이고 답답한 인상을 보이는 인상을 심어주게 된다. 이러한 두 가지 불편함을 해소시켜주는 리프팅이 바로 '템플리프팅'이다.

　'템플리프팅'은 헤어라인 부위에 매우 작은 절개를 통해 관자놀이 처진 근육을 제거하고 피부를 올려 주름을 교정하는 시술로 눈가와 팔자주름 개선은 물론 볼살리프팅의 효과를 얻을 수 있다. 상안검수술, 하안검수술로 없애기 힘든 눈 옆 깊은 주름을 개선하는 효과가 뛰어나 중년층은 물론, 볼처짐과 팔자주름의 개선 효과가 있어 젊은 층에서도 인기가 많다. 또한, 두피 최소 절개 기법으로 시술하여 흉터, 머리카락 손실, 통증 붓기 등이 적어 빠른 일상생활 복귀가 가능하다.

TIP_템플리프팅 시술정보				
시술시간	마취방법	입원여부	회복기간	체류기간
1시간	수면마취	필요없음	7~10일	7~10일

실리프팅

특수한 돌기가 있는 녹는 실(PDO)을 수술 없이 피부 진피층에 삽입하여 얼굴 전체 주름을 팽팽하게 당겨주는 비절개 시술이다.

녹는 실을 이용한 V라인 만들기

　기존의 표피층 시술에 비해 피부 진피층에 시술하여 시술효과가 매우 빠르게 나타나며, 시술 직후부터 눈으로 확인할 수 있을 정도의 드라마틱한 효과를 나타낸다. 늘어지고 처진 피부를 원하는 방향으로 리프팅하게 되므로 턱선을 갸름하게 만들거나 입체감 있는 얼굴을 만드는데 매우 효과적이다.

　이때 사용하는 실은 콜라겐 형성과 함께 녹는 실이라 실이 삽입된 부위는 콜라겐이 재생이 되고, 진피 내 섬유화의 진행으로 피부에 탄력을 주어 리프팅 효과를 얻게 된다. 이로 인해 늘어졌던 피부가 당겨져 V라인이 되는 효과를 볼 수 있으며 리프팅을 유지한 그대로 실은 녹아없어져 이물감이 없다.

20~30대가 선호하는 '실리프팅'

　피부에 의료용 실을 삽입하는 실리프팅은 처진 피부를 당겨 올려준 뿐만 아니라 콜라겐 형성과 탄력 증진, 주름 개선의 효과가 있다. 특히 20~30대 젊은 층은 피부의 처짐 정도나 탄력이 중년층에 비해 비교적 노화가 덜 진행되었기 때문에 절개를 이용한 '페이스리프팅'보다는 실리프팅을 선호하고 있다.

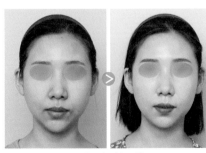

실리프팅 시술 전후

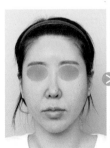
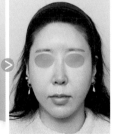

실리프팅 시술 전후

'실리프팅'은 일상생활로의 복귀가 빠르면서 비교적 빠른 시간 내에 간단하게 시술할 수 있고, 즉각적인 효과를 볼 수 있어 중장년층은 물론 20~30대의 젊은 층에서 큰 인기를 끌고 있다.

시술 후 바로 일상생활이 가능

국소마취를 통해 10~20분 가량의 짧은 수술시간과 특수 바늘을 이용하여 실을 삽입하므로 단 1mm의 절개도 없이 확실하게 리프팅 효과를 완성시켜 준다. 물론 흉터 또한 남지 않으며 부기도 거의 없다. 일상생활이 바로 가능하여 지장을 주지 않으며 2년 이상 효과가 지속된다. 처진 볼살, 턱선 개선, 주름 개선, 탄력, V라인 형성, 미백 등 다양한 효과를 볼 수 있다.

TIP_실리프팅 시술정보

시술시간	마취방법	입원여부	회복기간	체류기간
30~40분	국소, 수면마취	필요없음	5일	5일

주름의 원인, 노화만은 아니다

피부의 탄력 감소는 꼭 노화 때문만은 아니다. 최근에는 노화 이외에도 무리한 다이어트로 인한 체중 감소와 바쁜 일상에서 오는 스트레스, 불규칙한 생활습관 등 여러 가지 환경적 요인으로 인한 피부의 탄력 감소가 나타나고 있다.

특히 피부의 탄력이 감소하게 되면 볼살이 점점 아래로 처지게 되어 얼굴라인이 변형되고, 팔자주름이나 눈가, 이마주름이 더욱 깊게 부각되어 보인다. 때문에 나이가 들어 보이는 노안과 사나운 인상으로 보이기 마련이다.

과거의 리프팅 시술은 중년층이 노화로 인해 잃어버린 피부의 탄력과 주름을 제거하는 안티에이징의 이미지가 강했지만, 최근에는 리프팅 시술이 단순 주름이나 피부 처짐 개선뿐만 아니라 얼굴형을 갸름하게 만들어 주는 V라인의 효과가 있어 피부의 탄력과 갸름한 얼굴형을 원하는 20대부터 주름 개선과 어려 보이는 얼굴

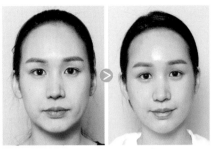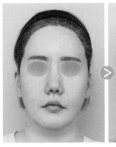

20대 리프팅 시술 전후   30대 리프팅 시술 전후

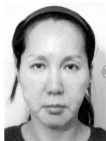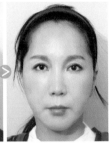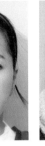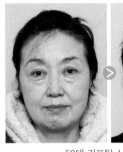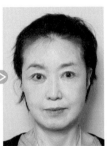

40대 리프팅 시술 전후   50대 리프팅 시술 전후

을 원하는 중년층까지 광범위한 연령대에서 리프팅 시술로 동안을 완성하고 있는 추세이다.

시대가 변함에 따라 그에 대한 미의 기준은 조금씩 달라지고 있지만 남녀노소를 불문하고 조금 더 제 나이보다 어려 보이는 동안에 대한 관심은 변하지 않고 있다. 최근 동안 외모 만들기에 대한 관심이 높아지면서 피부를 더 젊게 하고 탄력적으로 만드는 미용의료 시술이 함께 발전하고 있다. 그러나 의사의 숙련도에 따라 수술 결과가 크게 달라지기 때문에 반드시 임상 경험과 노하우가 풍부한 전문의에게 수술받는 것이 중요하다.

성공적인 '리프팅'을 하려면

주름은 사람에 따라 정도 차이도 매우 큰 복합적인 증상이다. 옷을 입더라도 키, 몸무게, 둘레를 맞춰야 하는 것처럼, 리프팅 시술을 받을 때도 현재 나의 피부 상태는 어떤지, 개선하고자 하는 주름은 어느 부위인지, 본인 주름의 원인이 무엇인지를 꼼꼼히 따져봐야 만족도를 높일 수 있다. 성형수술의 목적은 본인에게 가장 자연스러우며 이상적인 얼굴에 찾는 것에 있다. 얼굴의 노화 정도를 나이와 생활습관 등의 상관관계를 통해 주름의 근본적인 원인을 밝혀 과하지 않은 시술을 하는 것이 중요하다.

동일한 수술이라도 환자에 따라 그 결과는 다르게 나타난다. 실 리프팅은 피부의 탄력이 비교적 양호하고 주름의 정도가 심하지 않은 경우에 효과가 있는 시술이다. 그 외의 탄력이 떨어지고 주름의 정도가 심한 경우에는 효과가 떨어질 수밖에 없으며 무리하게 시술을 하면 얼굴의 전체적인 불균형을 초래할 수밖에 없다. '페이스리프팅'은 박리의 범위, 지방과 근육을 당겨주는 정도에 따라 리프팅 효과 및 유지 기간 등이 매우 다양할 수 있다. 따라서 단순히 입소문 또는 광고를 통해서 수술을 결정하기보단 풍부한 시술 경험과 노하우를 가진 숙련된 전문의와 충분한 상담을 통해 자신에게 맞는 수술법을 찾는 것이 무엇보다 중요하다.

07 While opposing the age, 'the lifting' is the secret and the right answer

Wanting to get young is a basic desire of people

There is the story that, for the skin, Cleopatra used milk, rose water, and even the venom of the snakes. And it has been conveyed that Yang, Kuei-fei, a beautiful woman of China was promiscuous of the things that are good for the skin care, including the swallow's next, the pomegranate, etc. Although it is difficult to confirm whether all the stories that are passed down in this way are real, it is clear and distinct that it is a part with which one can know how much the people pursued the youth regardless of all ages and countries.

Especially, with the development of the modern, medical field, such anti-ageing was reborn. 'Anti-ageing' means 'preventing getting old'. It has the meanings of 'the prevention of the ageing' and 'the rejuvenation'. In these latter days, in relation to anti-ageing, there are the diverse functional products, including the cosmetics, foods, etc. that slow down the ageing and regenerate the cells. But, even if such things prevent, to a certain extent, the generations of the wrinkles, the continuous sagging of the skin due to the wrinkles that were already created on the face and the gravity cannot be prevented perfectly. The surgical procedure for improving the sagging of the skin and the phenomenon of the farsightedness due to old age that occurred because of such ageing is, indeed, lifting.

| Face Lifting

It is the most definite operational method that recovers the elasticity of the skin by improving the overall ageing phenomena of the face, including the nasolabial folds, the cheek deflection, the perioral folds, the gular sutures, etc., by improving from the fundamental causes.

The magical Face lifting that restores the youth once again

Regarding the fine wrinkles that were generally created by the life habits or the facial expressions, there are the many methods which can solve them simply and quickly, including the Botox, the filler, etc. But, regarding the deep nasolabial folds, the cheek deflections, the nasojugal folds, the forehead wrinkles, the Cheek Meat that is off, etc. which are created while getting older with the passing of time, it is difficult to improve the wrinkles if the fundamental causes are not solved. The deep wrinkles due to ageing occur with the ligaments of the fat, muscles, skin, etc. of the face getting loosened and sagged due to the gravity. The surgical procedure method that solves such fundamental causes and improves the wrinkles naturally is, indeed, the Face lifting.

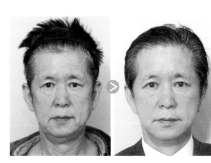
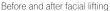
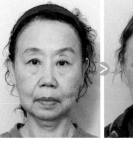
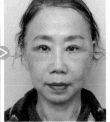

Before and after facial lifting   Before and after facial lifting

Facial lifting is one of the most effective lifting operations. It's not just a skin enhancement procedure, it's a direct solution to the root cause of the skin and SMAS layers. It is an operation to improve sagging skin and wrinkles. It has a high effect of improvement and can see the effect of natural lifting.

Although the general lifting that simply pulls the skin only can temporarily improve the wrinkles, the natural results cannot be obtained. And, when the time passes, the skin gets saggy again. In contrast, a big, special feature of Face lifting is the natural maintenance for a long period of time by separating and moving the saggy fat pads through the FAME technique which pulls the saggy fats and muscles on the lower side of the skin together. Its effect is the best in improving the entire wrinkles of the fact and not a certain portion.

The Face lifting is fundamentally an operation for the improvement of the wrinkles. Because the age, the wrinkles, the condition of the ageing of the skin, etc. are different with every patient, engaging in a diagnosis that suits each and every individual by closely and accurately understanding these precedes.

Afterwards, after separating a part of the fascial plane (SMAS) tissue, which is pointed out as the biggest element among the causes of the wrinkles through a minimal incision of the contours of the ear of which the scar cannot be seen the most, eliminate it and suture it.

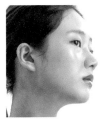 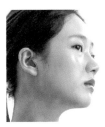 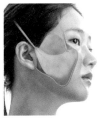 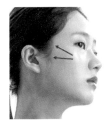

Step 1
Diagnose the facial lines that fit the conditions of the customer.

Step 2
Incise about 1~2cm on the front side of the ear that has already been designed.

Step 3
After separating the fascial plane (SMAS) tissue within the range of the part indicated with the solidus, eliminate it and suture it.

Step 4
Separate and eliminate the fascial plane (SMAS) tissue, suture it, and cover the skin.

The operation time should be short. The youth should be long

Because it is an operation that adds the elasticity by understanding the cause of the wrinkles and by definitely improving the wrinkles, there is no worry regarding the recurrence of the wrinkles, and one can see the semi-permanent wrinkles improvement effects. Also, because the minimal incision is done on the part that cannot be seen the most, the scar nearly cannot be seen with the eyes. So, there is no blemish caused by the operation. And, as the time of the surgical procedure and the time of the recovery are short, the return to the daily life is very quick.

The lifting done more by the young generation

The trend is such that the young-looking face is completed through the lifting surgical procedure performed for the wide-ranging age groups, from those who are in their 20s who want a slender facial shape to the middle-aged who want an improvement of the wrinkles and the young-looking face.

TIP_Information on Face Lifting

Operation time	Anesthetizing method	Hospitalization	Convalescent period	The length of one's visit
3~4 hours	Sleep anaesthesia	According to whether or not bleeding	7~10 days	7~10 days

| Temple Lifting

It is an operational method that improves, at once, from the functional part of the saggy eyes to the saggy, periorbital wrinkles, to the nasolabial folds, to the Cheek Meat lifting, and to the cosmetic complex.

Not only the improvement of the wrinkles around the eyes, but also the effect of the lifting of the Cheek Meat

Although the phenomenon of the drooping of the upper eyelids and the lower eyelids mainly appear with the progress of the ageing, there are the cases, too, in which the eyelids droop innately.

The drooping of the eyelids cause a big discomfort with regard to not only the cosmetic part but, also, with regard to the functional part, too. With the eyelids covering the view, not only are there the functional discomforts, including the lowering of the eyesight, the creation of the forehead wrinkles by using the muscles of the forehead in order to open up the eyes, etc., but also the impression that looks sleepy and stifling gets implanted. The lifting that alleviates such two kinds of discomforts is, indeed, temple lifting.

The temple lifting is a surgical procedure that eliminates the drooping muscles of the temples through a very small incision of the hairline part, pulls up the skin, and corrects the wrinkles. One can obtain not only the improvements of the eye rims and the nasolabial folds but also the Cheek Meat lifting effect. Because the effect of improving the deep wrinkles on the sides of the eyes, which are difficult to be eliminated through the upper eyelid operation and the lower eyelid operation, is extraordinary, and because there are the effects of improving the cheek drooping and the nasolabial folds, there is a lot of popularity among the middle-aged and the young.

Also, because the surgical procedure involves the technique of the minimal incision of the scalp and, therefore, there are small scars, loss of the hair, painful swelling, the quick return to the daily life is possible.

TIP_Information on Temple Lifting

Operation time	Anesthetizing method	Hospitalization	Convalescent period	The length of one's visit
1 hour	Sleep anaesthesia	No need	7~10 days	At least 3 days

| Thread Lifting

It is a non-incision surgical procedure that pulls tight the wrinkles of the whole face by inserting a melting thread that has a special swelling (PDO) into the skin layer of the skin without an operation.

Making a V-line using a melting thread

Compared to the previously existent, outer-layer-of-the-skin surgical procedure, the effect of the surgical procedure appears very quickly by operating on the skin layer of the skin. It shows the dramatic effects to the extent that they can be confirmed with the eyes from right after the surgical procedure. As the loosened and saggy skin is lifted in the direction desired, it is very effective in making the jaw lines slender and making a face with the cubic effect.

Because the thread that is used at this time is a thread that melts, together with the formation of a collagen, the part into which the thread was inserted regenerates the collagen. And, due to the progress of the fibrosis within the thick skin, the lifting effect is obtained by giving the elasticity to the skin. Because the skin that was loosened due to this gets pulled, the effect of becoming a V-line can be seen. And, the thread that maintained the lifting just the way it was melts and disappears, and, therefore, there is no foreign body sensation.

The thread lifting preferred by those who are in their 20s and 30s

Not only does the thread lifting which inserts a medical-purpose thread into the skin pull up the saggy skin, but, also, it has the effects of the formation of the collagen, the promotion of the elasticity, and the improvement of the wrinkles. Especially, because the ageing of the extent of the drooping and the elasticity of the skin of the young bracket in their 20s and 30s has been proceeded less relatively, they prefer the thread lifting rather than the face lifting that uses the incision.

As, regarding the thread lifting, because the return to the everyday life is quick, the surgical procedure can be done within a relatively quick time and simply, and the immediate effects can be seen, it has been very popular not only among the middle-aged class but also among the young bracket in their 20s and 30s.

The everyday life is possible right after the surgical procedure.

As the thread is inserted by using the short operation time of about 10~20 minutes and by using a special needle while the patient is undergoing the local anaesthesia, the lifting effect is completed definitely even without an incision of 1mm. Of course, no scar remains, also, and there is nearly no swelling.

The everyday life is possible right away, there is no trouble, and the effect continues over 2 years. The diverse effects can be seen, including the saggy Cheek Meat, the improvement of the jaw lines, the improvement of the wrinkles, the elasticity, the formation of the V-line, the whitening, etc.

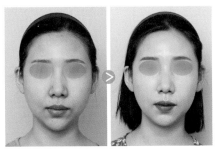

Before and after Thread Lifting

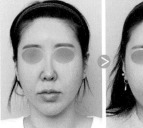

Before and after Thread Lifting

TIP_Information on Thread Lifting				
Operation time	Anesthetizing method	Hospitalization	Convalescent period	The length of one's visit
30~40 mins	Localized and Sleep anaesthesia	No need	5 days	No need

Aging is not the only cause of the wrinkles

The reduction of the elasticity of the skin is not only because of ageing. Recently, the reduction of the elasticity of the skin due to the many kinds of the environment factors have been appearing, including the reduction of the weight due to an excessive diet, the stress coming from the busy everyday life, the irregular life habits, etc. other than the ageing.

Especially, if the elasticity of the skin gets reduced, the facial lines get transformed because the Cheek Meat gradually droops below and the nasolabial folds, the eye rims, and the forehead wrinkles look even more deeply carved. Because of this, it is a matter of course that the farsightedness due to old age and the fierce impression are seen.

Although, regarding the lifting surgical procedures of the past, the image of the anti-ageing that removes the elasticity and the wrinkles of the skin that were lost due to the ageing of the middle-aged had been strong, because, recently, the lifting surgical procedure has been having the effect of the V-line which not only improves the simple wrinkles and the skin laxity but, also, makes the facial shape slender, the trend has been that the young-looking faces have been completed through the lifting surgical procedure performed on the wide-ranging age groups, from those who are in their 20s, who desire the elasticity of the skin and the slender facial shape, to the middle-aged, who want the improvement of the wrinkles and a young-looking face.

Although, according to the changes of the era, the standard of beauty has been getting different by little bits, the interest in the young-looking face that looks a little bit younger than the age has not been changing, regardless of the males, the females, the elderly, and the children.

Recently, with the interest in making the outward appearance with a young-looking face getting higher, the cosmetic, medical procedures that make the skin younger and elastic have been developing together. However, because the results of an operation become very much different according to the level of the skill of the doctor, it is important to receive an operation by a medical specialist whose clinical experiences and

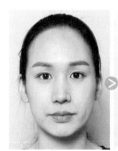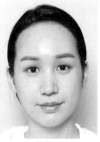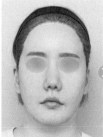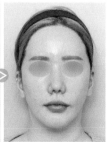

Before and after 20s Lifting   Before and after 30s Lifting

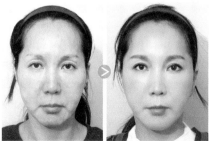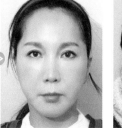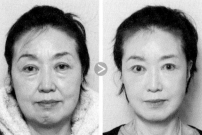

Before and after 40s Lifting   Before and after 50s Lifting

know-how are abundant, without fail.

The successful 'Lifting'

The wrinkles are a symptom of which the differences of the extents are very big and complex according to the person. Just as, when wearing the clothes, they must fit the height, body weight, and girth, when receiving a lifting surgical procedure, too, the level of satisfaction can be heightened only by carefully examining how my skin conditions is now, what part has the wrinkles to be improved, and what the cause of the wrinkles of the person concerned is. The purpose of plastic surgery lies in getting the most natural and ideal face for the person concerned. Regarding the extent of the ageing of the face, it is important to carry out a surgical procedure that is not excessive by disclosing the fundamental cause of the wrinkles through the correlations between the age, the life habits, etc.

Even if they are the same operations, the results appear differently according to the patient. The thread lifting is a surgical procedure that has the effects in case the elasticity of the skin is relatively good and the extent of the wrinkles is not extreme. In the case in which the other elasticity decreases and the extent of the wrinkles is extreme, the effect has no choice but to decrease, and, if the surgical procedure takes place excessively, the entire imbalance of the face will be caused and there is no other choice.

Regarding the face lifting, the lifting effect, the time period of the maintenance, etc. can be very diverse according to the range of the desquamation and the extent of the pulling of the fats and the muscles.

As a result, instead of making the decision on an operation simply through the word of mouth or advertisements, it is more important than anything else to find an operational method that fits oneself through the sufficient counseling by a skilled medical specialist who has the abundant surgical procedure experiences and know-how.

녹는 실 리프팅(Dissolvable Thread Lifting)
비절개/절개 탄력밴드 리프팅(Non-incisional/Incisional Elastic Band Lifting)
안면거상술(Face lifting)
엔도타인 이마거상술(Endotine Forehead Lifting)

동안 성형, 얼굴과 함께 삶의 태도를 바꾸는 기술

Anti-aging Surgery, Changing Life Attitudes Together

사람은 누구나 나이가 들면 중력의 영향으로 인해 연부 조직이 밑으로 처지게 된다. 또 이런 처짐은 주변 피부와 인대, 근막들도 같이 처지게 한다. 늘어난 연부 조직 및 인대 조직을 원래의 위치대로 돌려놓는 것이 '리프팅' 수술이다.

As people age, the effects of gravity cause connective tissues to sag downwards. This sagging also affects the surrounding skin, ligaments, and fascia. The surgical procedure that restores the loosened connective tissues and ligaments to their original positions is called 'lifting' surgery.

바노바기성형외과
Banobagi Plastic Surgery Clinic

www.banobagi.com

반재상(Barn-Jae Sang)

• 성형외과 전문의, 의학박사(M.D., PhD Board Certified Plastic Surgeon)
• 서울대학교 의과대학 졸업(Seoul National University College of Medicine)
• 서울대학교 성형외과 외래교수
(Invited Professor, Dept of Plastic and Reconstructive Surgery, Seoul National University Hospital)
• 대한성형외과학회 정회원(Active member, Korean Society of Plastic and Reconstructive Surgeons)
• 대한미용성형외과학회 정회원(Active member, Korean Society of Aesthetic Plastic Surgery)

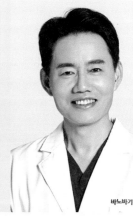

바노바기 성형외

08 마음까지 젊어지는 동안 성형, '리프팅'의 모든 것

장생(長生)의 비법 안티에이징 시술

　시간의 흐름에 역행하려는 염원은 인류의 꿈이다. 세상 모든 권력을 거머쥐었던 진시황도 불로장생(不老長生)을 위해 불로초를 얻기 위한 모든 방법을 동원했다는 것만 봐도 알 수 있다. 고령화 시대에 접어들면서 오래 살고 싶지만 늙고 싶진 않다는 이율배반적 욕구는 안티에이징 같은 개념을 탄생시켰다. 어떤 병에도 걸리지 않고 언제나 청춘으로 산다는 것은 불가능하지만, 의료와 과학의 발달은 인간에게 많은 가능성을 열어주었다. 불로(不老) 해법을 발견하지는 못했지만 장생(長生)의 비법은 찾아냈다. 늙는 것을 막을 수는 없지만 어느 정도 늦출 수는 있게 된 셈이다.

　사람이 늙는 이유는 세포가 노화하기 때문이다. 세포가 노화하면 세포 분열이 정지되고 노화된 세포가 신체에 축적된다. 노화된 세포가 쌓이면 쌓일수록, 노화 속도도 빨라지게 된다. 성형 수술은 쉽게 말해 이러한 노화 현상을 지연시키는 것이다. 성형외과에서 진행하는 안티에이징 시술은 단순히 늘어난 피부를 당기는 것만이 아니다. 종합적으로 노화 현상을 어떻게 되돌리는가에 초점을 맞춘다. 리프팅 같은 수술부터 부기나 흉터가 남지 않는 간단한 보톡스, 필러 주사 등을 적재적소에 적용해야 효과적인 결과를 가져다준다.

| 녹는 실 리프팅

피부 아래에 실을 몇 가닥 넣고 피부를 끌어올리는 실리프팅은 보통 녹는 실과 녹지 않는 실을 이용한다.

충분한 두께의 녹는 실, 인장력 우수

상담을 하다 보면 리프팅이란 개념을 사람마다 다르게 이해하고 있는 것을 알 수 있다. 대개 연령별로 차이가 나는데, 아직 탄력 문제로 큰 고민을 하지 않는 20대의 경우 리프팅을 갸름하게 만드는 '슬리밍 시술'로 생각한다. 반면 30대 이상이 되면 주름이나 처짐을 해결하는 '동안 시술'로 받아들인다. 모두 틀린 것은 아니다. 쉽게 말해 리프팅 시술은 '나이보다 어려 보이게 만드는 방법'이라고 이해하면 된다.

얼굴 리프팅은 크게 ▲레이저를 이용한 리프팅 ▲실리프팅 ▲안면거상술 등으로 구분된다. 처짐이 심하지 않다면 레이저 리프팅 정도로 처짐 현상을 개선할 수 있다. 특히 레이저 리프팅은 시술 후 바로 일상생활이 가능하고 흉터에 대한 걱정이 적다. 하지만 효과가 점진적으로 나타나며 노화 정도가 미미한 경우에만 충분한 효과가 있다.

피부 아래에 실을 몇 가닥 넣고 피부를 끌어올리는 '실리프팅'은 레이저 리프팅만으로 효과를 기대하기 어려운 경우 대안이 될 수 있다. 리프팅용 실에는 녹는 실과 녹지 않는 실이 있다. 현재 리프팅에 사용되는 녹는 실은 PDO(polydioxanone)를 재료로 하는 경우가 대부분이다. 충분한 두께를 가진 실이라면 녹아 없어지면서도 조직을 당기는 인장력이 강하고, 감염이 일어나는 경우가 드물어 안전하다. 실들마다 원사는 동일하나 돌기를 만드는 기술과 모양을 만드는 방식이 다르기 때문에 종류가 다양하다.

TIP_녹는 실 리프팅 시술정보

시술시간	마취방법	입원여부	회복기간	체류기간
30분~1시간	국소, 수면마취	입원없음	1~2일	2~3일

비절개/절개 탄력밴드 리프팅

유지 기간이 짧은 실리프팅과 회복 기간이 오래 걸리는 안면거상술의 장점만 살린 시술이다.

비절개 탄력밴드 리프팅

녹는 실을 이용한 리프팅은 유지 기간이 짧다는 단점이 있다. 짧으면 6개월, 길어도 2년이면 피부가 다시 처지는 경우가 많다. 시간이 경과함에 따라 피부를 끌어올리는 실의 장력(張力, 당기는 힘)이 약해지기 때문이다. 이에 비해 안면거상술은 효괴기 확실하고 반영구저이지만, 피부 절개·박리 부위가 넓고 회복에 오래 시간이 걸려서 환자에게 부담이 된다. 또 피부 박리 시 들어 올린 연부 조직의 혈액순환장애로 피부 괴사나 혈종 등의 부작용이 발생할 수 있다.

이러한 단점을 줄이기 위해 등장한 수술이 '탄력밴드'를 이용한 리프팅이다. 기존 실리프팅과 안면거상술의 장점만 뽑아낸 수술이다. 시간이 지나면 장력을 잃는 실 대신 탄력밴드라는 특수 소재를 사용한다. 탄력밴드는 가운데가 실리콘이며, 실리콘 양옆으로는 폴리에스테르 돌기가 붙어있다. 기존 실과는 달리 몸속에서 흐물흐물해지지 않아 잡아당기는 힘을 반영구적으로 유지한다. 원래 무릎 등 관절 인대 재건수술에 쓰이는 의료재료였던 만큼, 몸속에서 인대 역할을 대신한다. 피부 처짐 정도가 심하지 않고 탄력이 어느 정도 좋다면 비절개 방식으로 탄력밴드 리프팅을 하면 효과를 볼 수 있다.

TIP_비절개 탄력밴드 리프팅 시술정보				
시술시간	마취방법	입원여부	회복기간	체류기간
30분~1시간	국소, 수면마취	입원없음	1~2일	3일

절개 탄력밴드 리프팅

피부가 많이 늘어나 남는 양이 많다면 절개식 탄력밴드 리프팅이 필요할 수 있다. 탄력밴드 리프팅의 또 다른 장점은 절개 범위나 삽입 위치 등에 따라 다양하게 응용 가능해 여러 가지 효과를 기대할 수 있다는 것이다.

귀 뒤쪽으로 미세절개만 해 수술하면 턱 라인 늘어짐을 개선하는 데 효과적이고 수술 후 부기가 적어 회복이 빠르다. 기존 안면거상술에 응용하면 훨씬 적은 부위의 박리만으로도 리프팅이 가능하기 때문에 부작용 위험은 크게 줄이고 수술 효과는 그대로 유지할 수 있다.

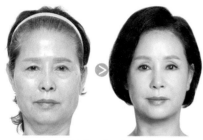

절개 탄력밴드 리프팅 시술전후

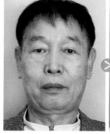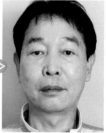

절개 탄력밴드 리프팅 시술전후

TIP_절개 탄력밴드 리프팅 시술정보				
시술시간	마취방법	입원여부	회복기간	체류기간
2시간	국소, 수면마취	입원없음	7일	7일

중안면부 리프팅

중안면부 리프팅은 눈 밑주름부터 중앙면부에 나타나는 복합적인 처짐을 한번에 개성하는 수술이다.

눈 아래 미세한 절개를 통해 피부와 처진 조직을 당겨주는 중안면부 리프팅

중안면부는 눈 밑에서부터 입꼬리까지 범위를 나타내며 이 부분의 노화는 부정적인 인상을 주며 노안의 원인이 되기 때문에 개선하는 것이 좋다. 중안면부는 지방이 무겁기 때문에 엔도타인을 이용하거나 탄력밴드를 이용한 안면 리프팅과 하안검 수술을 동시에 진행한다.

눈 밑을 절개하고 절개창을 통해 전체적인 중안면부 조직들을 고르게 박리해 당겨주는 것이다. 이때 눈 밑주름의 원인이 되는 지방, 근육, 피부까지 함께 수직으로 당기는 것이 수술의 핵심이다. 당겨진 조직은 엔도타인을 통해 단단히 고정하면 중안면부가 올라간 상태로 뼈에 달라붙기 때문에 시간이 지나도 다시 처지지 않는다. 이는 눈 밑의 노화는 중안면부 노화로 연결되어 있기 때문이라고 할 수 있는데, 중안면부 리프팅의 경우 일반 하안검보다 드라마틱한 결과를 기대할 수 있으며 지속 기간이 길다. 중안면부 리프팅은 하안검만을 시행했을 때 생길 수 있는 어색함과 부작용을 예방하는 상호보완적인 수술로 근육까지 고려하는 수술이기 때문에 더욱 자연스러운 효과를 볼 수 있다.

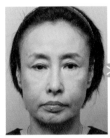 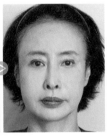
중안면부 리프팅 시술전후

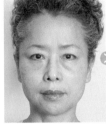 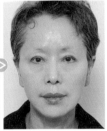
중안면부 리프팅 시술전후

TIP_중안면부 리프팅 시술정보

시술시간	마취방법	입원여부	회복기간	체류기간
1~1시간 30분	정맥마취	없음	3~5일	5일

| 안면거상술

안면거상술은 볼처짐, 입가주름, 목주름 고민 해결을 위한 시술이다.

드라마틱한 주름 개선 효과를 기대할 수 있는 안면거상술

주름, 꺼짐 현상, 처짐 현상은 우리가 흔히 말하는 노안의 구성요소라고 할 수 있다. 주름과 꺼짐 현상의 경우에는 아테콜 필러 등의 시술을 진행하기도 하는데

처짐 현상의 경우에는 리프팅이 보다 드라마틱한 효과를 가져올 수 있다. 이번에 살펴볼 시술은 안면거상술인데 특히 볼 처짐 현상, 입가 주름, 목 주름 해결이 가능하다. 볼, 입가, 목 등 얼굴 중 하단에 해당하는 부분의 주름 혹은 처짐 현상은 근막층(SMAS)이 힘을 잃는 경우에 생기게 된다. 근막층(SMAS)은 얼굴 표정 근육, 결체 조직, 근막혈관과 같이 피부를 구성하는 요소를 포함하고 있기 때문에 비교적 간단한 시술만으로는 해결이 어려운 경우가 많다. 그렇기 때문에 많은 환자들이 안면거상술에 대해 관심을 가지고 문의를 하고는 한다.

안면거상술은 노화한 피부의 근본적인 원인인 처진 근막층(SMAS)을 귀 앞쪽의 절개를 통해 박리하여 늘어진 피부 전반을 직접적으로 당겨주는 동시에 남은 피부를 제거하여 주름을 없애는 방식으로 진행된다. 이러한 과정을 거치는 만큼 안면거상술은 보다 확실하고 드라마틱한 결과를 얻을 수 있다.

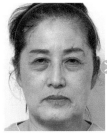 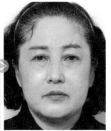 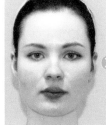 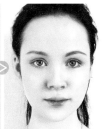

안면거상술 시술전후　　　　　안면거상술 시술전후

TIP_안면거상술 시술정보

시술시간	마취방법	입원여부	회복기간	체류기간
2~2시간 30분	정맥마취	없음 또는 경우에 따라 1일	3~5일	5일

| 엔도타인 이마거상술

엔도타인 이마거상술은 엔도타인이라는 보형물을 이용해 눈·이마의 주름을 한 번에 해결하는 시술이다.

내시경을 이용해 최소 절개로 진행하는 엔도타인 이마거상술

탄력밴드 수술이 주로 볼과 턱의 리프팅에 이용된다면 눈과 이마의 주름은 각각 상안검 수술·이마거상술을 실시한다. 문제는 상안검 수술의 경우 처진 눈두덩을 올려주는 과정에서 눈과 눈썹 사이가 좁아지고, 이로 인해 인상이 사나워질 수도 있다는 것이다.

이마거상술은 수술 부담이 크다는 단점이 있다. 이런 단점을 개선하기 위해 눈·이마 부위에도 새로운 기술이 도입됐다. 내시경과 '엔도타인'이라는 보형물을 이용해 눈·이마의 주름을 한 번에 펴는 방식이다. 기존 이마거상술처럼 이마 전체를 절개, 박리하는 대신 두피에 세 군데 정도 작은 절개를 하고 내시경을 넣어 피부 조직을 잡아 올린다. 끌어올린 피부는 엔도타인이라는 일종의 걸개로 고정한다. 미국 식품의약국(FDA) 승인을 받은 이 보형물은 위로 당겨진 피부가 연부 조직에 고정되는 동안 장력을 유지하다가 완전히 유착된 9~12개월 후면 체내에 흡수된다.

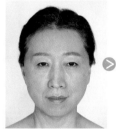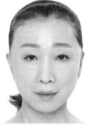
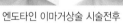
엔도타인 이마거상술 시술전후

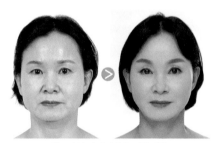
엔도타인 이마거상술 시술전후

TIP_엔도타인 이마거상술 시술정보				
시술시간	마취방법	입원여부	회복기간	체류기간
1시간	수면, 전신마취	1일	5일	5일

우리 얼굴에는 표정을 만들어주는 20여 개의 근육이 존재하는데 이마 부위의 상안면부 턱 부위의 하안면부에 위치한 근육들을 많이 사용할수록 주름과 나쁜 인상을 만들기 쉽다. 가령 무엇에 집중할 때 본인도 모르게 미간을 찌푸리며 인상을 쓰는 습관은 상안면부의 눈썹 주름근을 발달시켜 사납고 어두운 인상을 만든

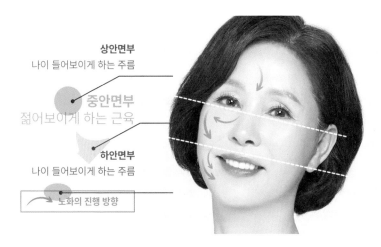

상안면부
나이 들어보이게 하는 주름

중안면부
젊어보이게 하는 근육

하안면부
나이 들어보이게 하는 주름

노화의 진행 방향

다. 또한 평소 일상생활에서 입을 꽉 다물고 있는 습관은 턱 부위의 입꼬리 내림근과 턱끝 근육을 발달시켜 무겁고 나이 들어 보이게 한다.

반대로 젊고 호감 가는 인상에 영향을 미치는 부위는 중안면부로, 특히 광대 부위의 근육들이 활발하게 운동을 하면 전체적으로 얼굴의 탄력이 올라가 주름을 예방하는 데 효과적이다. 이러한 광대 부위의 근육들을 발달시키기 위해서는 꾸준히 밝은 미소와 웃는 표정을 많이 짓는 것이 중요하다.

얼굴 광대 부위인 중안면부의 근육을 강화시키는 것을 '동안(童顔) 운동'이라고 불린다. 동안 운동에서 가장 중요한 부분은 입에 힘을 빼는 것이다. 입술과 입 주변 근육의 힘을 최대한 빼고 치아가 약간 보이도록 벌리며 '흐'라고 소리 낸다. 이어 입을 최대한 양옆으로 벌려 '리'라고 발음하며 광대에 힘을 주는 동작을 반복하면 된다. 꾸준히 하면 입꼬리가 올라가 온화한 이미지로 보이고 입 주변의 잔주름을 예방하며 애플존이라고 부르는 앞 광대 부분에 리프팅 효과도 볼 수 있다. 운동 초기에는 최소한 하루 4시간 정도 의식적으로 근육을 움직여줘야 주름을 만드는 습관을 바꿀 수 있다.

그러나 꼭 기억해야 되는 것은 아무리 동안이라고 해도 평생 늙지 않는 것은 아니다. 애초에 절대 안 늙겠다는 목표를 잡는 것이 아니라 건강하고 자연스럽게 늙겠다는 마음가짐이 무엇보다 중요하다.

08 Face Lifting Surgery that Makes Your Mind Younger : Everything About Lifting

Longevity Secrets anti-aging Treatment

The desire to reverse the passage of time is a human's natural desire. Even the all powerful Qin Shi Huang, who ruled the world, spared no effort to obtain the elixir of immortality, as evidenced by historical records. As we enter the age of aging, the desire to live longer without getting old has given rise to concepts like anti-aging. While it may be impossible to remain forever young and disease-free, the advancements in medicine and science have opened up many possibilities for humanity. Although we haven't discovered the elixir of immortality, we have found the secrets to longevity.

While we can't stop aging altogether, we can delay it to some extent.

The reason why people age is that cells undergo aging. When cell ages, their division ceases and these aging cells accumulate in the body. As aging cells accumulate, the rate of aging accelerates. anti-aging surgery, in simple terms, is a way to delay this aging process. anti-aging procedures performed in plastic surgery go beyond merely tightening loose skin. They focus on how to reverse the aging process comprehensively.

This includes surgeries like facelift and the strategic use of non invasive treatments such as Botox or dermal fillers to achieve effective results without leaving swelling or scars.

| Dissolvable Thread Lifting

Thread lifting, which involves inserting several threads beneath the skin to lift it, typically uses both dissolvable and non-dissolvable threads.

Adequate thickness of dissolvable thread, excellent tensile strength

During the consultation, it's apparent that people have varying interpretations of the concept of lifting. This generally varies by age; with those in their 20s, who aren't greatly concerned with elasticity issues, perceive lifting as a 'slimming procedure' to make them appear more slender. On the other hand, those aged 30 and above tend to view it as an 'anti-aging procedure' to address wrinkles and sagging. Neither perspective is entirely incorrect. Simply, one can understand the concept of lifting procedures as a way to 'appear younger than one's age.'

Facial lifting can be broadly categorized into ▲laser lifting ▲thread lifting ▲facelift surgery, among others. If sagging is not severe, laser lifting can be sufficient to improve the sagging. Laser lifting, in particular, allows for immediate resumption of daily activities after the procedure and has minimal concerns about scarring. However, the results appear gradually and are only sufficient when signs of aging are minimal.

Thread lifting, which involves inserting several threads beneath the skin to lift it, can serve as an alternative when expecting results solely from laser lifting is challenging. Threads used for lifting can be either dissolvable or non-dissolvable. Currently, most dissolvable threads used in lifting are made of PDO(polydioxanone). These threads, when of sufficient thickness, have strong tensile strength to pull the tissues while gradually dissolving and are relatively safe with a low risk of infection. While the core material is the same for all threads, the variety arises from the techniques used to create the barbs and the shapes of the threads.

TIP_DissolvableThread Lifting Procedure Information

Procedure Time	Anesthetizing method	Hospitalization	Recovery Period	Length of Stay
1~1 hour 30 mins	Local anesthesia, Sedation	No hospitalization	1~2 days	2~3 days

Non-incisional / Incisional Elastic Band Lifting

The advantages of a short-lasting thread lift and facelift with long recovery period have been combined into the Elastic Band Lift procedure.

Non-incisional Elastic Band Lifting

Thread lifting using dissolvable threads has a drawback of a short-lasting power. In some cases, the effect may last as shortas 6 months, and even at its longest typically up to only 2 years. This is because the tension(the pulling force) of the threads used to lift the skin weakens over time. In contrast, facelift surgery offers a more definite and permanent solution, but it involves larger skin incisions and dissections, resulting in a longer and more burdensome recovery period for patients. Additionally, there is a risk of side effects such as skin necrosis or hematoma due to impaired blood circulation in the underlying tissues when lifting the skin during the procedure.

The surgical procedure that has emerged to address these shortcomings is the 'Elastic Band Lift.' This surgery extracts the advantages of both traditional thread lifting and facelift procedures. Instead of using threads that lose tension over time, the Elastic Band Lift utilizes a special material known as an elastic band. This band features a silicone core with polyester barbs on either side. Unlike conventional threads, it maintains its pulling force permanently without becoming loose or saggy inside the body. Originally, this medical material was used for ligament reconstruction in knee and joint surgeries, so it serves as a substitute ligament within the body. If the skin sagging is not severe, and if the skin still has reasonable elasticity, the Elastic Band Lift can be performed in a Non-incision manner to achieve noticeable results.

TIP_Non-incisional Elastic Band Lifting Procedure Information				
Procedure Time	Anesthetizing method	Hospitalization	Recovery Period	Length of Stay
30 mins~ 1 hour	Local anesthesia, Sedation	No hospitalization	1~2 days	3 days

Incisional Elastic Band Lifting

If there is a significant amount of excess and loose skin, an incisional Elastic Band Lift may be necessary. Another advantage of the Elastic Band Lift is its versatility, as it can be adapted in various ways based on the extent of incisions, insertion locations, and other factors, offering the potential for achieving multiple desired effects.

Surgery performed through tiny incisions behind the ears is effective for improving jawline sagging, with minimal post-operative swelling and a faster recovery. When applied to traditional facelift procedures, it allows for lifting with minimal dissection in smaller areas, significantly reducing the risk of side effects while maintaining the surgical benefits.

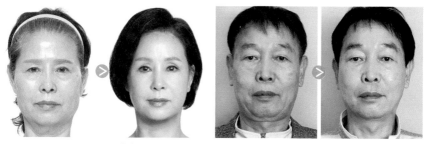

Before & After of Incisional Elastic Band Lifting

TIP_Incisional Elastic Band Lifting Procedure Information				
Procedure Time	Anesthetizing method	Hospitalization	Recovery Period	Length of Stay
2 hour	Local anesthesia, Sedation	No hospitalization	7 days	7 days

| Midface Lifting

Midface lift is a surgical procedure that simultaneously addresses complex sagging from under-eye wrinkles to the midface area.

Midface lift with subtle incisions below the eyes, which tightens the skin and

sagging tissues

The midface region encompasses the area from below the eyes to the corners of the mouth, and addressing the aging in this area is essential as it can create a negative impression and serve as a cause of aging. Given the presence of substantial fat in the midface, procedures often involve a combination of endotine, elastic band facelift, and lower eyelid surgery.

It involves making an incision below the eye and dissecting the entire midface tissue through the incision site, evenly pulling the underlying tissues. The core of the surgery lies in vertically tightening the factors responsible for under-eye wrinkles, including fat, muscle, and skin. The tightened tissues are firmly secured with endotine, allowing them to attach to the bone and preventing them from sagging over time. This is attributed to the connection between under-eye aging and midface aging, making midface lift surgery capable of producing more dramatic and longer-lasting results compared to regular lower eyelid procedures.

Midface lift is a mutually complementary surgical procedure that takes into account even the facial muscles, aiming to prevent the potential awkwardness and side effects that can arise when performing only lower eyelid surgery. As a result, it provides a more natural and harmonious outcome.

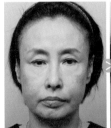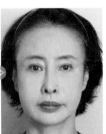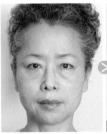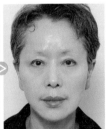

Before & After of Midface Lifting

TIP_Midface Lifting Procedure Information

Procedure Time	Anesthetizing method	Hospitalization	Recovery Period	Length of Stay
1~1hour 30mins	Intravenous anesthesia	No hospitalization	3~5 days	5 days

| Face lifting

Face lifting is a surgical procedure to solve concerns about sagging cheeks, wrinkles around the mouth, and neck wrinkles.

Face lifting, the surgery that can give you a dramatic effect expectation of wrinkle improvements

Wrinkles, sunken areas are the components of what we commonly refer to an aging process In the case of wrinkles and sunken areas, procedures like Artecoll filler can be performed, but in the case of sagging, lifting can bring a more dramatic effect The surgical procedure, about what we are going to speak up now, is a face lifting, which can make improvements of sagging cheeks, wrinkles around the mouth, and neck wrinkles possible.

Wrinkles or sagging of the lower face parts, such as jawlines mouth, and neck, occur when the SMAS layer loses its strength Since the SMAS layer includes the elements, such as facial muscles, connective tissues, and fascial blood vessels, it is often difficult to solve the problem with a simple procedure That is why many patients are interested in face lifting surgery.

Face lifting is performed by lifting up the sagging SMAS layer, which is a fundamental cause of skin aging, and by removing the remaining skin to eliminate wrinkles through an incision in front of the ears By going through this process, more certain and dramatic results can be achieved with the face lifting.

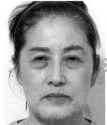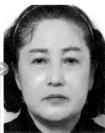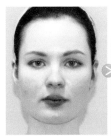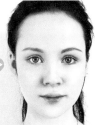

Before & After of Face Lifting

| Endotine Forehead Lifting

Endotine Forehead Lifting is a surgical procedure done to improve forehead and eyes wrinkles at once by using implant called Endotine.

Minimally invasive Endoscopic Endotine Forehead Lifting

Elastic Band surgery usually works for cheeks and jaw line lifting, while Upper Blepharoplasty and Forehead lifting surgeries are useful for eyes and forehead lines. In case of Upper Blepharoplasty after getting rid of sagging eyelids, the space between the eye and brow might get narrower, which can cause a harsher impression.

The disadvantage of Forehead lifting is that it might make you feel more pressure about undergoing it. But, in order to solve this disadvantage, the new technique was developed. It is an Endoscopic method with using implant called Endotine , which can improve eyes and forehead wrinkles at once. The Classic Forehead lifting required the big incision across the top of forehead, while with the Endoscopic technique the skin

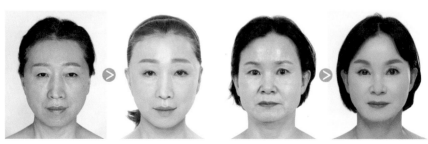

Before & After of Endotine Forehead Lifting

and tissues can be lifted up just through three small incisions. Lifted skin gets fixed on some kind of hanger called Endotine. This implant is FDA approved; it maintains the tension of lifted skin and absorbs in 9~12 months after the fixation to soft tissues is completed.

TIP_Endotine Forehead Lifting Information

Procedure Time	Anesthetizing method	Hospitalization	Recovery Period	Length of Stay
1 hour	Sedation, General anesthesia	1 day	5 days	5 days

Upper face
Wrinkles that make you look older

Midface
Muscles that make you look younger

Lower face
Wrinkles that make you look older

Aging Process

There are about 20 muscles that create our facial expressions, and they can be divided into three parts depending on their location. These parts are upper face (forehead area), mid-face (cheeks area), and lower face (chin area).

The more you use the muscles located in the upper and lower face, the easier you can get wrinkles and a bad impression. For example, when you concentrate on something, the habit of frowning even without realizing it develops the corrugator muscles of the upper face, creating a fierce and depressed impression.

In addition, in everyday life while using a smartphone or watching TV, the habit of keeping your mouth tightly closed develops the depressor muscles of the corners of the mouth and the muscles of the chin, making you look dull and older.

On the other way, the area that affects a youthful and attractive impression is the mid-face. In particular, if the cheek area's muscles are actively exercised, the overall elasticity of the face increases, which is effective in preventing wrinkles.

In order to develop these cheek area's muscles, consistently smiling and laughing brightly is very important. The habit of making smiling facial expressions may seem easy, but it is difficult unless you practice. That's why, it is very helpful to consciously exercise to strengthen the muscles of the mid face area.

Exercise, that strengthen the mid face muscles, is called 'anti aging exercise', because it makes you look younger This exercise is a method that can effectively prevent wrinkles and maintain skin elasticity by considering the movement direction and function of each facial muscle

The most important part of the 'anti aging exercise' is relaxing of your mouth Relax your lips and the muscles around as much as possible, open your mouth, slightly showing your teeth, and make a 'sound Then, make a wide smile as much as possible and say ' and repeat the movement of applying strength to your heek bones with the previous movement If you keep doing this exercise, the corners of your mouth will rise up, giving you a gentle look, preventing fine wrinkles around the mouth, and also providing a lifting effect of front cheek area, called an apple zone.

Exercising as much as possible is effective in preventing wrinkles, and when you just start your exercise, it is better to consciously move your muscles for at least 4 hours a day in order to change the habits, which cause wrinkles.

However, you shall remember, that no matter how young you are, it does not mean that you will never age Rather than setting a goal of never getting old in the first place, the most important thing is to have the mindset of aging healthily and naturally.

복합 안면거상수술(Stem Cell-Integrated Complex Face-Lifting)
모발이식수술(Stem Cell Treatment combined Hair Transplantation)

"

줄기세포 이용한 항노화수술

Representative Anti-Aging Surgery Using Stem Cells

"

나이에 비하여 젊게 보이는 것은 바로 풍성한 머리카락과 주름살 없는 얼굴입니다.

To look younger than one's age is to have a full head of hair and a wrinkle-free face.

글로벌성형외과
Global Aesthetic Plastic Surgery

www.globalps.co.kr

최오규(O-Kyu Choi)

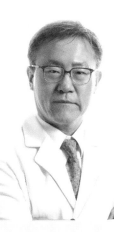

• 성형외과 전문의(Plastic Surgery Specialist)
• 가톨릭대학교 의과대학 의학박사(Doctor of Medicine, Catholic University School of Medicine)
• 대한미용성형외과학회 원로회원
(Senior Member, The Korean Society for Aesthetic Plastic Surgery)
• 전) 대한미용성형외과학회 회장
(Former President, The Korean Society for Aesthetic Plastic Surgery)

09

탈모, 피부 처짐…
100세 시대를 준비하는
'항노화 치료'

줄기세포를 이용한 대표적 항노화 수술

최근에 항노화(Anti-aging)라는 용어가 보편화되면서 성형외과 분야도 비약적인 발전을 거듭해 오고 있다. 그중 항노화 성형수술(Anti-aging plastic surgery)의 꽃은 누가 뭐라 해도 안면거상수술(Face-lifting)과 모발이식수술(Hair Transplatation)이라고 생각한다.

노화의 과정에서 나타나는 현상 중에 두드러지는 증상은 바로 주름살의 증가와 모발의 감소이다. 노화는 누구나 피해 갈 수 없는 삶의 여정인 동시에 누구에게나 찾아오는 손님과도 같다. '늙는다'는 것을 어차피 피해 갈 수 없다면 보다 건강하고 활력 있게 노후의 삶을 영위하는 것. 그것이 바로 이상적인 노년의 모습일 것이다.

실제로 환자와 상담을 나누다 보면 "안면거상술과 모발이식 수술은 언제쯤 받으면 좋을까요"라는 질문을 곧잘 받게 된다. 그때마다 "언제라고 단정할 수 없는 것이고, 환자 개인에 따라서, 또한 각자의 필요에 따라서, 결정되는 무한 시기의 선택만 있을 뿐이지만, 필자의 생각은 가급적 빨리하면 할수록 효과와 지속되는 시간은 좋다"라고 말한다. 100세 시대! 나이에 비하여 젊게 보이는 경우는 주름살 없는 얼굴과 풍성한 머리카락이기 때문이다.

복합 안면거상수술

나이가 들수록 근막층(SMAS)을 더 이 얇아지고 탄력도도 떨어진다. 이 경우 단순한 안면거상수술로는 한계가 있으며, 이때 줄기세포 시술을 복합적으로 적용하는 것이 가장 좋은 방법이라고 볼 수 있다.

나이가 들수록 근막층(SMAS)을 더 이 얇아지고 탄력도도 떨어진다. 이 경우 단순한 안면거상수술로는 한계가 있으며, 이때 줄기세포 시술을 복합적으로 적용하는 것이 가장 좋은 방법이라고 볼 수 있다.

안티에이징하면 성형 수술 또한 빼놓을 수 없다. 요즘 안티에이징 성형의 핵심은 예뻐 보이는 것이 아니라 한 듯 안 한 듯한 자연스러움이다. 이를 위해 글로벌 성형외과에서는 대표적인 항노화 수술인 안면거상 수술에 줄기세포 시술을 복합적으로 접목하고 있다.

안면거상 수술에 있어 줄기세포 시술을 복합적으로 적용하여 기대하는 효과는 다음과 같다.

①진피층의 콜라겐 조직 합성이 활발하게 되어 ②피부의 탄력과 두께가 젊었을 때처럼 회복되며 ③표피층의 재생 과정이 빨라져 피부의 톤이 맑아지고 ④피부표면 텍스처가 매끄럽게 되는 것은 물론 ⑤피부 전반적인 수분 함유량의 증가로 ⑥화장이 잘 받게 되는 부수적인 결과도 얻게 된다.

글로벌성형외과에서 안면거상 수술을 할 때 특별하게 강조하는 것은 두가지이다. 첫째는 흉터를 줄이기 위하고, 둘째는 흉터가 눈에 잘 띄지 않게 하는 것이다. 이

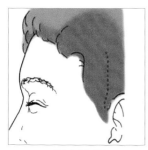

머리 속 절개선

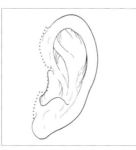

귀 앞 절개선

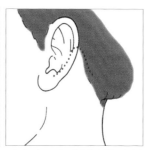

귀 뒤 및 목주름 개선을 위한 절개선

를 위해 피부 절개를 아래 그림과 같이 시행하여 흉터를 극소화하고 보이지 않도록 다양한 방법으로 연구하였다.

안면거상 수술 시 흉터를 방지하기 위한 방법 다음으로 주의해야 할 점은 합병증인 "칼귀"(Pixie ear/요정귀) 예방이다. 칼귀란 귓불의 형태가 둥그스름하지 않고 직선의 형태로 생긴 귀를 말하는데 2차, 3차 안면거상 환자들 중에 가장 흔히 볼 수 있다. 이러한 합병증을 예방하기 위해서는 안면거상수술(Face lift) 마지막 단계인 남는 피부와 연부조직 절제할 때 주의해야 한다.

실패 없는 안면거상 수술을 위해서는 가장 먼저 귓밥이 위치하는 곳에 표시를 하고, 귓밥을 중심으로 피부절제를 시작히여 머리쪽–귀앞–귀 뒤–목의 순서로 당기면서 마무리하는 것이 중요하다. 특히 귓밥은 얼굴의 다른 어느 부분보다도, 동양 철학의 관상학에서 '장수유복'의 상징으로 중요하게 생각하는 부위기에 그 모양에 각별히 신경을 쓰는 편이다.

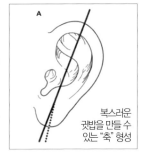

귀 뒤와 목이 만나는 선상에서 축을 만들어서 그림같이 당기면서 적당한 긴장을 이용하면 안면거상수술의 가장 흔하고 치명적 부작용이라고 필자가 생각하는 "칼귀(Pixie ear)"를 예방할 수 있음은 물론 필자가 원하고 환자들이 대부분 좋아하는 비교적 복스럽고 통통한 아름답고도 탐스러운 "귓불" 모양을 얻을 수 있다.

필자가 강조하는 방법은 복합적인 안면거상수술이다. 즉 주름의 정도에 따라 안면부 피부를 피하에서 분리하게 되는데, 위쪽으로는 눈꼬리 가까이 안와부와 광대뼈까지 박리하고, 아래쪽으로는 입 가장자리 가까이까지 박리하며, 목의 주름을 없애기 위해서는 턱 아래 부분까지 연장하기도 하여 기존의 방법보다 더욱 광범위하게 박리하게 된다(More wide dissection). 과거에는 여분의 피부만을 절제하였으나 최근에 필자는 피부와 근육 사이에 있는 얼굴 피부의 긴장을 유지하여 주는 일종의 근막성분(SMAS)도 같이 적절하게 피부와 동시에 당겨서 절제함으로써 수술 효과를 극대화 시킬 수 있고, 주름이 펴진 상태를 오랫동안 지속시킬 수 있다.

그리고 또한 뺨과 아래턱 부위에 지방이 고여, 중력에 의해 밑으로 처질 경우 더욱 나이 들어 보이는데, 이때는 최근 개발되어 각광받는 듀얼 모드(Dual Mode) 레이저(표 1, 2)를 이용한다. 즉 지방 분해 흡인술과 레이저 리프팅을 병행하여 지방을 제거하고 당김으로써 특히 뺨에서 턱을 지나 목으로 이어지는 선을 부드러우면서도 젊고 아름답게 할 수 있다.

표1 : The two wavelengths have different physical properties

1470nm/ 980nm dual wavelength
1470nm lipolysis – destruction or melting of fat tissue
980nm causes contraction of tissue through proper thermal injury
face lifting
correction of breast ptosis, buttock lifting, remediation of abdominal stretch marks

초음파 지방분해 흡인술을 병행하면서 특히 코 옆에서 입으로 이어지는 깊은 골이나 눈 아래에 깊이 주름이 나 있는 곳에는 자기 지방이식수술도 같이하여 보충하기도 한다. 또한 턱을 앞으로 나오게 하는 수술로서 턱에서 목으

표 2

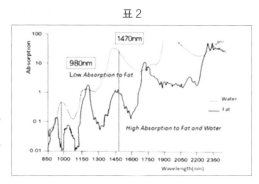

로 이어지는 선을 젊게 할 수 있다. 특히 목의 주름을 없애기 위해서는 목 부분의 박리를 세밀하고 철저하게 하여 목을 이루는 상층부의 근육을 절제함으로써 목이 갸름하게 만들어 한층 젊게 보일 수 있다.

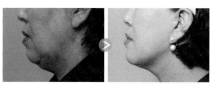

줄기세포 안면거상 수술전후

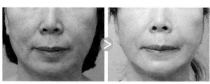

줄기세포 안면거상 수술전후

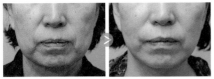
줄기세포 안면거상 수술전후

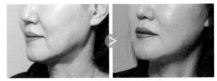
줄기세포 안면거상 수술전후

TIP_줄기세포 안면거상 수술 정보				
수술시간	마취방법	입원여부	회복기간	체류기간
4시간	수면마취	당일	2주	2주

┃ 모발이식수술

모발이식 후 줄기세포 치료를 병행할 경우 모낭의 생착률을 높여주고, 손상된 조직의 재생과 분화를 도와 모발이 빠르게 자라도록 도와준다.

줄기세포 치료는 말 그대로 신체에 존재하는 줄기세포를 이용하는 방법이다. 필자는 실제로 줄기세포 모발이식수술을 셀프(Self) 수술받은 대상 환자이기도 하다. 또한 끊임없이 줄기세포 시술로 수술 후 다양한 환자를 관리하고 있는 경험자로서 그 누구보다도 줄기세포를 이용한 모발이식수술에 대해 자신이 있다.

여성은 두말할 필요도 없고 남성들에게서 까지도 앞머리에 머리털이 없는 대머리 같은 경우에는 왠지 나이가 들어 보이고 겉늙어 보여 대인 관계나 사회생활까지 지장을 받는 경우가 흔하다. 이런 남성들은 외모뿐 아니라 사업상 보다 젊고 활기차게 보이려는 목적 때문에 성형외과를 찾는 경우가 급증하는 추세다.

특히 최근 들어서는 스트레스에 시달리는 젊은 미혼의 남녀가 빠지는 모발 때문에, 관리나 모발이식을 위하여 글로벌성형외과를 찾는 경우가 늘고 있다. 이런 남성 여성들의 고민은 "모발(모낭)이식수술"로 해결할 수 있다. 모발이식수술은 머리 뒷쪽에서 모낭을 얻어다가 환자와 수술 전에 상담하여 원하는 부위에 필요한 만큼 마치 모내기를 하듯이 모낭을 하나하나 심어 주는 방법이다.

이 수술에서 환자가 숙지해야 할 것은 일단 처음 심은 모낭에 붙어 있는 털은 8~12주에 걸쳐서 떨어져 나간 다음에, 새로 생착된 모낭으로부터 다시 털이 난다는 것과, 처음에는 굵기나 크기, 모양, 촉감 등에서 원래의 음모와는 다르고 머리털에 가까우나, 6개월~1년 정도 지나면 그 성향이 점점 원래의 머리카락에서 음모 쪽을 닮아 간다는 사실이다. 모발이식수술에 있어서 가장 중요한 것은 생착률을 높이는 것이다. 심은 모발이 강하게 뿌리 내리기 위한 방편으로 줄기세포시술을 모발이식수술과 함께하여 획기적인 효과를 거두고 있다.

줄기세포시술 방법

줄기세포시술 방법은 모낭이식수술 하는 부위에, 즉 모판의 상태를 좋게 하기 위하여 총 3회에 걸쳐서 시술하는데, 그 시기는 다음과 같다.

- 1차 : 모발이식수술 1주일 전에
- 2차 : 이식한 모발이 빠지기 시작하는 모발이식수술 8주 후에
- 3차 : 이식한 모발이 거의 빠지면서 이식한 모낭에서 생착한 새로운 모발이 나기 시작하는 모발이식수술 12주 후 진행

이렇게 총 3번에 걸쳐서 모낭이 위치하는 진피하부(subdermal area)에, 줄기세포를 주사, 시술하여 드라마틱한 결과를 낳고 있다. 특히 과거 1차 혹은 2차, 3차 모발이식수술 후에 기대치에 못 미치거나 실패한 경우, 별 뾰족한 대안이 없었으나 줄기세포시술 + 모발이식수술의 복합적인 방법이 중년 및 노년 대머리로 고민 중인 남성들의 희망이 되고 있는 것이다.

특히 기업체 대표, 의사나 변호사 같은 전문직 등 많은 고객을 만나면서 젊게 보여야 할 필요성이 있는 사람들에게는 획기적인 소식이 아닐 수 없다. 모발이식 수술의 성공률은 의사의 술기, 환자의 상태 등에 따라 큰 차이가 있으므로, 수술 전

에는 궁금한 점이나 의심나는 부분, 걱정스러운 사항에 대해 임상 경험이 풍부한 전문의와 충분히 상담 후 결정하는 것이 좋다.

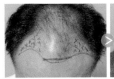 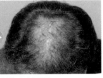

줄기세포모발이식 수술전후

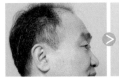

줄기세포모발이식 수술전후

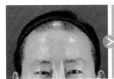 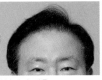

줄기세포모발이식 수술전후

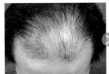 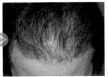

줄기세포모발이식 수술전후

TIP_줄기세포 모발이식 수술정보

수술시간	마취방법	입원여부	회복기간	체류기간
4시간	수면마취	당일	2주	2주

항노화의 미래 – 줄기세포

줄기세포 치료는 항노화 수술의 모든 영역에서 다양하게 함께 치료 적용될 수 있다. 이미 남여성의 다양한 원인을 가진 탈모에 적용하여 좋은 치료 결과를 보이고 있으며 얼굴 피부 진피층에도 줄기세포 치료를 적용, 주름제거나 리프팅 치료에 효과를 보이고 있다.

줄기세포 치료 효과는 약물이나 독소, 화장품, 호르몬 등과는 달리 단 한 번의 치료만으로도 상당 기간 그 효과를 유지할 수 있다. 또한 조화로운 피부 기능의 회복으로 과거 많이 사용했던 성장 호르몬 치료처럼, 특정 기능만의 상승으로 인해 생기는 여드름과 같은 피부 질환이 발생되는 부작용을 최대한 피할 수도 있다.

줄기세포는 사람의 피부를 포함, 모든 장기와 조직에는 정상적으로 존재하며 이들의 기능은 조직과 장기의 기능 유지, 활성화, 수명 결정 등의 핵심적인 기능을 수행한다. 그런데 나이가 들어감에 따라 줄기세포의 자가 복제 능력이 서서히 떨어지고 기능이 약화되면서 각 조직과 장기의 전반적인 기능이 떨어지게 되고 노화를 거쳐 결국에는 그 수명을 다하게 된다. 따라서 젊은 줄기세포를 질병의 치료나 항노화에 적용하면, 이상적일 것이라는 이론적 배경이 이미 오래전부터 의학계에서 대두되어 왔다.

성형외과 지방흡입수술에서 얻을 수 있는 정상 성체지방세포에서 줄기세포를 얻는 방법은 줄기세포가 이미 어느 장기나 조직으로 분화가 끝난 상태이므로 안전성을 담보할 수 있고 윤리적으로 정당하다. 하지만 여러 질환의 치료는 불가능하며 필자의 병원에서는 미용 목적에 한정하여 항노화 성형수술 전 분야에 광범위하게 적용 및 시도하여 획기적인 결과를 얻고 있다.

마지막으로 줄기세포 중 정상 아기 분만 시 제대혈에서 분리되는 줄기세포가 있는데, 정상적인 발생이 끝난 안정적인 분화 능력을 가져 안전하게 여러 질환에 자유롭게 쓸 수 있다. 때문에 선진국을 비롯해 여러 나라에서 제대혈에서 줄기세포를 분리하고 배양하는 기술 분야에 치열한 경쟁을 하고 있는 상태이다. 이미 필자 병원에서 시도 중인 줄기세포를 이용한 성형외과적 진료는 탈모를 비롯 얼굴 피부 항노화, 주름제거, 리프팅 등 다양한 분야에 걸쳐 치료에 적용될 전망으로 건강한 100세 시대의 희망이 될 수 있다.

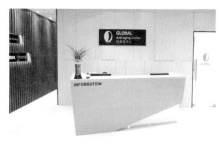
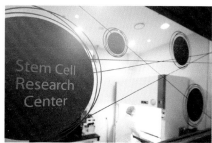

09

Hair loss, sagging skin... "Anti-aging treatments" to prepare for the era of centenarians

Recent Updating Anti-Aging Procedures Utilizing Stem Cells

As the term 'anti-aging' has become commonplace, our field of plastic surgery has also advanced significantly. In my opinion, the crowning glories of anti-aging plastic surgery are, indisputably, face-lifting and hair transplantation.

Prominent signs of the aging process are the increase of wrinkles and the thinning and removal of hair. Aging is an unavoidable journey of life and an uninvited guest that visits everyone. If aging is an inevitable journey, the goal is to lead a life in our later years that is healthier and more vibrant. That would indeed be the ideal vision of our golden years.

Hence, during consultations at my Global Plastic Group, the most frequent question I encounter is about the timing for face-lifting and hair transplantation combined with stem cell therapy. The answer is not definitive; it is infinitely variable, depending on the individual's circumstances and needs. However, my stance is that the sooner these procedures are performed, the better the outcome and longevity of their effects. Looking younger than one's age often involves having a wrinkle-free face and a full head of hair.

Stem Cell-Integrated Complex Face-Lifting

As we age, the submuscular aponeurotic system (SMAS) becomes thinner and loses elasticity. In such cases, simple facelift surgery may have its limitations, and the best approach is considered to be a combination of stem cell procedures.

As we age, the submuscular aponeurotic system (SMAS) becomes thinner and loses elasticity. In such cases, simple facelift surgery may have its limitations, and the best approach is considered to be a combination of stem cell procedures.

Indeed, when it comes to anti-aging, plastic surgery plays a significant role. Nowadays, the key focus of anti-aging plastic surgery is not just about looking beautiful, but also achieving a natural and subtle appearance. To achieve this, leading global plastic surgery practices are combining stem cell procedures with prominent anti-aging surgeries like facelifts.

The effects I expect from combining stem cell treatments with face-lifting include:

1) Active synthesis of collagen tissue in the dermis,

2) Restoration of the skin's elasticity and thickness to its youthful state,

3) Acceleration of the epidermal regeneration process, brightening skin tone,

4) Smoothing of the skin texture on the surface,

5) An overall increase in the skin's moisture content, resulting in

6) Makeup that looks more flattering and lasts longer.

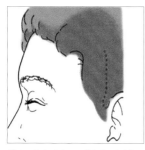 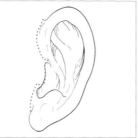 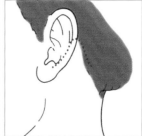

Figure 1. Incisions within the hairline   Figure 2. Incisions in front of the ears   Figure 3. Incisions behind the ears and along the necklines for neck wrinkle improvement

When performing facial rejuvenation surgery at global plastic surgery, two specific aspects are emphasized. The first is minimizing scars, and the second is ensuring that scars are not prominently visible. Extensive research has been conducted to achieve this by employing various techniques of skin incision, as shown in the diagram below, to minimize and conceal scars effectively.

To prevent scarring following face-lifting surgery, as illustrated in the figure above, careful attention must be paid during the final stage of a face-lift, specifically when excising excess skin and soft tissue, to avoid the common complication known as the "Pixie ear."

First, mark the location of the earlobe and begin the excision of skin centered around this point, proceeding in the order of head – front of the ear – behind the ear – neck while pulling to complete the process.

I mainly focus on preserving the shape of the "earlobe," which is considered a symbol of longevity and good fortune in Eastern physiognomy. By creating an axis at the point where the neck meets behind the ear and pulling along this line with appropriate tension, it is possible not only to prevent what I believe to be the most common and critical side effect of face-lifting, the "Pixie ear," but also to achieve the fuller, more youthful, and desirable "earlobe" shape that I and most patients prefer.

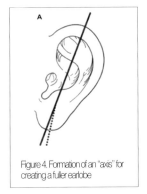

Figure 4. Formation of an "axis" for creating a fuller earlobe

The method I emphasize is a comprehensive face-lifting procedure. Depending on the extent of the wrinkles, the facial skin is detached from the underlying layers, with dissection extending near the corner of the eye to the orbital and zygomatic bone above and to near the corner of the mouth below, as well as under the chin to address neck wrinkles, involving a more wide dissection than traditional methods.

Previously, only excess skin was removed, but I now also appropriately excise a fascial component (SMAS) that maintains the tension of facial skin, thereby maximizing the surgical effect and maintaining a smooth appearance for a longer duration.

Additionally, if fat accumulates in the cheek and jaw areas, causing sagging due to gravity and an aged appearance, I employ the recently developed and popular Dual Mode laser (Table 1, 2) to perform lipolysis and laser lifting simultaneously, smoothing and rejuvenating the line that extends from the cheek to the neck.

Table 1: The two wavelengths have different physical properties.

1470nm/ 980nm dual wavelength
1470nm lipolysis – destruction or melting of fat tissue
980nm causes contraction of tissue through proper thermal injury
face lifting
correction of breast ptosis, buttock lifting, remediation of abdominal stretch marks

In conjunction with ultrasonic liposuction, autologous fat grafting with stem cell are also performed to fill deep furrows from the side of the nose to the mouth and under the eyes where deep wrinkles are present.

Table 2

Surgery that brings the chin forward can also rejuvenate the line from the chin to the neck. In particular, to eliminate neck wrinkles, a detailed and thorough dissection of the neck area is performed, excising the upper muscles of the neck, resulting in a more youthful appearance with a slender neck.

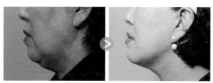

Stem Cell Facelift Before and After Photos

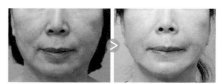

Stem Cell Facelift Before and After Photos

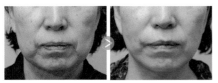

Stem Cell Facelift Before and After Photos

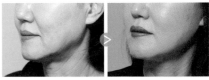

Stem Cell Facelift Before and After Photos

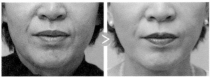
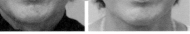

Stem Cell Facelift Before and After Photos

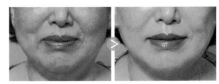

Stem Cell Facelift Before and After Photos

TIP_Stem Cell Facelift Procedure Information				
Surgery Duration	Anesthesia method	Hospital Stay	Recovery Period	Stay Duration
3-4 hours	IV sleeping Anesthesia – No pain	1 day	2 weeks	2 weeks

Stem Cell Treatment combined Hair Transplantation

When stem cell therapy is performed concurrently with hair transplantation, it can help increase the survival rate of hair follicles and facilitate the regeneration and differentiation of damaged tissues, ultimately promoting faster hair growth.

Stem cell therapy, literally, is a method that utilizes stem cells present in the body for treatment. As someone who has personally undergone stem cell-based hair transplantation and continuously manages the results through stem cell treatments, I confidently recommend and write from firsthand experience.

Notably, scalp hair has significant aesthetic and even fashion implications for both men and women. The absence of frontal hair or a balding head can age a person, impede social interactions, and affect professional life. This perception drives more men to seek cosmetic solutions, aiming for a youthful and vigorous appearance in their careers.

Lately, stress-burdened young unmarried men and women are visiting our Global Plastic Surgery for hair care and transplantation due to hair loss. Both men's and women's worries can be addressed with "follicular (follicle) unit transplantation." This surgery involves harvesting hair follicles from the back of the head and implanting them individually in the desired areas, like planting seeds.

Patients should understand that the hair initially attached to the transplanted follicles will fall out over 8 to 12 weeks, after which new hair will grow from the transplanted follicles. Initially, this hair may differ in thickness, size, shape, and texture from the original pubic hair, resembling scalp hair more closely.

Still, it will gradually adopt characteristics similar to the original hair after six months to a year. The most important aspect of hair transplantation surgery is to increase the graft survival rate. Stem cell therapy, combined with hair transplantation surgery, is being used as a means to promote strong hair root growth and has shown remarkable results.

The method of stem cell therapy

The method of stem cell therapy involves a total of three procedures performed on the area where hair follicle transplantation is done, in order to improve the condition of the scalp. The timing of these procedures is as follows:

- 1st - one week before the hair transplantation,
- 2nd - eight weeks after the hair transplantation, as the transplanted hair begins to shed,
- 3rd - approximately 12 weeks post hair transplantation surgery, when the transplanted hair has mostly shed, and new growth begins from the transplanted follicles, stem cell injections are performed into the subdermal area where the follicles are situated.

This has been done over three treatments to achieve groundbreaking surgical outcomes and effectiveness. Particularly for patients who have undergone primary, secondary, or tertiary hair transplantation without meeting expectations or those who have faced failure, and for those who have repeatedly undergone hair transplantation without alternative solutions, this combination of stem cell treatment and hair transplantation is becoming a beacon of hope for middle-aged and elderly male patients with baldness.

Specifically, corporate executives, doctors, lawyers, and other professionals who must maintain a youthful appearance while consulting with a clientele find this revolutionary news an excellent option. Since the success rate of hair transplantation surgery varies significantly depending on the surgeon's skill and the patient's condition, it is imperative to discuss any questions, doubts, or concerns with an experienced specialist before making a decision.

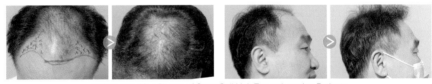

Before and After Photos of Stem Cell Hair Transplantation Patients

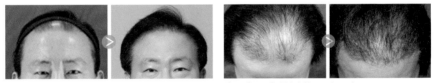

Before and After Photos of the Author's Own Stem Cell Hair Transplantation

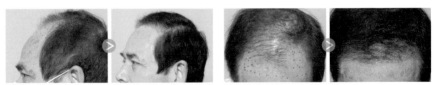

Before and After Photos of the Author's Own Stem Cell Hair Transplantation

TIP_Stem Cell Hair Transplantation Procedure Information				
Surgery Duration	Anesthesia method	Hospital Stay	Recovery Period	Stay Duration
4 hours	IV sleeping Anesthesia – No pain	Same Day	2 weeks	2 weeks

The Future of Anti-Aging – Stem Cells

Stem cell therapy, now being applied across all field of anti-aging surgery, has shown promising treatment outcomes for hair loss in both men and women of various causes and is advancing further. Applying stem cell treatments to the dermal layer of the skin has been successful in anti-aging efforts and wrinkle removal, as well as in achieving comprehensive facial lifting effects.

Stem cell therapy, unlike drugs, toxins, cosmetics, and hormones, can sustain its effects for a considerable period after just one treatment. It facilitates the restoration of harmonious skin functions, avoiding side effects such as acne, which can occur with the singular enhancement of certain functions, as was the case with widely used growth hormone treatments in the past.

Generally, stem cells are present in all organs and tissues, including the skin, where they play a vital role in maintaining and activating tissue and organ functions, as well as determining their lifespan. However, as we age, stem cells gradually lose their self-replication ability and become less functional, leading to the overall decline in organ and tissue function, aging, and eventually death. Hence, applying youthful stem cells in disease treatment and anti-aging has been a longstanding theoretical premise in the medical community.

In plastic surgery, a method of deriving stem cells from the average adult fat cells obtained during commonly performed liposuction procedures guarantees safety, as these stem cells have already differentiated into specific organs or tissues, thus being ethically justifiable.

However, this method is not feasible for treating various diseases. Therefore, in my

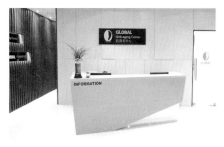 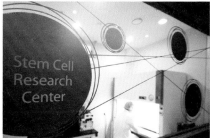

clinic, we apply this technique extensively and exclusively for cosmetic purposes across all fields of anti-aging plastic surgery, achieving groundbreaking results.

Lastly, stem cells from umbilical cord blood, obtained during normal childbirth, possess stable differentiation capabilities following normal development, allowing their safe use in various diseases.

This has led to intense competition in the technology of isolating and culturing stem cells from umbilical cord blood in advanced countries and worldwide. The use of stem cell therapy in cosmetic surgery, which is already being performed at our hospital, has the potential to be applied in various fields such as hair loss treatment, facial skin anti-aging, wrinkle removal, and lifting. It can become a beacon of hope in the era of healthy longevity, where people can live up to 100 years.

오타모반(Ota Nevus)
이소성 몽고반 & 이토모반(Ectopic Mongolian Spot & Ito Nevus)
흑자증(Lentigo)

피부색소 질환 치료는 정확한 진단이 첫걸음

피부에 생긴 오타모반 더 이상 콤플렉스가 아니다!

The first step in treating skin pigmentation disease is to have accurate diagnosis Ota nevus on the skin is no longer a complex!

화장으로도 가려지지 않는 오타모반과 색소 치료를 전문적으로 진료해오고 있다. 30년 넘게 쌓아온 전문성과 풍부한 경험, 노하우를 바탕으로 평생을 고통받아 온 환자들에게 희망이 되어주고 있다.

We specialize in treating nevus of Ota and pigmentation that cannot be hidden by makeup. Based on expertise, abundant experience, and know-how accumulated over 30 years, we are providing hope to patients who have suffered their entire lives.

라움성형외과
Raum Plastic Surgery

www.raumps.com

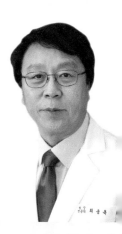

최응옥(Eung-Ok Choi)

• 성형외과 전문의(A specialist in plastic surgery)
• 고려대 의과대학원 의학박사(Doctor of Medicine at Korea University Graduate School of Medicine)
• 대한미용성형외과학회 정회원(A member of the Korean Society of Aesthetic Plastic Surgeons)
• 대한성형외과의사회 레이저성형연구회 회장 역임
(Former President of Laser Plastic Surgeons Research Society of Korean Plastic Surgeons
• 고려대/한양대 의과대학 외래교수
(An adjunct professor at Korea University/Hanyang University School of Medicine)

10

몸에 난 푸른 색 반점, 정확한 진단과 치료로 맑고 깨끗한 얼굴 만들기

난치성 피부 색소질환, 정확한 진단이 중요한 이유

얼굴에 생긴 크고 작은 피부질환은 생명에 큰 위협이 되지는 않지만 심한 스트레스를 가져와 자신감을 떨어뜨리고 심리적으로 위축되게 만든다. 특히 '오타모반'과 같은 피부 색소질환은 종류가 다양하고 구별이 쉽지 않아 치료시기를 놓치고, 잘못된 치료가 적용되는 일이 잦은 편이다.

선천성 피부질환 중 하나인 오타모반은 출생 시 진피층에 남아있던 멜라닌 세포가 시간이 지난 후에도 사라지지 않고 세포에서 멜라닌 색소를 분비해서 푸른색을 띄는 것을 말한다. 일반적으로 잘 알려진 몽고반점과 달리 시간이 지날수록 색이 짙어지고 부위가 점점 넓어진다는 특징을 가진다. 이마나 관자놀이, 눈꺼풀 위 아래, 볼 등 얼굴 위쪽 부위에 주로 발생하는 오타모반은 출생과 동시에 증상이 보이는 경우가 50%, 사춘기 전까지 발생하는 경우가 50% 정도다. 증상이 심하게 번지면 귀나 귀 뒤, 안구 흰자까지 퍼지게 된다.

오타모반은 서양인보다 동양인에게서 더 많이 나타나고 남성보다는 여성 환자 비율이 더 높은 편이다. 우리나라 국민은 1만 명당 약 3명 정도에게 발병한다는 통계 결과가 있어 희귀한 질환은 아닌 편이다. 하지만 오타모반은 색소가 분포한 위치에 따라 치료가 달리 적용될 수 있어 성공적인 치료 결과를 원한다면 무엇보다 정확한 진단이 우선 되어야 한다. 흑자와 양측성후천성오타양모반 등의 질환 역시 구분이 어려운 편으로 정확한 진단이 이뤄지지 않을 경우, 엉뚱한 곳에 엉뚱한 치료만 하는 불상사가 일어날 수 있다는 점을 염두에 둬야 한다. 그러므로 정확한 진단하에 맞춤형 치료가 가능한 의료기관, 피부 타입에 따라 신속하고 유연하게 대처할 수 있는 경력과 노하우를 가진 의료진을 선택하는 것이 중요하다.

오타모반

오타모반이란 눈 주위에 푸른색이 보이거나 검은색을 띠는 넓은 반점을 말한다. 주로 눈 주위, 관자놀이 이마, 광대뼈 부위, 콧등 등에 흔히 나타나며 자연 소실 되지 않는다.

선천성 오타모반

모든 오타모반은 선천성이다. 다만 그 발생 시기가 태아 때 발생하여 출생 시 보이는 경우도 있고, 출생 시에는 없다가도 생후 1달 이상이 지나면서 멍이 든 것처럼 나타나서 점차로 크게 번지는 경우가 45% 정도이고, 55%는 소아 때는 전혀 없다가 사춘기 때 나타날 수 있다. 이 경우도 발현 시기가 늦어진 것일 뿐 선천성으로 보아야 한다. 치료 후 보습과 선크림 바르기 등 사후관리를 철저히 해야 한다.

발생원인

현재까지 원인 규명이 명확히 이루어지지는 않았으나 널리 인정되고 있는 가설로는 아래와 같다.

- 태생기 멜라닌 세포는 태아 발생 8주까지 신경능선(neural crest)으로부터 표피에 도달한다.
- 멜라닌 세포는 발생 3~4개월경에 발견이 되고 발생 4~5개월이 되면서 가지돌기가 생기며 멜라닌 소체를 합성하여 주위 각질 형성 세포로 이동하게 된다. 정상 피부에는 출생 시 멜라닌 세포가 두피, 손등, 천골 부위의 진피에 존재할 수 있는데, 이들은 큰 아메바모양 세포로, 출생 후 곧 사라지나 일부에서는 소실되지 않고 진피 멜라닌 세포 병변을 초래한다. 이러한 원인으로 나타나는 진피 멜라닌 세포 병변으로 오타모반, 이토모반, 이소성 몽고반 및 몽고반을 들 수 있다.
- 일본, 한국 등 동양인에 많이 발생하고 백인종과 흑인종에는 드물다.
- 남 : 여 = 1 : 5의 비율로 여성에게서 많이 나타나는 통계를 보이나, 본원의 통계 조사 결과 한국인에서는 남 : 여 = 1 : 3의 비율로 나타남을 보이고 있다.
- 한국에서는 인구 10,000명당 3명의 발생 빈도를 보이고 있다.

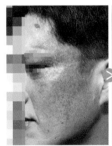
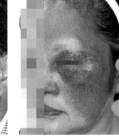
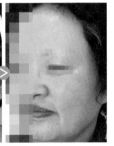

선천성 오타모반 치료전후   선천성 오타모반 치료전후

TIP_선천성 오타모반 치료정보

치료가능시기	치료시간	마취방법	입원여부	치료간격	치료횟수
생후12개월 이후	30분~1시간	수면, 연고, 국소마취	입원없음	1~2개월	4~8회

소아 오타모반

선천성으로 소아에게서 나타나는 오타모반을 말하며, 출생 시에는 대부분 작은 부위에 마치 멍이 든 것처럼 보이다가 점차 번지면서 색깔이 진해지는 양상을 띤다.

영유아기에 번지는 경우 대개 출생 후 1년 정도 내에 많이 번지게 된다. 소아 오타모반의 경우 성인에 비해 치료 효과가 훨씬 빠르고, 아무리 심한 소아 오타모반일지라도 치료를 잘 받으면 완치가 된다. 부모님의 인내심과 노력이 필요하며, 유능

하고 경험 많은 의사의 치료법에 따라 결과에 많은 차이가 있다

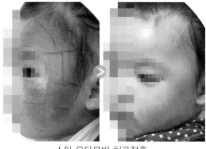
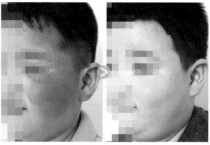

소아 오타모반 치료전후   소아 오타모반 치료전후

TIP_소아 오타모반 치료정보					
치료가능시기	치료시간	마취방법	입원여부	치료간격	치료횟수
생후12개월 이후	30분~40분	수면. 연고. 국소마취	입원없음	6주	4~7회

후천성 오타양모반

10대 후반부터 20대 초반에 걸쳐, 오타양모반이 얼굴 대칭적으로 나타나는 모반이다. 양쪽 광대뼈 부위에 둥글게 나타나며, 관자놀이, 이마, 콧등, 콧볼 등에 대칭으로 발생한다. 색깔은 갈색으로 보이고 시간이 지나면서 점차 진해진다.

흔히 '기미'로 착각하고 치료를 하지만, 이런 치료법으로는 완치가 안된다. 어머니가 후천성 오타양모반이 있는 경우, 딸에게서도 나타나는 경우가 흔하다.

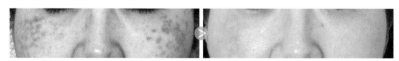

후천성 오타양모반 치료전후

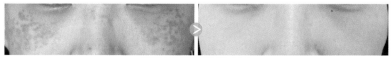

후천성 오타양모반 치료전후

치료가능시기	치료시간	마취방법	입원여부	치료간격	치료횟수
증상발현시기부터	10분	연고, 국소마취	입원없음	4~8주	3~5회

TIP_후천성 오타양모반 치료정보

치료가능시기	치료시간	마취방법	입원여부	치료간격	치료횟수
증상발현시기부터	10분	연고, 국소마취	입원없음	4~8주	3~5회

│ 이소성 몽고반 & 이토모반

이소성 몽고반점은 손목이나 발목 등 다른 부위에 나타나는 몽고반점을 말한다. 이토모반의 경우 계속 진행하여 더 진해지므로 적극적인 치료가 필요하다.

아시아계 민족에게 매우 빈도가 높게 발생하는 모반으로 출생 시 아기의 엉덩이 부위에 파란색의 반점을 몽고반이라 한다. 엉덩이 이외의 부위에도 몽고반이 생기는 경우가 있는데 이를 이소성 몽고반이라 한다.

몽고반이나 이소성 몽고반은 만 3~4세 경이 지나면 대부분 자연 소실되는 경우가 많지만, 이소성 몽고반의 쇠퇴율이 몽고반보다는 적은 비율로 소퇴된다.

이토모반이란 어깨, 목, 쇄골상부, 상지에 청색반으로 나타나는 모반으로 오타모반보다 더 광범위하게 나타나며 조직학적으로 차이는 없다. 이토모반은 몽고반과는 달리 자연 소실 되지 않기 때문에 치료가 필요하다.

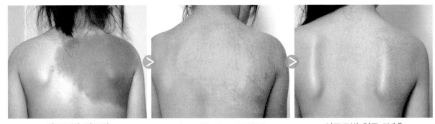

이토모반 치료전   이토모반 치료 16개월후   이토모반 치료 5년후

TIP_이소성 몽고반 & 이토모반 치료정보

치료가능시기	치료시간	마취방법	입원여부	치료간격	치료횟수
생후12개월 이후	30분~40분	수면, 국소마취	입원없음	6주	4~6회

흑자증

햇빛의 자외선 노출과 피부노화 등으로 나타나는 짙은 갈색 점(얼룩)이다. 멜라닌의 침착증가에 의해 생기며, 표피 피부접합부에 멜라닌 함유세포가 증가하여 발생된다. 흑자증에는 군집성 흑자증, 일광성 흑자증, 단순 흑자증으로 나뉜다.

군집성 흑자

피부 상피층에 멜라닌 색소의 증식으로 나타나는 모반이다. 후천적으로 발생되며 얼굴의 어느 부위든 나타난다. 흑자가 집단으로 군집을 이루어 나타나는 것과 모반이 번지는 특징이 있다. 치료하면 일시적으로 없어진 것처럼 보이지만, 시간이 지나면 다시 일부분 재발된다. 치료에 대한 반응은 개인차가 있다.

※ 치료법 : 4주 간격 2~3회 치료에 깨끗하게 된다.

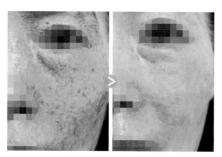

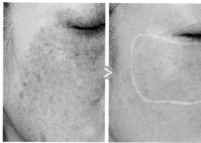

군집성 흑자 치료 전후   군집성 흑자 치료 전후

일광성 흑자

자외선에 노출된 피부에 흔히 발생하며 표피성 색소 질환이다. 얼굴에 광범위한 범위에 경계가 둥글게 나타난다. 검버섯과 비슷해 보이지만, 검버섯과 달리 표면이 매끄러워 보인다. 얼굴, 목 등 몸 전체에 나타날 수 있다.

치료하면 깨끗해지지만, 3~5년이 지나면 다시 일부분 재발된다. 치료에 대한 반응은 개인차가 있다.

※ 치료법: 1회 치료에 80% 정도 치료되고, 4주 후 2회 차 치료에 깨끗하게 된다.

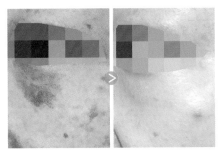
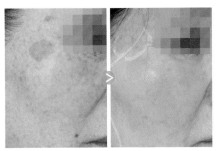

일광성 흑자 치료 전후   일광성 흑자 치료 전후

난순 흑자

자외선에 노출된 피부에 흔히 발생하며 표피성 색소 질환이다. 얼굴에 광범위한 범위에 경계가 둥글게 나타난다. 검버섯과 비슷해 보이지만, 검버섯과 달리 표면이 매끄러워 보인다. 얼굴, 목 등 몸 전체에 나타날 수 있다.

치료하면 깨끗해지지만, 3~5년이 지나면 다시 일부분 재발된다. 치료에 대한 반응은 개인차가 있다.

• 치료법: 1회 치료에 80% 정도 치료되고, 4주 후 2회 차 치료에 깨끗하게 된다.

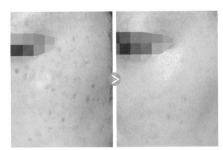
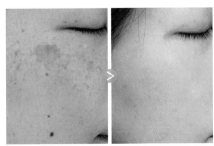

단순 흑자 치료 전후   단순 흑자 치료 전후

TIP_흑자증 치료정보

치료가능시기	치료시간	마취방법	입원여부	치료간격	치료횟수
증상발현시기부터	10분	수면, 연고, 국소마취	입원없음	4~8주	2~3회

흑자증 치료 후 주의사항

• 스크럽, 각질제거, 때밀이 타월은 시술 부위 주변에 절대 사용하면 안 된다.
• 사우나는 2주 지나서 갈 수 있지만, 치료 기간 동안은 자제하는 것이 좋다.
• 스키장, 해수욕장은 피해야 한다.
• 실내, 실외 수영장(소독약 성분)은 가급적 이용을 피하는 것이 좋다.
• 치료 후 7일 지난 후부터 자외선 차단 철저히 한다.

진단이 중요, 정확한 진단에 따른 치료 필요

얼굴에 생기는 점은 검은점, 빨간점, 흰점, 푸른점, 흑자, 기미, 주근깨, 잡티 등 색과 모양과 형태가 다양하다. 빨간점은 혈관종이라 하며 출생 때부터 또는 후천적으로 혈관이 많이 늘어나서 얼굴 등에 붉은색 또는 자주색으로 피부가 울퉁불퉁하게 또는 평평하게 변하는 것을 말한다. 흰점은 탈색모반이라 하여 선천적으로 생기는 것과 백납(백반증)이라고 하는 후천적으로 생기는 것이 있다.

푸른점의 경우, 점이 생기는 위치가 피부의 깊은 부위이므로 색깔이 푸른색으로 변하는 것이다. 청색모반은 검은 점과 비슷하지만 약간 더 크고 푸른색을 가지는 점이 특징이다. 푸른점의 또 다른 점인 오타모반은 얼굴의 한쪽 면에 생기는 선척적인 점과 후천적으로 얼굴 양쪽에 기미처럼 점이 생기는 후천성 오타모반이 있다.

점의 치료 방법은 각각의 점의 종류에 따라 제거하는 방법이 다양하다. 점이 아주 큰 경우에는 피부를 절제해 내는 수술법이 이용된다. 작은 경우는 전기소작술, 화학박피술, 레이저 등의 방법이 있다. 점을 뺀 후에 흉터가 남지 않는 것이 레이저이므로 많은 경우 레이저를 이용하여 점을 제거한다.

검은점 이외의 점들은 대개의 경우 레이저 치료를 한다. 라움성형외과에서는 흑자증, 오타모반, 이토모반 등 갈색(흑갈색)점과 푸른색 점은 루비레이저로 치료한다.

10 Blue spots on the body, Create a clean face through accurate diagnosis and treatment

Intractable skin pigmentation disease
Important reason for accurate diagnosis

Skin diseases large or small that appear on the face do not pose a major threat to life, but they cause severe stress, lowering self-confidence and causing psychological weakness. In particular, there are various types of skin pigmentation diseases such as 'Ota's nevus' and it is not easy to distinguish them, so treatment timing is often missed and the wrong treatment is often applied.

Nevus of Ota, one of the congenital skin diseases, is a condition in which melanin cells remaining in the dermal layer at birth do not disappear over time and secrete melanin pigment, giving the baby a blue color. Unlike the well-known Mongolian spot, it has the characteristic that the color becomes darker and the area becomes wider over time. Ota's nevus, which mainly occurs on the upper part of the face, such as the forehead, temples, upper and lower eyelids, and cheeks, shows symptoms at birth in 50% of cases and occurs before puberty in about 50% of cases. If the symptoms become severe, they may spread to the ears, behind the ears, or to the whites of the eyes.

Nevus of Ota appears more often in Asians than in Westerners, and the proportion of female patients is higher than that of male patients. Statistics show that it affects about 3 out of 10,000 Koreans, so it is not a rare disease. However, Ota's nevus may be treated differently depending on where the pigment is distributed, so if you want a successful treatment result, an accurate diagnosis must come first. Diseases such as lentigo and bilateral acquired nevi of Ota are also difficult to distinguish, so it is important to keep in mind that if an accurate diagnosis is not made, an unfortunate event may occur where the wrong treatment is given in the wrong place. Therefore, it is important to select a medical institution that can provide customized treatment under accurate diagnosis and a medical staff with the experience and know-how to respond quickly and flexibly according to skin type.

| Ota Nevus

Ota nevus refers to a wide spot with bluish or black color around the eyes. It usually appears around the eyes, the temples, the forehead, the cheekbone area, and the bridge of the nose, and does not disappear naturally.

Congenital Ota Nevus

Every Ota nevus is innate. However, there are cases where the occurrence period occurs during the fetus and is visible at birth. Even if they are not at birth, about 45% of them appear bruised after more than a month of birth, and they gradually spread significantly, and 55% can appear during puberty without any childhood at all. In this case, it should also be viewed as congenital, only that the onset period has been delayed. After treatment, follow-up care such as moisturizing and applying sunscreen should be thoroughly proceeded.

Causes of Occurrence

Although the cause has not been clearly identified so far, the widely accepted hypotheses are as follows:

- Genital melanocytes reach the epidermis from the neural crest up to eight weeks of fetal development.

- Melanocytes are discovered around 3-4 months after their occurrence, and branch bumps are formed at 4-5 months after their occurrence, and melanosomes are synthesized and moved to surrounding keratinocytes. In normal skin, melanocytes may be present in the dermis of the scalp, back of the hand, and sacral dermis at birth, which are large amoeba-shaped cells that disappear soon after birth, but in some cases do not disappear, resulting in dermal melanocyte lesions. Ota nevus, Ito nevus, Ectopic Mongolian spot, and Mongolian spot are examples of dermal melanocyte lesions that appear as such causes.

- It occurs a lot in Asians such as Japan and Korea, and is rare in Caucasian and African-American.

- Male:Female=1:5 ratio shows statistics that are common in women, but as a result of our statistical survey, Male:Female=1:3 ratio is shown in Koreans.

- In Korea, the frequency of occurrence is 3 per 10,000 people.

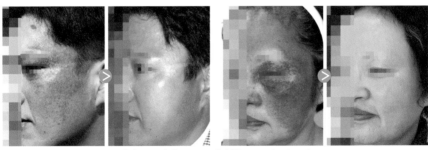

Before and after congenital Ota nevus treatment

TIP_Information on the treatment of congenital Ota nevus					
Possible time for treatment	Treatment duration	Anesthetic method	Hospitalization status	Treatment interval	Number of treatments
After 12 months of age	30 minutes~ 1 hour	Topical ointment, local infiltration anesthesia	n/a	1~2 months	4~8 times

Ota Nevus in Children

It refers to Ota nevus, which occurs congenital in children due to birth, and at birth, most of the small areas look as if they are bruised, and then gradually spread and the color becomes darker.

When it spreads in infancy, it usually spreads a lot within one year or so of birth. In the case of Ota nevus in children, the treatment effect is much faster than that of adults, and no matter how severe it is, they can be cured if the treatment is proceeded well. It requires patience and effort from parents, and the outcomes will be different a lot depending on the treatment of competent and experienced doctors.

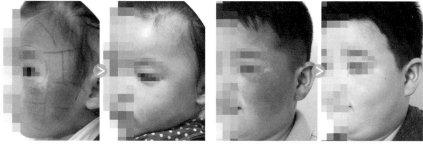

Before and after Ota nevus in children treatment

TIP_Informations on the treatment of Ota Nevus in children					
Possible time for treatment	Treatment duration	Anesthetic method	Hospitalization status	Treatment interval	Number of treatments
After 12 months of age	30~40 minutes	Sleep, topical ointment, local infiltration anesthesia	n/a	6 weeks	4~8 times

Acquired bilateral nevus of ota like macule(ABNOM)

From their late teens to early 20s, Ota nevus reveals symmetrically in their faces. It appears round on both cheekbones and occurs symmetrically on the temples, the forehead, the bridge of the nose, and the tip of the nose. The color looks brown first and gradually darkens over time.

They are often misunderstood as freckles and people try to treat it with treatment of freckles, but it cannot be cured with this treatment.

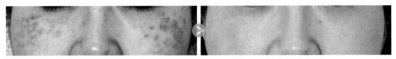

Before and after acquired Ota nevus treatment

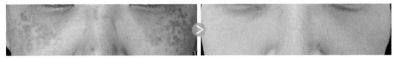

Before and after acquired Ota nevus treatment

TIP_Informations on the treatment of acquired Ota Nevus

Possible time for treatment	Treatment duration	Anesthetic method	Hospitalization	Treatment interval	Number of treatments
From the onset of symptoms	10 minutes	Topical ointment, local infiltration anesthesia	No hospitalization	4~8 weeks	3~5 times

| Ectopic Mongolian Spot & Ito Nevus

Ectopic Mongolian spots refer to Mongolian spots that appear on other parts of the body, such as the wrists or ankles. In the case of Ito nevus, it continues to progress and become darker, so active treatment is necessary.

Ota nevus refers to a wide spot with bluish or black color around the eyes. It usually appears around the eyes, the temples, the forehead, the cheekbone area, and the bridge of the nose, and does not disappear naturally.

It occurs frequently among Asian ethnic groups, and the blue spot on the baby's hip at birth is called the Mongolian spot. Mongolian spot may also occur in areas other than the hips, which is called ectopic Mongolian spot. Most of the Mongolian or ectopic Mongolian spot disappear naturally after the age of 3 to 4, but the rate of decline of ectopic Mongolian spot is less than that of Mongolian spot.

Ito nevus is a birthmark that appears as a blue mark on the shoulder, neck, upper clavicle, and upper extremity, and appears more widely than the Ota nevus, and there is no histological difference.

Ito nevus, unlike Mongolian spot, does not disappear naturally, so it needs treatment.

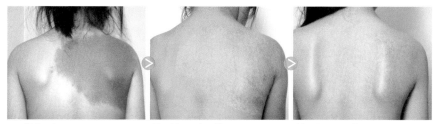

Before Ito nevus treatment   After 16 months of Ito nevus treatment   After 5 years of Ito nevus treatment

TIP_Informations on the treatment of ectopic Mongolian spot & Ito nevus

Possible time for treatment	Treatment duration	Anesthetic method	Hospitalization	Treatment interval	Number of treatments
After 12 months of age	30~40 minutes	Sleep, local infiltration anesthesia	No hospitalization	6 weeks	4~6 times

| Lentigo

It is a dark brown dot(spot) caused by exposure to ultraviolet rays of sunlight and skin aging. It is caused by an increase in melanin deposition, and it it's caused by increase in melanin-containing cells at the skin junction of the epidermis. Lentigo is divided into agminated lentigenous nevus, solar lentigo, and simple lentigo.

Agminated Lentigenous Nevus

It is a nevus caused by the proliferation of melanin pigments in the skin epithelial layer. It occurs acquiredly and appears in any part of the face. There is a characteristic that clusters appear in groups and nevus spreads.

When treated, it seems to be temporarily gone, but it partially recurs over time. The response to treatment varies from person to person.

※Treatment : It will be cleaned for 2-3 treatments every 4 weeks.

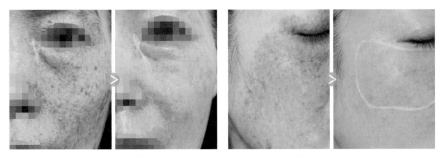

Before and after treatment for clustered lentigo

Solar Lentigo

It is common on skin exposed to ultraviolet rays and is an epidermal pigment disease. The boundaries appear round over a wide range of the face.

It looks similar to age spots, but unlike age spots, its surface looks smooth. It can appear all over the body, including the face and neck.

It becomes clean when treated, but it partially recurs after three to five years. The response to treatment varies from person to person.

※Treatment : About 80% can be treated in one treatment, and it will be cleaned in the second treatment after 4 weeks.

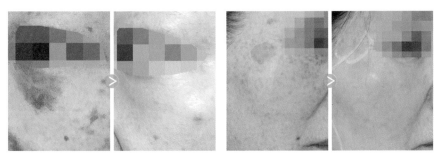

Before and after solar lentigo treatment

Simple Lentigo

It is characterized by melanin pigment proliferation in the epithelial layer of the skin independently of areas (face, arms, legs) exposed to ultraviolet rays.

It becomes clean when treated, but it partially recurs after 1 to 2 years. The response to treatment varies from person to person.

※Treatment: About 80% can be treated in one treatment, and it will be cleaned in the second treatment after 4 weeks.

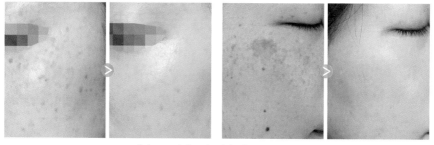

Before and after simple lentigo treatment

TIP_Information on the treatment of lentigo					
Possible time for treatment	Treatment duration	Anesthetic method	Hospitalization status	Treatment interval	Number of treatments
From the onset of symptoms	10 minutes	Sleep, topical ointment, local infiltration anesthesia	n/a	4~8 weeks	2~3 times

Precautions after treatment for lentigo

- Scrubs, exfoliation, and scrubbing towels should never be used around the treatment area.

- You can go to the sauna after two weeks, but it is better to refrain from it during the treatment period.

- Ski resorts and beaches should be avoided.

- It is recommended to avoid using indoor and outdoor swimming pools (disinfectant ingredients) as much as possible.
- After 7 days of treatment, UV protection is thoroughly applied.

Diagnosis is important,
Treatment is required according to accurate diagnosis

The spots on the face vary in color and shape such as black spots, red spots, white spots, bluish spots, lentigo, freckles, and blemishes.

A red spot is called a hemangioma, which refers to a large increase in blood vessels from birth or acquired, making the skin uneven or flat in red or purple on the face or around areas. White spot has two different types. One is innate and called achromic nevus, bleached one, and the other is acquired and called vitiligo (leukoplakia).

In the case of bluish spots, the color changes to blue because the place the spot is formed is deep in the skin. Blue nevus is similar to black spot, but is characterized by slightly larger and more bluish. Another spot of the bluish spot, Ota nevus, has an innate spot on one side of the face and an acquired Ota nevus, which is acquired like freckle on both sides of the face.

The treatment method of spots varies depending on the type of each spot. If the spot is very large, surgery to remove the skin is used. If the spot is small cases include methods such as electric ablation, chemical ablation and laser, etc. Since it is a laser that does not leave a scar after removing the spot, in many cases, the spot is removed using a laser.

Other than black spots are usually laser treated. In Raum Plastic Surgery, brown (black brown) spots and bluish spots such as lentigo, Ota nevus, Ito nevus are treated with Ruby lasers.

지방흡입술과 5D 지방조각술(Liposuction & 5D liposculpture)
지방흡입 재수술(Revision liposuction)

완벽한 아름다움을 추구하는 전신 지방조각술은 완벽을 추구하는 예술이다

To achieve a perfect and stunning figure through whole-body liposculpture, it takes an artist's touch and expertise

지방흡입술은 지방을 단순하게 뽑아내는 것으로 그치지 않는다. 지방은 조각의 대상이다.
그러므로, 지방흡입술을 '지방조각술'이라고 부른다.

Liposuction is more than just removing fat. The fat is the object to be sculpted.
That's why liposuction has to be called "liposculpture."

리디안의원
Lydian Cosmetic Surgery Clinic

www.lydianc.com

안경천(Kyung-Chun An)

- 고려대학교 의과대학 외래교수(Clinical Professor of Korea University, College of Medicine)
- 리디안의원 원장(Director of Lydian Clinic)
- 대한 미용의학회 티칭 펠로우
(Teaching Fellow of Korean College of Cosmetic Surgery and Medicine)
- 한국미용의학회 홍보 이사
(Director of Public Relations, Korean Society of Cosmetic Medicine and Surgery)
- 아시아 지방의학의회 학술의장(Asia Fat Congress Scientific Chair)

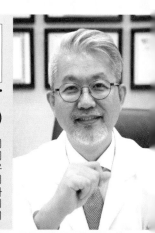

11 지방을 조각하여 아름다운 몸매를 창조한다

아시아인과 지방흡입수술

동양인들에게 있어서 지방흡입은 쉽지 않다. 일단 동양인의 지방 조직에는 섬유질이 매우 많고 흉터가 잘 생긴다. 이러한 문제점을 고려해 새로운 지방흡입수술 방법이 개발되었다. 고전적으로 2~5mm 굵기의 관을 이용하여 지방을 흡입한다. 방법은 비슷하겠지만 빨리 많이 뽑아내는 것이 쉬운 기기, 지방 이식을 하기에 더 쉬운 기기, 리프팅 효과를 내기 위한 고주파 지방 흡입 기기, 지방을 분쇄하고 세밀한 수술을 할 수 있게 도와주는 초음파 기기, 지방을 녹이는 기능을 가진 레이저 지방 흡입 기기 등이 지금까지 개발된 기기들이다.

간혹 병원에 비치 되어있는 지방흡입 기기가 환자의 관심사가 된다. 하지만, 그보다 중요한 점은 의사의 예술성과 미용 의학적 지식이다. 미용수술 결과는 의사의 예술작품이다. 자신을 수술할 의사를 선택할 때는 수술하는 의사가 내어놓는 전후 사진들의 예술성에 초점을 맞추고 자신이 선호하는 작품을 선택하는 지혜로움이 필요할 것이다. 포토샵으로 전후 사진을 보정하는 것이 난무한 현재, 무보정 전후 사진으로 현실적인 감각으로 의사의 실력을 평가하는 것이 바람직할 것이다.

┃ 지방흡입술 & 5D 지방조각술

지방흡입 수술의 범위는 광범위하다. 머리부터 발까지 모든 부위가 포함된다. 거의 모든 지방흡입수술은 특별한 수술 후 관리 방법을 통해 바로 신속한 회복이 가능하다.

마취와 수술 후 통증

수술 후 통증은 마치 운동 하지 않던 사람이 20~30개의 윗몸 일으키기를 한 후에 배가 당겨서 아파하는 정도의 통증을 수반하는 정도가 전부이다. 통증은 수술 중에 근육이 캐뉼라에 많이 찔리면 심하게 아플 수 있다. 그러므로, 의사의 숙련도에 따라 통증의 정도 차이가 크다. 처음 한 달은 붓기가 남아 있으며 부자연스러울 수 있으나, 약 3개월 정도 지나면 전체적으로 부드럽고 아름다운 곡선이 만들어진다.

지방흡입수술을 하기 위해서는 투메선트라는 용액을 주입하게 되는데 이 용액 안에 국소 마취제가 포함되어 있다. 이때 통증은 볼펜으로 쿡쿡 찌르는 정도의 아픔이 있을 수 있다. 하지만, 약간의 통증도 두려워하는 경우가 많아서 수면 마취나 전신마취를 통하여 수술하는 경우가 많다.

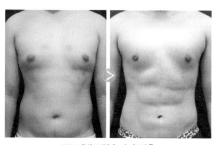

5D 지방조각술 수술전후

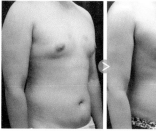

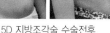
5D 지방조각술 수술전후

얼굴

얼굴은 다양한 부위에 지방이 존재한다. 볼, 이중 턱과 같은 부위가 주 수술 부위가 되겠다. 얼굴과 목 부위의 지방은 몸보다 지방세포의 크기가 작고 혈관이 많을 뿐 아니라 안면이라는 특수성 때문에 여러 가지 조심해야 할 부분들이 많다.

수술 후 약 일주일 정도 많이 붓게 되며, 멍이 들 가능성이 있다. 얼굴의 지방을 제거할 때 가장 중요한 점은 피부가 처질 수 있다는 것이다. 그래서, 나이가 든 환자에 있어서는 안면거상 술을 같이 하거나 코그실을 이용하여 피부를 당겨주면서 수술을 해야 하는 경우가 많다. 안면의 신경 손상과 같은 부작용 때문에 얼굴의 특정 부위에 일시적인 마비가 올 수 있으나 대부분 2~3개월 이내에 돌아온다. 얼굴은 레이저, 고주파, 초음파 기기를 이용해 수술하는 것이 효과적이다. 이러한 기기를 사용하지 않으면 지방이 거의 흡입되지 않는다. 기기의 종류에 따라 약간의 특성이 다르지만, 저자는 수술 속도가 가장 빠른 초음파 기기를 사용하는 것을 선호한다.

팔

대부분의 경우에는 위팔(어깨부터 팔꿈치까지)을 수술하게 된다. 팔을 수술할 때는 뒤쪽, 안쪽과 바깥쪽을 수술한다. 앞쪽을 같이 수술하게 되는 경우는 매우 드물다. 팔이 두꺼워 보이는 원인 중에는 겨드랑이와 그 아래쪽 지방이 팔을 바깥쪽으로 밀게 되어 더 두꺼워 보이는 결과를 초래한다. 그러므로, 팔의 지방흡입을 고려한다면 겨드랑이, 겨드랑이 아래 부위 등의 지방의 양을 고려하여야 하며 필요하다면 이러한 부위를 동시에 수술해야 만족스러운 결과를 얻을 수 있다.

팔 피부의 처짐 현상을 막아주기 위해서 고주파나 초음파 기기가 많은 도움이 된다. 수술 시 절개 부위는 보통 겨드랑이에 작은 절개 구를 통해 수술한다. 필요에 따라서는 팔꿈치에도 절개 구가 필요할 수 있다. 이 흉터는 팔꿈치 주름을 잘 이용하면 노출 부위지만 잘 보이지 않는다.

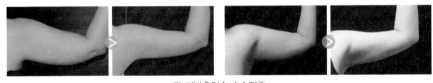

팔 지방흡입술 수술전후

하체 지방흡입

허벅지를 수술하는 데 있어서 핵심은 흉터가 잘 보이지 않아야 한다는 것이다.

필자의 경우 60cm가 넘는 긴 캐뉼러를 통해 2개의 절개만으로 수술한다. 필요에 따라 4개의 절개로 수술하기도 한다. 그래서 흉터가 눈에 띄는 경우가 거의 없다. 허벅지는 너무 많은 양의 지방을 뽑으려고 욕심을 부리다가는 울퉁불퉁한 결과를 초래하기 십상이다. 반듯한 다리를 얻는 것, 처진 엉덩이의 모습이 올라가 보이게 하는 것, 바깥쪽에 튀어나온 허벅지를 편평하게 해 주는 것, 두께를 줄여주는 것의 순서가 올바른 하체 지방흡입의 목표이다. 엉덩이가 처져 보이는 경우 엉덩이 상부에 지방 이식을 통해 리프팅을 유도하기도 한다. 복부와 옆구리 부위에서 흐르는 곡선을 고려하여 함께 수술한다면 훨씬 더 아름다운 모양의 몸매를 얻을 수 있다.

종아리 지방흡입을 하기 위해서는 보통 오금에 있는 주름위에 절개하게 된다. 근육이 큰 경우라면 신경차단술이나 보톡스, 또는 PDO 실을 이용한 근육퇴축술을 같이 해 주는 것이 추천된다.

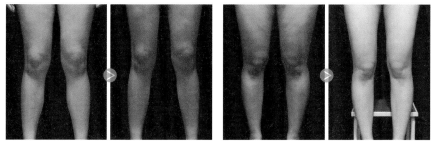

하체 지방흡입술 수술전후

여성–가슴축소

유방이 너무 크고 처진 모습의 여성은 지방흡입을 통해 유방을 축소하고 리프팅 시킬 수 있다. 흔히 시행되는 유방축소수술은 'ㅗ' 자 형태의 아주 큰 흉터를 동반하기 때문에 지방흡입으로 수술을 받기 원하는 여성들이 늘어나는 추세다. 유방의 처진 정도가 심하면 유륜절개를 통해 흉터를 최소화하면서 수술하기도 한다.

가슴 지방이식

등에 지방이 많은 경우에 유방에서 등으로 이어지는 곡선에 지방이 많이 축적되어 가슴이 왜소하게 보일 수 있다. 이런 때에는 등과 겨드랑이 아래 부위의 지방을 흡입하여 가슴이 돋보이게 수술하기도 하며 필요에 따라 줄기세포를 이용하여 지방 이식을 유방에 같이 하기도 한다. 최근 발표되는 논문에 의하면 지방 이식에 의한 유방확대술이 유방암 발병률에 미치는 영향이 없다고 한다. 그러므로, 안심하고 유방 자가지방이식수술을 받아도 될 것 같다.

여성형 유방증

유선을 파괴하기 위해서는 초음파 장비를 사용해야만 딱딱한 유선을 파괴할 수 있다. 유선외 양이 너무 많은 경우에는 유선 제거가 필요하기도 하다. 필자는 젖꼭지를 절개하는 방법으로 하기 때문에 흉터가 전혀 보이지 않는다. 남성에게도 수술 후에 눈에 띄는 흉터는 그 누구도 원하는 바가 아니기 때문이다.

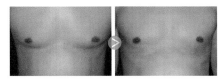 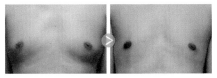

여성형 유방증 수술전후

복부

임신이나 체중감량을 통해 피부가 늘어지고 튼 살이 동반되는 경우가 많아서 피부의 두께가 불규칙적이고 늘어진 경우가 많기 때문에 깔끔한 수술결과를 만드는 것이 매우 어렵다.

일반 지방흡입

일반적인 방법은 복부에 잡히는 지방 덩어리를 줄이려는 목표로 수술하는 경우를 말한다. 흉터가 잘 보이지 않고 울퉁불퉁하지 않으면서 지방량을 줄였다면 좋은 결과라고 할 수 있을 것이다. 필자의 경우 복부, 옆구리, 뒷구리를 포함하는 지방흡입을 하는 경우 앞뒤로 한 개씩, 단 2개의 절개부위를 통해서 수술하기 때문에 흉터가 눈에 띄지 않는다는 장점이 있다.

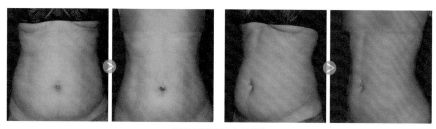

일반 지방흡입 수술전후

복부 성형

이 수술은 튼 살이 심하거나 피부가 과도하게 늘어져 있는 경우에 선택하게 되는 수술이다. 팬티 안으로 긴 흉터가 생기기 때문에 걱정하는 환자들이 많이 있다. 하지만, 일반 지방흡입으로는 늘어진 피부 때문에 편평한 결과를 얻을 수 없다. 임신 후에 복부 근육이 같이 늘어져서 복부 근육도 팽팽하게 묶어주게 된다.

음모 부위에서부터 배꼽까지의 복부 피부를 절개하고 배꼽보다 위쪽의 피부를 아래로 잡아당겨 봉합하게 되면 기적처럼 편평한 복부를 만들 수 있게 된다. 복부성형을 하는 대부분의 경우에 복부 지방흡입을 같이한다. 흉터는 약 2년 정도 지나면 얇은 흰 선으로 남게 되며 팬티 안에 자리 잡기 때문에 비키니를 입는 것도 가능하다.

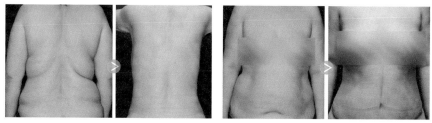

▲ 54세 여성, 복부, 팔 등에 파워 지방흡입(총 12L) 복부성형 수술전후 – 수술횟수 : 2회 분할

TIP_복부성형술 수술정보					
수술시간	마취방법	입원여부	샤워가능	회복기간	체류기간
4~6시간	수면, 전신마취	필요없음	3~7일	4~7일	7~14일

5D 지방조각술

5D(5 dimensions)는 5개의 층, 즉 1) 피부, 2) 표층 지방, 3) 중간층 지방, 4) 깊은 층 지방, 5) 근육을 고려해 아름답고 탄력 있는 몸매를 만들어주는 수술을 말한다.

첫째, 피부의 상태가 다양하므로 피부의 두께와 탄력도를 고려해야 한다. 수술하게되는 모든 위치에 따라 지방의 해부학적 형태가 다르고 특성이 다르며 수술 방법 또한 달라지기 때문에 3개 층을 모두 고려한 수술방법 선택이 필요하다.

둘째, 근육의 모양을 고려하여 복근의 형태가 잘 드러날 수 있게 수술을 하는 것이다. 수술 디자인부터 간단하지 않다. 초음파 진단기를 이용해 피부와 지방 아래 감추어진 근육의 모양을 면밀하게 관찰한 후에 수술 디자인을 하게 된다. 남자 환자의 경우에는 '王' 자, 여자의 경우에는 '川' 자의 형태로 직복근의 형태가 도드라져 보이게 만들며 외복사근의 모양까지도 고려하여 디자인하고 수술한다. 환자의 선호도에 따라 진하게 할 수도 있고 부드럽게 할 수도 있다.

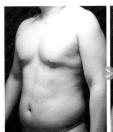

▲ 45세 남자, 5D 지방조각술 수술전후
수술부위 : 가슴라인, 복부, 옆구리, 등

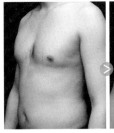

▲ 43세 남자, 5D 지방조각술 수술전후
수술부위 : 가슴, 복부, 옆구리

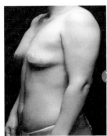
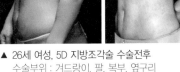

▲ 26세 여성, 5D 지방조각술 수술전후
수술부위 : 겨드랑이, 팔, 복부, 옆구리

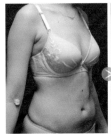
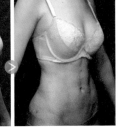

▲ 50세 여성, 5D 지방조각술 수술전후
수술부위 : 팔, 겨드랑이, 등, 복부 , 옆구리, 엉덩이,
허벅지 줄기세포, 가슴 지방이식

지방흡입 재수술

실패한 지방흡입수술은 재앙과도 같다. 한 번 잘못된 지방흡입수술을 복원하는 것은 매우 어려운 과정이다. 하지만 2~3회의 재수술을 통해 다시 편평하게 수술하는 것이 가능하다.

잃어버린 자신감을 되찾는 작업 : 지방흡입 재수술

　피부가 얇은 사람, 너무 마른 사람, 피부가 많이 처진 사람, 튼 살이 많은 사람의 경우엔 지방흡입이 매우 어렵다. 울퉁불퉁한 결과가 나오는 경우는 지방을 편평하게 뽑아주지 못해 발생하게 된다. 멍이 너무 많이 들었을 때도 해당 부위에 섬유질이 많이 생겨 옴폭하게 파이는 경우도 있다. 특정 부위 피부의 진피가 많이 손상을 받게 되면 피부가 딱딱해져서 전체적인 모양이 틀어지기도 한다. 울퉁불퉁하게 된 원인과 상황에 따라 처치 방법이 다르며 단 한 번의 수술로 모든 것을 교정하기는 매우 어렵다. 보통 첫 수술 6~12개월 후에 재수술하게 된다. 보통 2개월에 한 번씩, 2~3회의 수술이 필요한 경우가 많다.

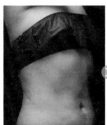 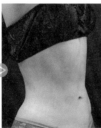

▲ 43세 여성. 복부 지방흡입 재수술

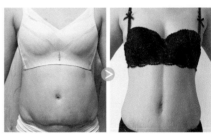

▲ 35세 여성. 복부 성형 재수술
2년전 복부 지방흡입과 복부성형 수술 후 복부 표면이 편평하지 못하고 복부성형 흉터가 팬티 위로 올라와 있어 재수술을 시행함.

TIP_지방흡입술 수술정보

수술시간	마취방법	입원여부	샤워가능	회복기간	체류기간
1~2시간/부위	국소. 수면. 전신마취	필요없음	2일	2일	3~7일

11 Sculpting fat to create a beautiful body

Asians and liposuction

Liposuction can pose a challenge for individuals with Asian heritage. Traditional liposuction has some drawbacks, especially when it comes to removing fat from Asian adipose tissue, which is fibrous and tends to scar easily. To tackle these issues, innovative methods have been developed. While the basic method of removing fat using a cannula remains the same, newer devices have been invented to make the process faster and more efficient. These include devices for fat grafting, radiofrequency liposuction for lifting, ultrasound devices for more precise surgery, and laser liposuction to melt the fat.

Patients may be concerned about the quality of the liposuction machines used in a clinic. However, it's important to remember that the surgeon's skills and knowledge of aesthetic medicine are more crucial in achieving the desired results. Cosmetic surgery is a form of art, and when choosing a surgeon for your procedure, it's important to focus on their artistry based on their before and after photographs. In this age of digital retouching, it's best to evaluate a surgeon's skills by considering unretouched before and after photos to ensure that you make a wise and realistic choice.

| Liposuction & 5D liposculpture

The scope of liposuction is extensive, covering all areas from head to toe. Most liposuction procedures ensure a rapid recovery with specialized post-operative care.

Anesthesia and post-operative pain

After undergoing a surgical procedure of liposuction, it is common to experience post-operative pain that can be compared to the soreness and tightness you feel in your stomach after doing several sets of 20 or 30 sit-ups, especially if you don't exercise regularly.

The level of pain can be severe if the muscles have been prodded by numerous movements of cannulas during the surgery. The pain can be described as a ballpoint pen prick. However, many people are afraid of even a little pain, so the procedure is often performed under sleep sedation or general anesthesia. The intensity of the pain may vary depending on the surgeon's level of expertise.

Swelling may persist for the first month, which may appear unnatural, but after about three months, the final outcome is a smooth and aesthetically pleasing contour.

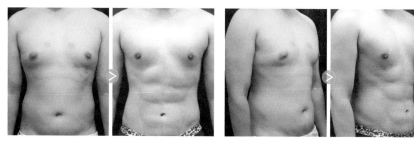

5D liposculpture (men) before and after surgery

Face

Special considerations must be made when removing fat from the face, as this area has smaller fat lobules and more blood vessels than the rest of the body. The main surgical areas for fat removal are the cheeks and double chin, but it's important to be cautious as the skin can sag after surgery, especially in older patients. In these cases, a facelift or cogged threads may be necessary to lift the skin.

It's normal for patients to experience swelling for about a week and bruising is also possible after surgery. However, any numbness in certain areas of the face due to facial nerve damage usually returns within two to three months.

Various devices such as laser, radiofrequency, ultrasound, and plasma devices are used to remove fat from the face. However, fat removal is rarely performed without the use of these devices. While each device has slightly different characteristics, the author prefers to use ultrasound as it is the fastest

Arms

When it comes to liposuction of the arms, the focus is typically on the upper arm from shoulder to elbow. The surgery is performed on the back, inside, and outside of the arm, with the front being rarely treated. It's important to consider the amount of fat in the armpits and underarms when deciding on liposuction of the arms, and these areas should be treated at the same time if necessary to achieve a satisfactory outcome.

To prevent sagging skin on the arms, plasma, radiofrequency or ultrasound devices can be used effectively. The procedure is typically done through small incisions in the armpits, and if necessary, an incision may also be made near the standing elbow. Although the resulting scar is visible, it can be concealed within the elbow crease.

The author takes great care to ensure that scars are minimal and results are of high quality when performing armpit liposuction. This is achieved by using only one incision at the back of the armpit, which is hidden when the arms are down.

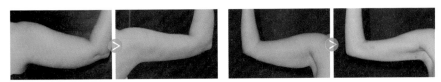

Arm liposuction before and after surgery

Lower body liposuction

During lower body liposuction, the main objective is to ensure that any resulting scars are not visible. For the thighs, the surgeon uses a cannula that is over 60 centimeters (23.6 inches) long, which requires only two incisions - one inside the navel and the other at the coccyx. This technique results in almost scarless liposuction of the thighs.

To achieve a smooth and lumpy-free result, the surgeon must be cautious when removing fat from the thigh area. The aim of proper lower body liposuction is to obtain a smooth skin contour, lift sagging buttocks, reduce the size of the thighs, and flatten outwardly protruding thighs. In cases where the buttocks appear saggy, fat grafting to the upper buttocks may be performed to lift them. When combined with the liposuction of the abdomen and flanks, a perfect hourglass figure can be achieved.

During calf liposuction, the surgeon usually makes a single incision at the ankle folds. For patients with larger muscles, the surgeon recommends a combination of nerve blocks, Botox, or muscle reduction with PDO threads.

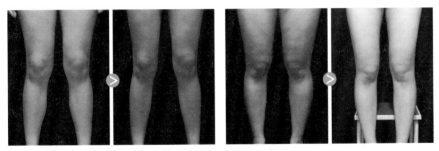

Lower body liposuction before and after surgery

Women - Breast Reduction

Women with large and saggy breasts can opt for liposuction to reduce and lift them without needing to undergo conventional breast reduction surgery that leaves a large scar. In cases where the sagging is severe, a regular mammoplasty must be done with minimized scarring suture techniques.

Breast fat grafting

Breast fat grafting can be an effective solution for those who lack sufficient fat in their breasts. Some individuals may have excess fat deposits on their back and sides of their chest, which can make their breasts appear smaller. In such cases, removing the fat from these areas, along with liposuction, can improve the shape of the breasts. Additionally, fat grafting using stem cells can be used to enhance the breasts. Recent studies have shown that breast augmentation through fat grafting is safe and does not increase the risk of breast cancer.

Gynecomastia

Gynecomastia treatment involves the use of ultrasound machines to destroy hard glands. In some cases, excision of glandular tissues and/or nipple lifting surgery may be necessary for better results. Meanwhile, for male breast liposuction, I make an incision inside the areola area that typically leaves minimal scarring, which is not noticeable for any race. Visible scarring after breast surgery is not desirable, particularly for men.

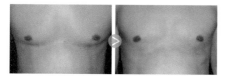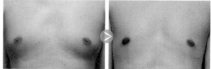

Before and after gynecomastia surgery

Liposuction of the Abdominal area

Liposuction in the abdominal area is challenging because of the presence of loose skin and irregular stretch marks. Loose skin makes achieving a neat result difficult.

General type of liposuction of the abdominal area

In general, liposuction aims to reduce fatty lumps in the abdomen. The outcome of abdominal liposuction is considered successful if there are no prominent scars, or bumps, and the noticeable fat volume is reduced. When it comes to liposuction involving the abdomen, flanks, and back, I perform the procedure through only three incisions, resulting in one invisible scar at the navel, one in the pubic area, and one at the coccyx. None of these scars are easily noticeable.

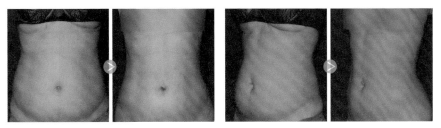

Before and after general liposuction surgery

Abdominoplasty

Abdominoplasty is the recommended procedure for patients with severe stretch marks and loose skin. Regular liposuction may not be enough to achieve a smooth and flat result due to the presence of excess skin. In cases where the abdominal muscles have separated horizontally, creating a condition called diastasis recti, the muscles must be tightened together.

The abdominoplasty procedure involves making a single incision in the abdominal skin that runs from one side of the pelvic bone to the other. The surgeon then pulls down the skin above the navel, removes any excess skin and sutures both ends to create a flat abdomen. In many cases, liposuction is also performed on the abdomen. Although a thin white line scar is left after the surgery, it usually fades over time and becomes almost

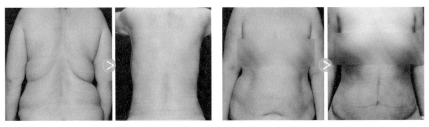

▲54 years old woman, power liposuction on abdomen, arms, etc. (total 12L) before and after abdominoplasty surgery - Number of surgeries: 2 splits

invisible within two years. The scar may be noticeable with certain types of clothing but should not be visible when wearing a bikini.

TIP_Abdominoplasty Information					
Operation time	Anesthsia	Admission	Take Shower	Recovery time	Stay in Korea
4~6 hours	Topical, Sleep, general anesthesia	None	3~7 days	4~7 days	7~14 days

5D Liposculpture

When talking about 5D or 5 dimensions surgery, it means that the surgeon takes into account five different layers of the body, namely : 1) skin, 2) superficial layer fat, 3) medial layer fat, 4) deep layer fat, and 5) muscle to create a toned and beautiful body.

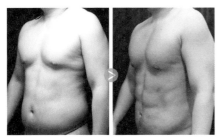

▲ 45 years old man, 5D liposculpture before and after surgery
Surgical area : chest line, abdomen, flanks, back

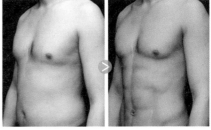

▲ 43 years old man, 5D liposculpture before and after surgery
Surgical area: chest, abdomen, flanks

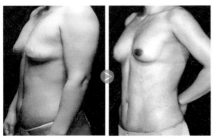

▲ 26 years old female, 5D liposculpture before and after surgery
Surgical area : armpits, arms, abdomen, flanks

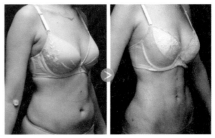

▲ 50 years old woman, before and after 5D liposculpture surgery
Surgical areas : arms, armpits, back, abdomen, flanks, buttocks, thigh stem cells, breast fat transplant

When talking about 5D or 5 dimensions surgery, it means that the surgeon takes into account five different layers of the body, namely : 1) skin, 2) superficial layer fat, 3) medial layer fat, 4) deep layer fat, and 5) muscle to create a toned and beautiful body.

The shape of the muscles is also important, especially for defining the abdominal muscles. The surgical design is not easy, as it requires the use of an ultrasound diagnostic device to closely observe the shape of the muscles hidden under the skin and fat. The shape of the rectus abdominis muscle is emphasized in the form of a "王(wang : means king)" for men and a "川(chuan: means stream" for women. The shape of the external oblique muscle is also taken into account when designing and operating. Depending on the patient's preference, the burrows could be emphasized or made to blend with the surrounding area.

TIP_General Information about liposuction					
Operation time	Anesthsia	Hospitalization	Take Shower	Recovery time	Stay in Korea
1~3 hours	Sleep anesthesia, general anesthesia	0-2 days	1-2 days	2 days	3~7 days

| Revision liposuction

Liposuction is a cosmetic procedure that, if not done correctly, can have disastrous consequences. Unfortunately, reversing the effects of a bad liposuction is often very difficult. However, there is hope for those who have experienced unsatisfactory results. With two or three revision surgeries, it is possible to achieve the desired smooth outcome.

Regaining lost confidence: liposuction revision surgery

For many people, undergoing liposuction can be a life-changing experience that boosts their confidence and self-esteem. However, for those with thin skin, an overly thin body type, excessive sagging skin, or a high number of stretch marks, liposuction can be particularly challenging. In such cases, lumpy or uneven results can occur due to the inability to remove the fat evenly, and severe bruising can result in fibrous tissue and undulations. In addition, if the dermis of the treated area is heavily damaged, the skin can become hard and lose its shape.

To address these issues, the treatment plan will depend on the cause of the unevenness and the individual's situation. It is often difficult to correct everything in a single surgery, and a second surgery may be required 6 to 12 months after the first. In some cases, a series of two to three surgeries may be necessary, with each surgery performed every two months. Fat transfers to the depressed areas may be needed to restore smooth contours.

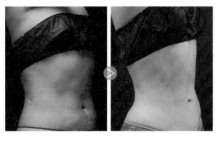 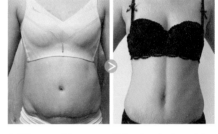

▲ 43 years old woman. Abdominal liposuction revision surgery

▲ 35 years old woman. Abdominoplasty revision surgery
Reoperation was performed due to the uneven surface of the abdomen and the high scar line above the panties. The scar is hidden under the panties after the reoperation.

비수술 필러제거(Non surgical filler removal)
두상 필러 시술(Scalp volume augmentation)

필러 부작용과 두상 모양을
비수술로 자연스럽게 해결한다!

Filler side effects
and head shape are naturally
resolved without surgery!

자연스럽고 건강한 아름다움을 위해 필러를 맞은 사람들이 많았지만 그만큼 부작용을 겪는 사람들도 많다. 이를 해결 가능한 것이 다이오드 레이저 시술로 필러 녹이는 주사와 절개 제거 수술로도 해결이 어려운 이물질 제거도 가능하다.

There have been many people who have taken fillers for natural and healthy beauty, but there are also many people who suffer from side effects. This can be solved by Diode laser treatment, and it is also possible to remove foreign substances that are difficult to solve even with filler-dissolving injections and operation.

큐오필 앤 결의원
Q.O.Fill & Gyul Clinic

www.qofill-clinic.com

최철(Chul Choi)

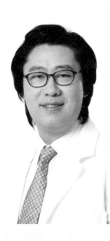

- 전, 분당제생병원 과장(Former Director, Bundang Jesaeng Hospital)
- 대한 두피모발학회 정회원(Member of the Korean Scalp and Hair Society)
- 대한 미용외과학회 정회원(Member of the Korean Society of Aesthetic Surgeons)
- 한국 & 중국 COVIDEN사의 브이락 실리프팅 마스터닥터
  (Korea & China COVIDEN's V-Loc Thread Lifting Master Doctor)
- 이탈리아 GMV사의 핑거롤(니들 쉐이핑), 플라즈마 프렉사 아시아 키닥터
  (Asia key doctor for Plexr & needle shaping(Finger roll) of GMV in Italy)

12 비수술 필러, 지방이식 제거 & 두상 필러

이물질화된 필러, 이식된 지방을 비수술적으로 제거 가능한 다이오드 레이저

미용을 위해 많은 사람들이 병원에서 허가 받은 필러(filler)와 지방이식(fat transfer)을 시술받아 왔다. 그중 일부 사람들은 이른바 "야매(일본어에서 변형된 '암거래'의 속어)로 불리는 불법 무허가 시술을 받은 사람들도 있다. 필러 부작용이 생기더라도 제거하면 된다고 생각하는 사람이 많은데 그리 간단한 일이 결코 아니다. 절개수술을 하더라도 완벽하게 제거하기 힘들고 오히려 함몰 등 부작용이 생길 수 있기 때문이다.

필러는 작은 알갱이가 모여 있는 형태다. 시술이 마음에 들지 않거나, 뜻밖의 부작용이 발생한 경우 필러를 녹이는 시술이 필요하다.

하지만 이 알갱이들 중 일부가 이물질로 인식된 경우는 '골치덩이'로 돌변한다. 캡슐화, 섬유화 등의 조직 변성으로 인해 히알라제와 같은 녹이는 주사에 해결 되지 않고, 절개 제거 수술도 이물질화된 조직 변성 때문에 효과적으로 제거가 어렵다. 이를 조직의 손상이나 흉터없이 필러만 제거하고자 개발한 기술이 바로 다이오드 레이저이다.

▎비수술 이물질 제거술

다이오드 레이저는 수술이나 절개 없이 얼굴 지방 제거를 목적으로 개발되었지만, 이물질화된 필러 육아종, 이식된 지방 제거도 가능한 비수술 치료법이다.

필러나 지방이식의 주된 목적은 볼륨감을 회복시키는 것이고 이것은 노화된 인상의 개선에 필수적이다. 또한 젊은 나이라도 미적 개선을 위해 다양한 부위에 사용되고 있다. 하지만 가능한 문제로는 필러가 주입된후 이물질로 인식하게 되면 과민반응이 일어날 수 있다는 점이다. 과민반응이 있던 없던 면역 세포가 필러 입자에 달라붙어 막을 형성하게 되는데 이를 캡슐화(Capsularization)라고 한다.

이러한 과정에서 만성 염증 상태가 발생할 수 있고 이를 치료하라는 과다한 신호가 발생하면서 콜라겐이 주변에 과형성되는데 이를 섬유화(Fibrosis)라 한다. 이렇게 캡슐화, 섬유화가 반복되며 조직변성이 발생하게 되어 커지면 육아종(Granuloma)이라 한다. 이를 제거 하기 위해 절개 수술을 고려하는 이들도 있지만, 효과적으로 제거가 되지 않고, 수술 흉터에 대한 부담감과 수술 후 모양이 더 나빠지는 부작용도 간과할 수 없다.

다이오드 레이저 수술 절차

다이오드 레이저는 본체에서 광섬유가 나오는데, 이를 피부를 관통시켜 육아종 부위에 조사하는 방식이다. 필러 부작용을 겪고 있다면 다이오드 레이저 후 흡입을 고려할 수 있다.

다이오드 레이저 수술 절차를 간단하게 설명드리면 다음과 같다

01 초음파 검사를 통하여 육아종의 크기, 위치 등을 미리 파악한다.
02 필러 입자들을 붙잡고 있는 캡슐화, 섬유화 같은 조직 변성을 다이오드 레이저로 해체시키고, 외부로 흡입해서 제거한다.

광섬유를 삽입하여 이러한 육아종 제거를 위해서는 기술과 풍부한 임상경험이 필요하다. 필러 부작용으로 인한 이물질 제거 수술을 고려하고 있다면 무엇보다 숙련된 의료진과 정밀 진단이 우선적으로 이뤄져야 할 것이다. 이물질 제거 노하우와 오랜 경험을 지닌 의료진이 필러 부작용의 상태를 정확히 파악한 후 필러를 제거하는 것이 중요하다.

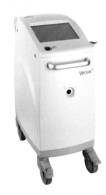

다이오드 레이저

장비에서 광섬유가 나오는 데, 이를 시술 부위 근방에서 삽입해서 조직에 레이저를 조사한다.

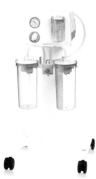

메델라 흡입기

다이오드 레이저가 육아종 주변 캡슐화, 섬유화를 해체하고, 이후 메델라 흡입기로 흡입해서 제거한다.

이물질 제거 후 모양회복을 위한 조직 재건

핑거롤(니들쉐이핑)

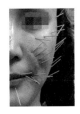

필러 육아종, 지방이식 부작용을 제거한다고 해서 필러 시술 이전의 모양으로 회복 되는 것은 아니다. 모양을 회복하기 위해서는 조직 재건술(핑거롤)이 필요하다. 핑거롤(Finger Roll)은 유럽 이탈리아의 GMV사에서 개발한 니들쉐이핑 장비를 이용한 시술로써 무너진 콜라겐 구조를 복구시키는데 도움 주는 장비이다.

핑거롤 시술은 피부 진피층 밑으로 수평으로 얕게 바늘을 삽입하고, 이 바늘에 니들 쉐이핑 장비에서 나오는 직류 전기가 흐르는 상태에서 바늘을 회전시키면 콜라겐이 생성되고, 조직이 회복되어 필러 시술 이전의 모양으로 회복을 돕는다. 또한 바늘 주변의 섬유조직들이 전기적 힘에 의해 감기게 되며 주변 조직을 위 아래로 끌어당겨, 피부가 팽팽하게 만드는 리프팅 효과가 있다. 이와 더불어 피부 볼륨을 증가하는 효과도 있어 필러 부작용 이전의 얼굴 모양으로 회복시키는 효과가 있다.

다이오드 레이저 부위별 필러 부작용 개선 사례

필러의 대표적인 조직변성, 육아종 개선 시술 사례이다. 이마, 미간 볼 광대 등 다양한 부위의 시술로 만족감이 높다.

이마 필러 육아종

필러의 대표적인 부작용인 조직변성, 육아종(granuloma) 개선 시술 사례이다. 이마, 미간, 볼, 광대 등 다양한 부위의 시술로 만족감이 높다. 히알루론산 필러 생산과정에서 가교결합이 지나치게 많이 생성된 불량품을 맞은 경우에 육아종으로 발전하는데, 이런 불량 구조를 다이오드 레이저로 해체하고, 흡입해서 제거한다.

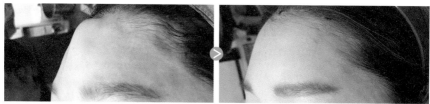

이마 히알루론산 필러 육아종 다이오드 레이저 제거 전후

미간 목주름 조직변성

미간은 필러 주위에 캡슐화, 섬유화 등의 조직변성이 심해, 피부 모양까지 변성이 된 경우이며, 다이오드 레이저로 성공적으로 제거했다. 목주름도 주름에 반영구 필러 시술 후 조직변성이 일어나며 밴드가 형성되어 다이오드 레이저 후 흡입으로 제거했다.

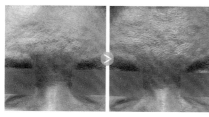 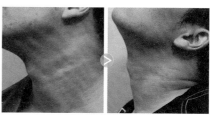

미간 부위 반영구필러 육아종 제거 전후　　　　목주름 부위 반영구 필러 육아종 제거 전후

입술 필러 육아종

오래 전 무면허 의사에게 야매(비합법적)로 필러를 맞은 경우다. 점차 육아종이 커져서 눈에 띄게 아래 입술 전체가 커지고, 튀어나와 다이오드 레이저로 제거했다.

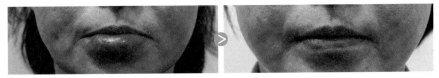

아랫 입술 영구 필러 육아종 제거 전후

볼 필러 육아종 & 조직 재건

우측 볼 영구 필러 육아종을 나이오드 레이저로 제기 추, 핑기롤(Needle shaping) 시술로 손상된 조직을 재건시켜 필러 시술 이전으로 얼굴 모양 회복한 케이스이다.

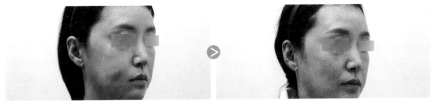

볼 필러 육아종 제거 & 핑거롤 조직 재건술 전후

애교 필러 육아종

오래전 히알루론산 필러를 시술 받았지만 점차 애교 모양이 변형된 모습이다. 이후 필러 녹이는 주사인 히알라제 주사를 3번 시도하였으나 우측 애교는 거의 변화가 없고, 좌측 애교 역시 일부가 녹았으나 눈꼬리 쪽은 여전히 남아있어 오히려 좌우 눈이 비대칭인 모습이다. 본인 스스로 너무 불만족스러운 외모 탓에 히알라제 주사 치료를 중단하고 본원 방문하여 다이오드 레이저로 제거한 케이스이다. 애교 부위는 조직이 약한 부위라서 다이오드 레이저로 제거 시 섬세한 기술이 필요하다.

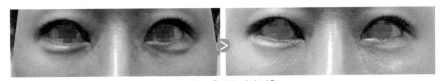

애교 필러 육아종 제거 전후

코, 미간 필러 육아종

코 성형 후 높이가 낮아 만족스럽지 못 해, 콧대 실리콘 보형물 위에 반영구 필러를 주입해 코를 높였다. 하지만 면역 거부 반응으로 부종 발적 통증을 호소하며 내원, 면역 억제 치료로 염증을 사라지게 만든후, 보형물 제거 없이 다이오드 레이저로 반영구 필러를 제거한 케이스이다.

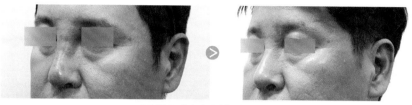

코, 미간 영구 필러 과민반응, 육아종 제거 전후

중앙안면부 지방이식 후 과다 볼륨

볼, 앞광대, 팔자 부위에 지방이식후 이식된 지방으로 과다한 볼륨을 다이오드 레이저로 제거한 후 핑거롤 시술로 모양 회복한 케이스이다.

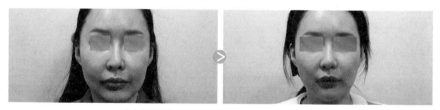

이식된 지방을 제거후 핑거롤로 모양 회복 시술 전후

TIP_다이오드 레이저 시술정보

시술시간	마취방법	입원여부	회복기간	체류기간
30분 ~1시간	수면, 국소마취	입원없음	7일	3~5일

▎두상 필러 시술

두상 모양 개선, 두상 볼륨 성형에 대한 요구는 많았던 부위다. 두상 필러는 두상 보형물 삽입과는 달리 비절개 방식으로 두상 어느 부위나 볼륨을 줄 수 있고, 일상생활로 복귀가 빠르며 보형물 수술이 주지 못하는 만족한 결과를 만들어 내고 있다.

두피 절개 후 본 시멘트 삽입을 하는 두상 보형물 수술 방법이 유일했지만, 두상 볼륨을 주는 데 한계가 있고, 절개를 한다는 측면에서 부담을 주었다. 하지만 이를 극복한 방법이 두상 필러다. 두개골 모양이 선천적으로 결함이 있거나, 뒤통수 등이 납작하여 콤플렉스를 느끼거나, 정수리, 측두부 등이 작아 얼굴이 커 보이는 경우에 두상필러가 적합하다.

대개 안면부의 황금 비율이 있는데, 이는 달걀을 세워 놓은 모양과 흡사하다. 달걀의 윗부분은 두상에 해당하며, 두상 볼륨이 전체적으로 좋아야 얼굴도 갸름하고 세련되게 보이는 것이다. 두상필러에 쓰이는 필러는 히알루론산 필러와 인체 유래 콜라겐 필러를 혼합해서 사용한다. 인체 유래 콜라겐 필러란 사후 인체 조직에서 추출하는 콜라겐을 원료로 한다. 또한 여기에 PRP를 혼합하여 필러 주변에 조직이 풍부하게 생성되도록 해 볼륨이 오래 유지되도록 한다.

두상 필러의 유지 기간은 3~5년 정도이다. 필러를 주입하는 층도 매우 중요한데, 안면부처럼 진피나 지방층에 주입하는 것이 아니고 근육층 아래와 뼈위쪽에 주입하는 것이 유지 기간도 길고, 혈관 침범이 없고, 모낭에 영향도 주지 않아 탈모 등의 부작용이 일어나지 않는다.

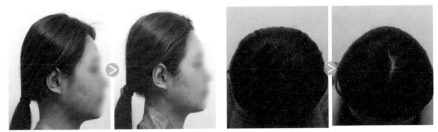

여성 뒤통수 두상필러 시술 전후_여성의 뒤통수가 볼륨이 나와서 예뻐 보이고 머리를 묶을 시 만족을 준다.

뒤통수의 볼륨을 만족스럽게 주려면 상부부터 하부까지 볼륨이 자연스럽게 나와야 한다. 특히 뒤통수 하부는 조직이 단단하여 필러로 볼륨 주기가 어렵다. 이를 극복하려면 필러 주입 시 기술과 경험이 중요하다. 뒤통수 상부만 볼륨이 나오고 하부는 볼륨이 안 생길 경우 만족도가 매우 떨어질 수 있다.

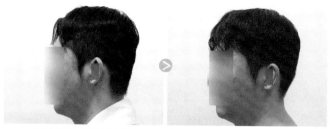

남성 뒤통수 전체 볼륨 증가 두상필러 전후, 특히 뒤통수 하부 볼륨 강조

측두부가 작아, 얼굴이 커 보이지만, 두상 필러후 두상 모양뿐만 아니라 얼굴도 작아보여 만족한 케이스이다.

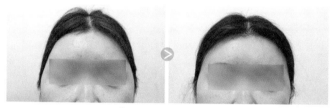

측두부 두상필러 시술 전후

이상적인 얼굴 황금비율은 1:1:0.8로 달걀을 세워 놓은 모양(Oval shape)인데, 달걀 윗부위가 두상에 해당되며, 두상볼륨이 좋아야 얼굴의 V라인이 돋보인다. 즉 정수리, 측두부, 이마 부위의 두상볼륨을 가져야 황금비율에 가깝게 된다. 아래 케이스는 하관과 턱이 길게 보이고 인상이 날카로운데, 정수리 측두부 이마에 볼륨을 풍족하게 주어서 하관이 길게 보이지 않고 인상이 부드럽고 세련되게 보인다.

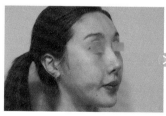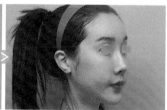

이마 정수리 측두부 두상필러 시술 전후

TIP_두상 필러 시술정보

시술시간	마취방법	입원여부	회복기간	체류기간
30분 전후	수면, 국소마취	입원없음	5일	3~5일

12

Non-surgical fillers, Fat graft removal & head filler

Diode Laser, a non-surgical method for removing foreign substances from fillers and transplanted fat

Many people have been getting approved fillers and fat transfers at hospitals for cosmetic purposes. Among them, some have received illegal, unauthorized procedures known colloquially as "Ya-mae"(a slang term derived from the Japanese word for illegal transactions). While some people think that side effects from fillers can be easily removed, it's far from a simple process.

Even with incision surgery, it is challenging to completely remove fillers, and it can even lead to complications such as dent. Fillers are formed by small pellets and if the procedure is unsatisfactory or unexpected side effects occur, a procedure to dissolve the fillers is necessary.

However, when some of these pellets are recognized as foreign substances, they transform into 'headaches.' Tissue changes like encapsulation and fibrosis make it difficult to effectively remove them through dissolving injections like hyaluronidase. Even incision removal surgery is not effective due to the foreign substance-induced tissue transformation. Diode laser technology has been developed to remove fillers without damaging tissues or leaving scars.

Non surgical filler removal

Diode laser was developed with the goal of removing facial fat without the need for surgery or incisions. However, it is also a non-surgical treatment method capable of removing foreign substance-transformed filler nodules and transplanted fat.

The primary purpose of fillers and fat transplantation is to restore volume, essential for improving the aged appearance. These procedures are used on various areas for aesthetic enhancement, even in younger individuals. However, a potential issue arises when the filler is recognized as a foreign substance, leading to the possibility of hypersensitivity reactions. Whether there is an immune response or not, immune cells can attach to filler particles and form a barrier, known as 'capsularization'.

During this process, chronic inflammation may occur, and excessive signals to treat it can lead to collagen overproduction in the surrounding area, termed fibrosis. Capsularization and fibrosis can repeat, causing tissue deformation, and if it progresses, it is called a granuloma. Some consider incision surgery for removal, but it is not always effective, and concerns about surgical scars and potential worsening of appearance after surgery cannot be ignored.

Diode laser Surgical Procedure

Diode Laser involves the emission of fiber optics from the main body, penetrating the skin to examine the area with granulomas. If experiencing filler complications, considering suction after Diode laser may be an option.

The Diode laser surgical procedure can be explained briefly as follows :

01 Use ultrasound examination to pre-determine the size and location of the granuloma.

02 Disrupt tissue transformations like capsularization and fibrosis, which hold the filler particles, with Diode laser, and suction externally for removal.

To successfully remove granulomas using fiber optics, technical expertise and extensive clinical experience are necessary. If considering surgery for foreign substance removal due to filler complications, it is crucial to prioritize skilled medical professionals and precise diagnostics. Experienced medical professionals with knowledge of foreign substance removal and extensive experience should accurately assess the condition of filler complications before removal.

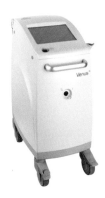

Diode laser

In the Diode laser equipment, fiber optics emerge, which are then inserted near the target area to examine the tissue with laser.

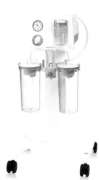

Medela Suction Device

Diode laser dismantles the encapsulation and fibrosis around the granuloma, and then, using the Medela suction device, suctions and removes it.

Tissue Reconstruction for Shape Recovery after Foreign Substance Removal

Finger Roll (Needle Shaping)

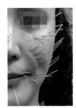

The restoration of the pre-filler procedure appearance is not automatic after removing filler granulomas or addressing fat transplantation side effects. To recover the shape, tissue reconstruction (Finger Roll) is necessary. Finger Roll utilizes equipment developed by GMV in Italy, aiming to restore collapsed collagen structures.

The procedure involves horizontally inserting a needle just below the skin's dermal layer. As the needle rotates in a state of direct current from the Needle Shaping device, collagen is generated, aiding in tissue recovery to achieve the pre-filler procedure appearance. Additionally, the fibrous tissues around the needle contract due to electrical forces, creating a lifting effect that tightens the skin. This process also increases skin volume, contributing to the restoration of the facial shape before filler complications.

Improvement Cases of Filler Complications by Diode laser in Various Areas

Presented are cases of improving tissue deformation, such as granulomas, which are common filler complications. High satisfaction is reported after removal procedures in areas such as the forehead, glabella, and cheeks.

Forehead Filler Granuloma

In cases where a defective product is encountered during the production process of hyaluronic acid filler, with an excessive formation of cross-linking, it can develop into a granuloma. To address such faulty structures, Diode laser is employed to dismantle and suction the problematic area for removal.

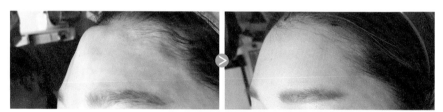

Before and After Diode laser Removal of Forehead Hyaluronic Acid Filler Granuloma

Glabella Tissue Deformation

Tissue deformation around the glabella, characterized by encapsulation and fibrosis, is effectively removed using Diode laser. Similarly, Diode laser is applied to suction and remove band formations causing tissue deformation after a semi-permanent filler procedure for neck wrinkles.

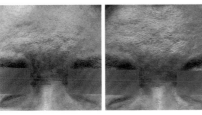

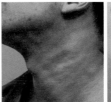
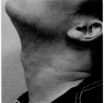

Before and After Removal of Semi-Permanent Filler Granuloma in the Glabella Area

Before and After Removal of Semi-Permanent Filler Granuloma in the Neck Wrinkle Area

Lip Filler Granuloma

In this case, the individual had received filler injections from an unauthorized practitioner (a.k.a. Ya-mae) a long time ago. Gradually, the granuloma grew, causing a noticeable enlargement of the entire lower lip, protruding outward. The solution involved using Diode laser for removal.

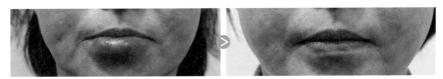

Before and After Removal of Semi-Permanent Filler Granuloma in the Lower Lip Area

Cheek Filler Granuloma & Tissue Reconstruction

On the right cheek, there was a semi-permanent filler granuloma, which was successfully removed with Diode laser. Subsequently, tissue reconstruction was

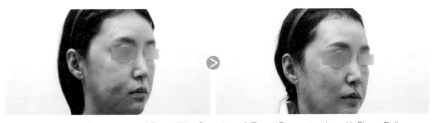

Before and After Removal of Cheek Filler Granuloma & Tissue Reconstruction with Finger Roll

performed using Needle Shaping (Finger Roll) treatment to restore facial shape to its pre-filler procedure state.

Bottom eyelid Filler Granuloma

After receiving hyaluronic acid filler injections for dimples a long time ago, the individual experienced gradual deformation of the bottom eyelid shape. Despite attempting hyaluronidase injections three times, minimal change occurred in the right bottom eyelid, and some melting occurred in the left bottom eyelid, but a portion near the eye corner remained. Dissatisfied, the individual discontinued hyaluronidase injections and opted for Diode laser removal. Given the delicate nature of the bottom eyelid area, precise technique is crucial for Diode laser removal.

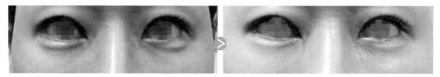

Case of bottom eyelid Filler Granuloma Removal with Diode laser

Nasal and Forehead Filler Granuloma

After undergoing nose surgery and being dissatisfied with the height, the individual opted to inject semi-permanent filler on top of a silicone implant to elevate the nose. However, due to an immune response, there were complaints of swelling, redness, and pain. After seeking medical attention and undergoing immune suppression therapy to eliminate inflammation, the semi-permanent filler was removed using Diode laser.

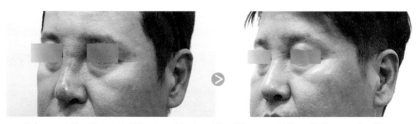

Before and After Removal of Nasal and Forehead Semi-Permanent Filler with Overreactive Response

Excessive Volume After Central Facial Fat Grafting

Following fat grafting to the cheeks, forehead, and temple areas, excess volume was reduced using Diode laser. Subsequently, the Finger Roll procedure was employed to restore the facial shape to its pre-fat grafting state.

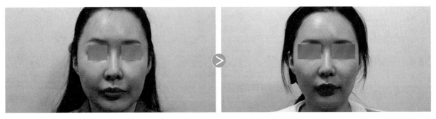

Before and After Removal of Grafted Fat and Shape Restoration with Finger Roll

TIP_Diode laser Procedure Information

Procedure Time	Anesthesia Method	Hospitalization	Recovery Period	Stay Duration
30 minutes to 1 hour	Sedation, Local Anesthesia	Hospitalization Not required	7 days	3~5 days

| Scalp volume augmentation

Head reshaping and volume enhancement have been areas with high demand. Unlike head implants involving scalp incisions, head fillers offer a non-invasive approach, providing volume to any head area. This method allows for a swift return to daily life and delivers satisfying results, especially when traditional implant surgeries fall short.

The traditional method involves an incision in the scalp, followed by cement insertion for cranial reshaping. However, this approach has limitations in providing volume to the cranial region, and the aspect of incisions poses concerns. Overcoming these challenges, head fillers present an effective solution.

They are suitable for cases where there are inherent flaws in the cranial shape, concerns about a flat occiput or other cranial features, causing a facial complex. Typically, achieving the golden ratio in the facial structure, akin to an upright egg, involves ensuring optimal cranial volume. The fillers used in cranial procedures are a combination of hyaluronic acid and collagen sourced from the human body. Additionally, the inclusion of Platelet-Rich Plasma (PRP) ensures rich tissue generation around the filler, contributing to long-lasting volume maintenance.

The duration of head filler effects typically lasts around 3 to 5 years. The injection depth is crucial, emphasizing injection below the muscle layer and toward the bone, providing extended duration, avoiding vascular invasion, and preventing complications like alopecia. In the case of a woman's head filler procedure enhancing volume in the occiput, satisfaction is derived from the visible volume that enhances the appearance when tying up the hair.

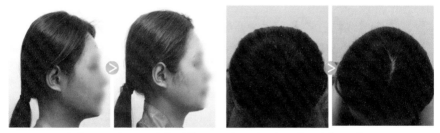

In the case of a woman's head filler procedure enhancing volume in the occiput, satisfaction is derived from the visible volume that enhances the appearance when tying up the hair.

Achieving satisfactory volume in the occiput involves ensuring a natural flow of volume from the upper to lower parts. Particularly challenging is the lower part of

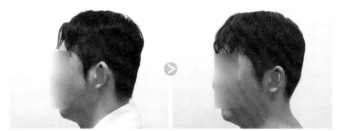

Enhanced Overall Volume in the Occiput for Men - Before and After Head Filler Procedure, Emphasizing Lower Occiput Volume

the occiput, with firm tissue making volume augmentation through fillers intricate. Overcoming this requires a skilled and experienced approach during filler injection. Dissatisfaction may arise if only the upper part of the occiput gains volume while the lower part lacks augmentation.

Small Temporal Region Making the Face Appear Larger; However, Satisfied with the Appearance of a Smaller Face After Heads Fillers

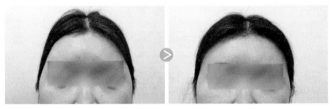

Side Temporal Region Head Filler Procedure - Before and After:

The ideal facial golden ratio is 1:1:0.8, resembling an oval shape with an upright egg. The upper part of the egg corresponds to the cranial region, and optimal cranial volume is crucial for highlighting the V-line of the face. In the presented case, where the lower face and jawline initially appeared elongated, giving a sharp impression, rich volume was strategically added to the forehead, temples, and the area around the crown. This resulted in a softened and sophisticated appearance, avoiding the elongated impression of the lower face.

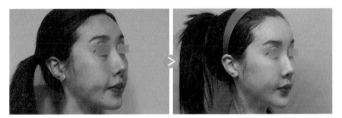

Forehead, Temple, Crown and Jawline, Head Filler Procedure - Before and After:

TIP_Diode laser Procedure Information

Procedure Time	Anesthesia Method	Hospitalization	Recovery Period	Stay Duration
30 minutes approximately	Sedation, Local Anesthesia	Hospitalization Not required	5 days	3~5 days

라미네이트(Laminates)
임플란트(Non-surgical implants)
치아교정(Orthodontics)

치아의 씹는 기능 회복 & 아름다운 미소,

자신감을 불어주는 심미치료

Restoration of chewing function of teeth Aesthetic treatment that gives you a beautiful smile and confidence

상실된 치아를 대신하는 임플란트를 비롯해 치아교정, 라미네이트 등의 시술이 기능적인 수복을 넘어 삶의 질까지 업그레이드해 주고 있다. 특히 내비게이션 임플란트는 통증 출혈이 적고 정확한 식립이 가능하다.

Procedures such as orthodontics and laminates, as well as implants to replace lost teeth, are not only restoring the function but also upgrading the quality of life. In particular, navigation implants have less pain and bleeding and can be placed accurately.

강남 임플라인치과
Gangnam Impline dentistry

www.impline.com

유종균(Jong-Gyun Yoo)

• 서울아산병원 의학대학원 구강외과 박사
(Doctor of Oral Surgery, Seoul Asan Medical Center Graduate School of Medicine)
• 대한치과교정학회 정회원(Regular member of the Korean Orthodontic Association)
• 대한임플란트학회 정회원(Regular member of the Korean Implantology Association)
• 하버드 치과대학 보철학 과정(Prosthodonics course in Havard school of dental medicine)
• 현) 임플라인 덴탈그룹 대표(now) Representative of Impline Dental Group)

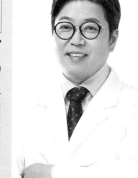

13 무삭제 라미네이트, 무절개 임플란트 치과 치료 새 패러다임 창조

기존 단점 극복한 교정장치와 임플란트

탈마스크 시대! 예전의 일상으로 돌아가 사람들과 밥을 먹고 여행을 즐기는 사람들. 특히 하늘길이 열리면서 해외 환자는 물론 고국을 찾아 미뤄왔던 치과 치료를 결심하는 사람들도 적지 않다. 치아는 대화할 때나 음식을 먹을 때 우리의 무의식 속에서 자연스럽게 노출되는 부분이다. 그만큼 입술이 열릴 때 보이는 치아의 모양은 상대방에게 보여지는 인상에 큰 작용을 한다.

그렇다면 내 치아에 적합하고 올바른 치료는 어떤 것들이 있을까? 앞니 모양을 개선하기 위해서는 크게 치아교정과 치아성형을 꼽을 수 있다. 치아교정은 치아의 손상 없이 자연적인 상태로 치아를 가지런하게 배열하는 방법이다. 치아에 손상이 없다는 장점이 있지만 치아에 교정장치를 붙여야 하고, 치료 시간이 길게 소요된다. 이러한 단점을 극복하기 위해 만들어진 것이 유라인(U-Line) 세라믹 브라켓으로 최소 내원 및 짧은 시간에 교정 마무리가 가능하다. 치아가 울퉁불퉁 튀어나오거나 변색된 앞니로 고민 주이시라면 라미네이트를 고려해 볼 수 있다. 임플란트는 다양한 이유로 손실된 치아를 인공치아로 대체하는 수술로써 시술 전 3D 컴퓨터 모의수술로 진단 및 수술과정을 예측해 절개 없이 안전하고 통증이 적은 시술이 가능하다. 몇 번의 방문만으로 시술이 가능해 외국에서 오신 분들에게 적합하다.

라미네이트

라미네이트는 치아시림 증상이나 신경에 관련한 많은 문제를 동반했던 것이 단점이다. 최근에는 치아를 삭제하지 않고 심미적 개선을 이루는 무삭제 방식의 라미네이트(제로믹)에 대한 관심이 높다.

라미네이트는 얇은 막 형태의 물질 일체를 지칭하는 것이고, 정확한 의학 용어는 '포셀린(자기류) 라미네이트(Porcelain Laminate) 시술'이다. 해외에서는 비니어(Veneers)라는 명칭이 보편화되어 있다.

라미네이트는 치아를 최소로 삭제하여 얇은 포셀린을 치아 앞면에 부착하는 치료로 심미치료 중 아주 짧은 시간 안에 치아의 모양, 크기, 색 등을 개선시킬 수 있다. 단, 치아를 많게는 0.7~1.0mm를 삭제해야 되는데, 이로 인해 치아 시린 증상 및 치아 내구도와 수명이 줄어들 수 있다. 이런 단점을 해소하기 위해 본 치과에서는 "제로믹"이란 무삭제 라미네이트를 개발하였다. 치아를 무삭제 또는 0.1mm 안팎의 최소 삭제를 통하여 치아시림 방지, 치아 내구도 강화, 수명연장, 탈락률 저하 등 단점을 극대화시킨 것이 장점이다.

그 결과 심미적인 아름다움을 더욱 중요시하는 외국인들로부터 인기다.

누런 치아(황니)를 라미네이트로 밝게 만든 케이스

치아미백으로는 한계가 있을 정도의 누런니를 가지고 있던 외국인 J 씨(35세)

치아 삭제 없이 무삭제로 진행했으며 치아색은 밝게 만들되 자연스러움을 주기 위해 치아의 팁부위는 투명하게 제작하였다.

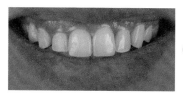 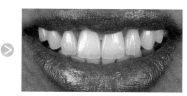

제로믹(무삭제 라미네이트) 시술전후.
4일간에 걸쳐 위아래 모두 16개 무삭제 라미네이트를 부착하였다.

치아우식(충치)으로 인한 레진 변색을 라미네이트로 밝게 만든 케이스

치아우식(충치) 치료 후 레진 변색으로 인하여 라미네이트 시술하였다. 불가피하게 0.1mm 내외로 치아 삭제를 통해 2차 우식 제거 및 변색 부위를 제거한 후 진행하였다. 추후 치아 변색 시 치아색이 비치지 않도록 라미네이트 안쪽에 얇은 흰 막을 입혀 밝은 톤을 유지하도록 하였다.

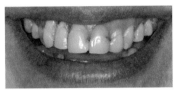 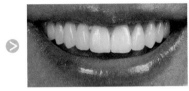

제로믹(무삭제라미네이트) 시술 전후. 3일 걸쳐, 10개의 무삭제 라미네이트를 부착하였다.

밝고 하얀 치아에 대한 니즈가 증가하면서 라미네이트 시술에 대한 관심이 높다. 하지만 라미네이트를 단순한 치료라고 생각하면 곤란하다. 개개인의 치아에 맞게 꼼꼼한 진단과 환자와의 많은 대화를 통해 원하는 부분을 최대치로 충족시켜야 함으로 매우 정밀한 치료이다.

또한 치아 신경이 예민한 사람이거나, 치아 삭제가 과도하게 이루어지는 경우엔 치아가 시리거나 통증을 느낄 수 있다. 치아의 바깥 부분만 접착하는 치료이므로 식습관도 탈락률을 매우 관여하므로 주의가 필요하다. 그러므로 라미네이트는 경험이 많고, 환자분의 원하는 부분을 충족시키는 치과를 선택하는 것이 중요하다.

TIP_라미네이트 수술 정보

수술시간	마취방법	입원여부	회복기간	내원 횟수	체류기간
30분	부분마취	없음	없음	2회	4일

▌무절개 임플란트

디지털, 무절개 임플란트는 잇몸절개 없이 임플란트만 2~3분 이내에 간단하고 빠르게 식립하는 방식으로 정확한 위치에 출혈 없이 심을 수 있다.

무절개 임플란트(Non-invasive Implant)란 기존의 방법과 달리 칼로 잇몸을 절개하지 않고 임플란트가 식립될 위치에 임플란트 픽스처 크기의 구멍을 뚫어 임플란트를 식립하는 술식이다.

잇몸을 열어 뼈를 노출하지 않아 출혈이나 통증에 대한 걱정을 덜 수 있어 회복 기간도 짧고 감염 위험도 상대적으로 낮다. 그렇다 보니 해외에 거주하시는 분, 멀리 지방에 살아 자주 치과 내원이 힘드신 분, 거동이 불편하신 분, 고령층, 당뇨나 고혈압이 있는 전신 질환을 앓고 있는 경우 고려해 볼 수 있다.

최근 임플라인 치과 강남본점에서 임플란트를 심고 미국으로 되돌아간 K 씨(80세)가 대표적 케이스다.

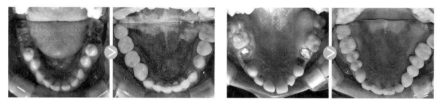

구치부 임플란트 수술전후

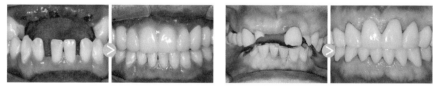

앞니 임플란트 수술전후

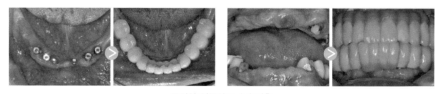

무치악 임플란트 수술전후

무절개 임플란트는 3D-CT 촬영과 3D 구강 스캐너 등 디지털 장비를 통해 신경 및 골조직을 미리 파악하고 정확하게 임플란트의 위치와 깊이를 정밀하게 계획할 수 있다. 수술 시간도 짧다. 임플란트 개당 수술 소요 시간이 빠르면 3분이라 한두 개의 임플란트는 하루 만에 치료를 모두 끝낼 수 있다.

시술 전 3D 컴퓨터 모의수술로 진단 및 수술과정을 예측해 절개 없이 안전하고 통증이 적은 시술이 가능하다. 몇 번의 방문만으로 시술이 가능해 외국에서 오신 분들에게 적합하다.

수술시간	마취방법	입원여부	회복기간	기간	체류기간
15~20분	부분마취	없음	2시간	1op 후 3개월 기다린 후 최종보철부착	1st-3day 2nd-4day

수술시간	마취방법	입원여부	회복기간	기간	체류기간
30~40분	부분마취	없음	3시간	1op 후 4개월 기디린 후 최종보철부착	1st 3day 2nd-4day

치아교정

기존 치아교정 장치의 단점을 극복하기 위해 만들어진 것이 유라인(U-Line) 세라믹 브라켓으로 최소 내원 및 짧은 시간에 교정 마무리가 가능하다.

일반적인 교정은 기간이 2~3년 간 걸리며, 매월 치과에 방문해야 하는 단점이 있다. 그 탓에 해외에 거주하시는 사람들의 경우 한국 교정의 우수성을 알면서도 쉽사리 교정을 할 엄두를 못하는 게 현실이다. 이러한 사람들을 위해 교정 기간이 짧고 병원 내원 횟수를 줄인 맞춤형 교정이 장치가 유라인(U-Line) 브라켓이다. 이 교정장치를 사용할 경우 교정 기간은 1년 미만이며, 내원 횟수는 4회로 교정을 끝낼 수 있다.

유라인 브라켓은 기존 교정 브라켓에 비해 굉장히 작고 투명해 치료 기간 중 눈에 잘 보이지 않는 장점이 있다. 또한 5~7개월의 비교적 짧은 기간에 교정 치

유라인 브라켓 부착 모습

료가 가능하며 환자의 상태에 따라 재교정이나 부분교정, 전체교정 등 다양한 범위의 치료를 빠르게 진행할 수 있다.

교정치료의 기본적인 정의는 치아들의 모양과 기능을 개선하기 위해 치아들을 움직이는 치료다. 즉 교정치료는 외모 개선뿐만 아니라 치아의 기능, 더 나아가 치아 자체의 보존 및 구강 건강을 위한 것이기도 하다.

앞니가 벌어진 경우

옛말에 '앞니가 벌어져 있으면 복이 새어 나간다'라는 말이 있다. 앞니는 사람의 인상에 있어서 가장 눈에 띄게 보이는 곳이기도 하다. 앞니가 벌어진 경우 발음이 부정확해지며, 말 또한 어눌해지게 진다. 또한 미관상 보기도 좋지 않다.

하지만 많은 분이 교정 자체를 어렵고 힘들게 생각하고 기간 또한 오래 걸릴 것으로 지레짐작하여 시도 조차 않으시는 분이 많은데, 꼭 그렇지가 않다. 앞니가 벌어진 교정 케이스 경우 내원 횟수가 많지 않고 짧은 기간 내에도 충분히 마무리 지을 수 있다.

1st _ 해외 거주 여성으로 치간이개(앞니 벌어짐)로 내원. 평소에 발음이 많이 세고 웃을 때 보이는 아랫니 사이에 빈공간이 콤플렉스였다. 진단 기간 6개월(3개월에 1회 내원 / 3회 완성)로 상담 후 교정을 시작! 첫 번째 치과 방문한 날 위아래 유라인 브라켓 장치 부착 후 14*14 Wire 착용 후 해외로 돌아갔다.

2nd _ 3개월 뒤 전반적 치아 레벨링(leveling)이 완성된 상태로 스페이스 클로징을 위해 교정용 파워체인(power chain)을 걸어 드리고 다시 해외로 돌아갔다.

3rd _ 6개월 뒤 내원 모습. 총 6개월 기간에 걸쳐 치아 레벨링은 완벽히 이루어 졌으며, 스페이스 클로징도 완벽하게 진행! 브라켓 제거 및 유지장치를 착용하고 마무리하였다.

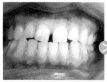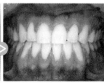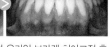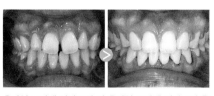

유라인 브라켓 치아교정 전 유라인 브라켓 치아교정 후 유라인 브라켓 치아교정 전 유라인 브라켓 치아교정 후

TIP_치아교정-유라인(U-Line) 브라켓 수술 정보					
교정기간	내원횟수	입원유무	회복기간	내원시 시간	일정
6개월	3회	없음	없음	1회 1시간, 2회 10분, 3회 1시간	각 1일

치열이 삐뚤빼뚤~ 덧니가 심한 크라우딩인 케이스

치열이 삐뚤빼뚤하면 양치가 잘되지 않아 치석이 많이 생기고, 잇몸 또한 고른 치아에 비해 빨리 안 좋아지게 되어 잇몸퇴축, 잇몸부음, 입냄새 등이 발현된다. 그라우딩이 심한 경우도 유라인 브라켓으로 짧은 시간과 최소 내원만으로 교정이 가능하다는걸 아래의 케이스로 알아본다.

1st _ 진단
치아들이 오밀조밀 모여드는 크라우딩(Crowding)으로 내원한 경우다. 크라우딩은 주로 앞니 쪽에 많이 존재하는데, 교정 진단 기간 8개월(2개월에 1회 내원 / 4회 완성)으로 상담 후 교정 진행 유라인 브라켓을 전체 부착 후 특수 와이어 삽입!

2nd _ 2월 후 치과 중간 체크, 크라우딩이 어느 정도 해소되었으며, 정밀함을 위해 굵은 특수와이어로 교체.

3rd _ 레벨링 완성. 완벽한 교합을 위해 고무줄 착용.

4th _ 총 8개월 기간에 걸쳐 치아가 가지런해지며, 교합도 완벽하게 진행! 브라켓 제거 및 유지장치를 착용하고 마무리함.

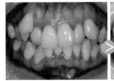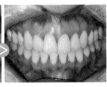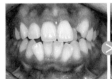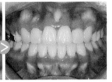

유라인 브라켓 치아교정 전 유라인 브라켓 치아교정 후　　유라인 브라켓 치아교정 전 유라인 브라켓 치아교정 후

TIP_치아교정-유라인(U-Line) 브라켓 수술 정보					
교정기간	내원횟수	입원유무	회복기간	내원시 시간	일정
8개월	4회	없음	없음	1회 1시간, 2회 10분, 3회 20분, 4회 1시간	각 1일

윗니가 아랫니를 과도하게 덮고 있거나 위아래 앞니 치아가 벌어진 케이스

개방교합은 어릴 적 손가락 빨기 및 혀내밀기 습관들로 많이 발생하는 케이스다. 과개교합은 앞니가 빨리 망가지는 원인이 되며, 인상 또한 답답한 이미지를 줄 수 있다. 이처럼 개방교합 및 과개교합도 유라인 브라켓을 이용하면 최소시간과 최소 내원으로 이를 해결해 줄 수 있다.

1st _ 진단
윗니와 아랫니가 제대로 맞물리지 못해 앞니가 떠 있는 형태의 개방교합(open-bite)과 윗니가 아랫니를 비정상적으로 많이 덮는 것을 과개교합으로 진단. 교정 진단 기간 8개월(2개월에 1회 내원 / 4회 완성)으로 상담 후 교정 진행. 유라인 브라켓을 전체 부착 및 특수와이어 삽입!

2nd _ 2개월 후 치과 중간 체크 및 굵은 특수와이어 교체 및 고무줄 착용.

3rd _ 교합 체크 및 고무줄 착용

4th _ 총 8개월 기간에 걸쳐 치아 교정 이루어 졌으며, 과개교합 및 개방교합이 완벽하게 정상교합으로 바뀜! 브라켓 제거 및 유지장치를 착용하고 마무리함.

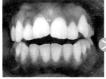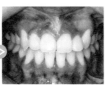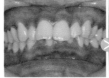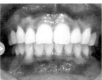

유라인 브라켓 치아교정 전 유라인 브라켓 치아교정 후   유라인 브라켓 치아교정 전 유라인 브라켓 치아교정 후

TIP_치아교정-유라인(U-Line) 브라켓 수술 정보					
교정기간	내원횟수	입원유무	회복기간	내원시 시간	일정
8개월	4회	없음	없음	1회 1시간, 2회 10분, 3회 10분, 4회 1시간	각 1일

다만 치아교정의 경우 평균적으로 기간이 2년 정도가 소요된다는 점과 교정 기간 동안 사용하는 교정장치는 오히려 심미적인 부분에서 부담이 될 수 있어 교정 치료를 망설이는 경우가 있는데, 이러한 단점을 극복한 장치가 유라인 브라켓이다. 앞으로도 지속적인 연구 개발과 새로운 술식으로 해외에 계시는 많은 분이 한국의 치아 교정의 혜택을 누릴 수 있도록 발전시켜 나가겠다.

13 Non-removal laminates, non-surgical implants... Creation of new paradigm in dentistry field.

Orthodontic devices and implants that overcome existing shortcomings

It's time to take off your mask! People are going back to their old daily lives. They enjoy eating and traveling with others. While there are foreigners who go on medical tourism to Seoul, there are people who decide to visit their home country Korea and get dental treatments that they have been putting off for a long time.

Teeth are a part that is naturally exposed in our daily life when talking or eating foods. The shape of the teeth that are visible when the lips are opened has a great influence on the impression given to others.

There are two major ways to improve the shape of your front teeth: orthodontics and tooth plastic surgery. Orthodontics is a method of aligning teeth in a natural position without damaging them. It has the advantage of not damaging the teeth, but requires the attachment of orthodontic appliances to the teeth and takes a long time to finish treatment. The U-Line ceramic bracket was created to overcome those shortcomings, allowing correction to be completed in a short amount of time and with minimal visits.

If you are annoyed from protruding or discolored front teeth, you may want to consider laminate. To address the shortcomings of existing laminates, there is also a non-removal laminate called "Zeromic". In addition, implant surgery, which replacing lost teeth by various reasons with artificial teeth, is also popular.

| Laminates

The downsides of laminate are that it is associated with many problems related to nerves and toothache. Recently, there is a lot of interest in non-removal laminate (Zeromic), which improves aesthetics without removing tooth structure.

Laminate refers to any material in the form of a thin film, and the correct medical term is 'Porcelain Laminate Treatment'. Abroad, the name Veneers is common.

Laminate is a treatment that removes the surface of tooth and attaches thin porcelain to the front of the teeth. During aesthetic treatment, the shape, size, and color of the teeth can be improved in a very short period of time. However, at most 0.7 to 1.0 mm of the tooth must be removed, which may cause symptoms of tooth sensitivity and reduce tooth durability and lifespan. To solve these shortcomings, our dental office developed a non-removal laminate called "Zeromic". It is extending lifespan through non-removal or minimal reduction of around 0.1 mm. Therefore, this minimizes problems of laminate such as toothache, sensitivity and maximizes the durability.

As a result, it is popular among foreigners who wants to improve their aesthetic beauty more.

A case of yellow teeth (yellow staining) patient are whitened with laminates (Zeromic)

Mr. J (35 years old), a foreigner who had yellow teeth which general whitening treatments are not worked enough.

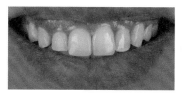 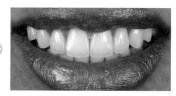

Before and after Zeromic (non-removal laminate) treatment. During the period of 4 days from first visit, 16 Zeromics were attached to both upper and lower.

The procedure was performed without any removal of teeth structure. Color of Zeromic is designed to be white when attached, but the tips of the Zeromic is made transparent to give a natural look to teeth.

A case of resin discoloration due to dental cavity (2nd caries) iswhitenedwith Zeromic

Laminate is performed due to resin discoloration after dental caries (cavities) treatment. Inevitably, the procedure was carried out after removing secondary caries and discoloration areas through tooth removal of approximately 0.1 mm. To prevent the teeth color change in case of teeth discoloration in the future, a thin white film was applied to the inside of the laminate to maintain a bright tone.

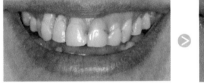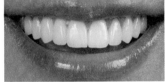

Before and after Zeromic (non-removal laminate) treatment. 3 days from first visit, 10 Zeromics were attached.

As the need for bright and white teeth increases, interest in laminate treatment is high. However, it is difficult to think of laminate as a simple treatment. It is a very precise treatment as it requires thorough diagnosis tailored to each individual's teeth and many conversations with a patient to meet the patient's needs as much as possible.

TIP_Laminate case information

Period of treatment	Anesthesia	Recovery period	Hospitalization	Number of visits	Length of stay
30 minutes	local aneathesia	None	No	2 visit	5 days

| Non-surgical implants

Non-surgical implant is a simple and quick way to install the implant within 2 to 3 minutes without making an incision in the gums, so they can be placed in the exact location with minimum bleeding.

Since the gums are not opened to expose the bone, there is less worry about bleeding or pain, so the recovery period is short and the risk of infection is relatively low. Therefore, it can be considered for those who live overseas, those who lives far away and having difficulty to visit the dentist frequently. Also who have difficulty moving, the elderly, or those suffering from systemic diseases such as diabetes or high blood pressure.

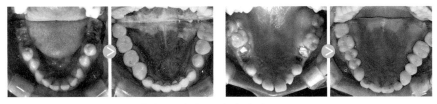

Before and after molar implant surgery

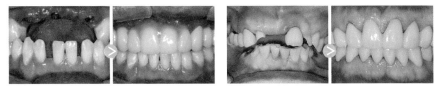

Before and after incisor implant surgery

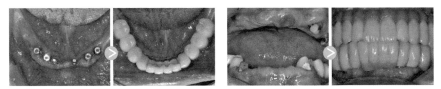

Before and after full case implant surgery

Non-surgical implants need to identify nerves and bone tissue in advance through digital equipment such as 3D-CT imaging and 3D intraoral scanners, and accurately plan the location and depth of the implant. The surgery time is also short. The surgery time for each implant is as fast as 3 minutes, so treatment for one or two implants can be completed in one day-single visit.

Period of treatment	Anesthesia	Recovery period	Number of visits	Residence in Country	Hos
15~20 minutes	Local anesthesia	2 hours	Final restoration delivery after 3months from surgery	1st. 3day 2nd. 4day	none

Period of treatment	Anesthesia	Recovery period	Number of visits	Residence in Country	Hos
30~40 minutes	Local anesthesia	3 hours	Final restoration delivery after 4months from surgery	1st. 3day 2nd. 4day	none

| Orthodontics

The U-Line ceramic bracket was created to overcome the shortcomings of existing orthodontic devices, allowing orthodontic treatments to be completed in a short period of time and with minimal visits.

Generally orthodontic treatment is considered to take 2 to 3 years to complete. And has the disadvantage of requiring monthly visits to the dentist.

Because of this, even though people living overseas knows the excellence of Korean orthodontics, they cannot easily get orthodontic treatment. Therefore, for those living overseas, we have developed an orthodontic device tailored to all ages with a short orthodontic period and fewer visits to the hospital.

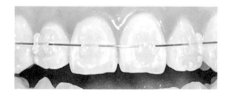

<Picture of U-line bracket attached>

U-Line brackets have the advantage of being much smaller and more transparent than existing orthodontic brackets, making them less visible during the treatment period. In addition, orthodontic treatment is possible in a relatively short period of 5 to 7 months, and a wide range of treatments such as re-orthodontic case, partial orthodontic case, or full orthodontic case can be performed quickly depending on the patient's condition.

The basic definition of orthodontic treatment is treatment that moves teeth to improve their position, angle and function. In other words, orthodontic treatment is not only for improving appearance, but also for the function of teeth, further preservation of the teeth themselves, and oral health.

In case of the front teeth are spaced apart (Diastema)

There is an old proverb in Korea saying that if your front teeth are wide open, your luck will leak away. The front teeth are very crucial part of a person's impression. If there is a space between front teeth, pronunciation becomes inaccurate and speech also becomes slurred. Also, it does not look good aesthetically. However, many people think that orthodontic treatment is difficult and will take a long time. So many people do not even try it, but this is not always true. In cases of correcting a space between front teeth, the number of visits is not that many and can be completed within a short period of time.

1st visit _ Visit with interdental diastema(frontteethspacing). The diagnosis period is 6 months (visiting once every 3 months /completed in 3 visits) and is started after consultation on the day of first visit. On the firstday of visiting the dentist, we attached upper and lower U-line orthodontic brackets and installed a special wire.

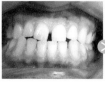 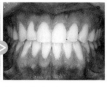 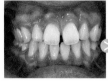 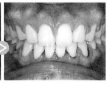

| Before orthodontic treatments done by U-line bracket | After orthodontic treatments done by U-line bracket | Before orthodontic treatments done by U-line bracket | After orthodontic treatments done by U-line bracket |

2nd visit _ 3months later, with over all tooth leveling complete, an orthodontic power chain is used to close the space.

3rd visit _ Teeth leveling was finished after a total period of 6 months, and space closing was also carried out perfectly! Treatment is completed by removing the bracket and delivering a retainer.

TIP_Orthodontic treatment. U-line bracket case information

Total period of treatment	Number of visits	Hospitalization	Healing period	Time taken for each visit	Recovery period
6 month	3 visit	No	None	1st 1H 2nd 10min 3rd 1H	1day each

In case of crooked teeth-severe crowding with snaggletooth

In the case of severe crowding, teeth cannot be brushed well, which leads to the formation of tartar, and the gums also deteriorate faster than aligned teeth. Causing gum recession, swollen gums and bad breath. We will show in the following cases that even in cases of severe crowding, Orthodontic treatments can be done with a U-line bracket in a short period of time and with a minimum visit to a dental office.

1st visit _ Diagnosis
This is a case where the teeth are crowded together due to lack of space(crowding). Crowding mainly exists on the front teeth, and orthodontic treatment is carried out after consultation with a diagnosis period of 8 months (visiting once every 2 months / completed in 4 visits). After attaching the entire U-line bracket, installed a special wire!

2nd visit _ After February, interim dental check-up, the crowding is somewhat resolved, and replaced with a thick special wire for precise adjustment.

3rd visit _ Leveling complete. Wearing an elastic band for perfect occlusion.

4th visit _ Over a total period of 8 months, teeth become aligned and molar teeth occludes perfectly! Completed by removing the bracket and delivering a retainer.

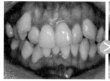
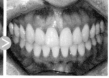
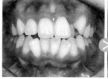
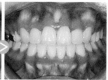

Before orthodontic treatments applying U-line bracket	After orthodontic treatments applying U-line bracket	Before orthodontic treatments applying U-line bracket	After orthodontic treatments applying U-line bracket

TIP_Orthodontic treatment. U-line bracket case information

Total period of treatment	Number of visits	Hospitalization	Healing period	Time taken for each visit	Recovery period
8 month	4 visit	No	None	1st 1H 2nd 10min 3rd 20min 4th 1H	1day each

Cases where the upper teeth excessively cover the lower teeth or the upper and lower front teeth are spaced apart

Openbite is a common case that occurs due to thumb sucking or tongue thrusting habits during childhood. Overbite causes the front teeth to break down quickly and can also give a frustrating image. Likewise, Openbite and overbite can be solved using U-line brackets in the minimum amount of time and visits.

Openbite is a term of the upper and lower teeth do not occlude properly, causing the front teeth to float. And the condition of upper teeth covering an abnormally large amount of the lower teeth is diagnosed as overbite.

1st visit _ Correction is carried out after consultation with an orthodontic diagnosis period of 8 months (visiting once every 2months/ completed in 4 visits). We attached U-linebrackets and installed special wire!

2nd visit _ After 2months, check-up at the dentist and replace into thick special wire and install a rubber band.

3rd visit _ Check occlusion and install elastic bands

4t visit _ Teeth correction was performed over a total period of 8 months, and overbite and open bite were completely changed to normal bite! Completed by removing brackets and delivering a retainer.

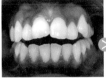 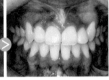 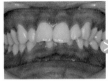 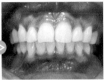

| Before orthodontic treatments applying U-line bracket | After orthodontic treatments applying U-line bracket | Before orthodontic treatments applying U-line bracket | After orthodontic treatments applying U-line bracket |

TIP_Orthodontic treatment. U-line bracket case information

Total period of treatment	Number of visits	Hospitalization	Healing period	Time taken for each visit	Period of residence
8month	4 visit	None	None	1st 1H 2nd 10min 3rd 10min 4th 1H	1day each

For someone who has malocclusion, it may difficult to chew foods well, which can lead to digestive problems, inaccurate pronunciation, and aesthetic satisfaction may be reduced. so active treatment is necessary. However, in the case of orthodontic treatment, it usually takes about 2 years on average and the orthodontic appliance used during the correction period can be rather burdensome in terms of aesthetics. Thus, many people hesitate to take orthodontic treatment. But these disadvantages can be overcome. The key device is the U-line bracket.

In the future, we will continue to develop and improve new techniques so that many people from abroad can take the benefits of Korean orthodontic treatment.

레이저여성성형수술(Laser female plastic surgery)

여성들이여, 출산 전으로 돌아가자!

Rediscover the joys of your pre-childbirth self and reclaim your fulfilling sex life with Vaginal Rejuvenation!

2001년 레이저질성형, 디자이너레이저여성성형, 레이저여성성형이라는 명칭을 사용하여 수술전문 병원으로 개원하였고, 현재까지 세계적으로 중국, 미국, 영국, 프랑스, 두바이, 아랍에미레이트, 독일, 이탈리아, 홍콩, 인도네시아, 싱가포르, 일본, 브라질, 아르헨티나, 러시아, 몽고, 키르키스탄 등 많은 환자들이 수술을 받고 있다.

Since its inception in 2001, our center has been at the forefront of innovative surgical technology, attracting patients from around the globe. Clients hailing from various countries.

리즈산부인과의원
RIZ Laser center

www.womanlaser.com

이형근(Hyung-Geun Lee)

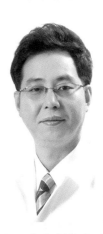

- 산부인과 전문의, 의학박사(M.D., Ph.D. , OB / GYN Specialist)
- 현, RIZ 네트워크 대표 이사(CEO, RIZ Network)
- 가톨릭대학교 의과대학 산부인과 조교수 역임
(Assistant professor, Catholic University Medical School OB/GYN department)
- 미국 베벌리힐스 앰뷸러티 수술 센터(Beverly Hills Ambulatory Surgery Center)
- 서울대학교 보건대학원 HPM 수료
(Completed Seoul National University Graduate School of Public Health HPM)

14 미인의 새로운 기준, 레이저여성성형!

질 노화 및 손상에 대한 관리, 개인맞춤형질관리치료시스템 PVT 개발

의학의 발전은 치료의학, 예방의학, 웰빙 의학으로 발전하여 인간의 수명을 100세 시대로 연장하고 있다. 모든 사람이 원하는 것은 수명연장과 더불어 건강하고 젊게 기능하면서 살아가는 것이다. 성생활은 순환을 활성화함으로써 심혈관 및 전신에 산소공급을 원활히 하여줌으로써 안티에이징에 큰 도움을 준다. 하지만 이러한 중요한 성생활에 걸림돌이 되는 것이 여성의 경우 질이완이다.

미혼의 경우 선천적이거나 다이어트, 운동 부족, 물렁살로 인해서 질 이완이 발생한다. 기혼의 경우 출산으로 인해 골반저근육의 손상으로 질 이완이 초래되기 때문에 질이완을 교정하지 않을 경우 사랑으로부터 멀어지거나, 급기야는 가정파탄에 이르는 게 현실이다. 또한 폐경 이후 질 이완은 골반장기탈출을 초래하여 생활의 질 뿐만 아니라 노령건강에 악영향을 미치므로 질 건강관리는 모든 여성이 필수적으로 신경 써야 하는 중요한 부분이다. 그리고 갱년기, 폐경을 맞이하면서 제일 많이 호소하는 증상이 질 건조증과 질 위축이다. 그래서 이러한 여러 문제점을 해결하기 위해서 수술적 방법 이외에 기능을 개선하고 질점막의 콜라겐을 생성함으로써 질의 탄력을 증진시키는 관리가 절실히 필요한 상태이다. 이에 이형근 박사가 출산 및 노화, 성생활, 질 건조증, 질 이완 등의 고민을 토로하는 여성들을 위해 PVT(Personal Vaginal Therapy)를 개발하였다.

레이저여성성형수술

레이저여성성형은 LVR(Laser Vaginal Rejuvenation · 레이저질성형수술), DLV(Designer Laser Vaginoplasty 디자인레이저여성성형수술 · 레이저소음순성형수술) 그리고 LMH(Laser Micro Hymenplasty · 레이저미세처녀막재생수술)로 나눌 수 있다.

LVR(Laser Vaginal Rejuvenation) : 레이저질성형수술

레이저질성형수술은 3가지로 표현할 수 있다.

- 출산 전 기능적인 질 구조로 되돌리는 수술
- 20~30대의 젊은 질구조로 되돌리는 수술
- 성적으로 매력 있는 여자로 태어나는 수술

레이저질성형은 선천적으로 이완되거나 출산을 통해 손상된 골반저근육을 기능적으로 재건하는 수술이다. 반면 이쁜이 수술은 늘어난 회음부(bulbocavenous, superficial perineal muscle)를 위쪽으로 올려주는 수술이다.

출산으로 인한 골반저근육의 손상

골반장기는 자궁, 방광, 직장으로 구성되어 있다. 이러한 골반장기가 중력에 의해서 밑으로 빠지는 것을 막기 위해 골반저근육이 골반장기를 받치고 있다. 골반저근육은 PR(puborectalis), PC(pubococcygeus), IC(Iliococcygeus) 근육으로 이루어져 있다. 임신말기에 자궁은 약 2천배 이상 커지며, 태아는 자궁경부가 10cm 열리고 얇은 IC 근육이 이완되면서 질 안쪽에 깊은 부분에 손상 없이 분만이 진행되지만, PC, PR 근육은 두꺼운 근육이므로 태아 머리가 통과할 경우 여러 방향으로 손상을 받게 된다. 그래서 회음절개를 시행하여 근육 손상을 최소화하지만, 급속분만이나 난산의 경우, 골반저근육의 손상은 피할 수가 없다. 그 밖에 만성 기침, 무서운 짐을 드는 것, 심한 운동, 나이, 비만 등도 골반근육을 늘어나게 하는 요인이 된다.

골반저근육의 손상은 요실금(incontinence), 질이완증후군(vaginal relaxation

syndrome)을 초래하며 직장탈(rectocele), 방광탈(cystocele), 자궁탈(prolapse uteri) 등 골반장기탈출증의 원인이 된다.

질이완증후군(Vaginal Relaxation Syndrome : VRS)은 질 입구나 질 안쪽을 감싸고 있는 골반저근육의 손상으로 탄력과 조여짐이 상실된 상태로 질염, 요실금, 질방

기존 수술과의 차이점

			WVR (웨이브질성형) (Wave, 3step Multilayer)	LVR (레이저질성형) (3step, 2layer)	P.P (이쁜이수술)
수술항목	일반	질점막박리술	○	○	○
		질근막박리술	○	○	○
		RVS 박리술 (Recto vaginal space)	○	○	○
	깊이	장 & PR / 장 & PC / 장 & IC / 근육박리술	All	장 & PR / 장 & PC 단계	장 & PR
		골반근육부위별 분리술 (PR, PC, IC)	All	장 & PC 단계	PR
	밀착력 탄력감 성감도	인대박리술	Ⅲ Positive	Ⅰ Positive	X
		신경차단술 (pudendal)	Ⅲ Positive	Ⅰ Positive	X
		혈관차단술	Ⅲ Positive	Ⅰ Positive	X
		인대성형술	Ⅲ Positive	Ⅰ Positive	X
		혈관성형술	Ⅲ Positive	Ⅰ Positive	X
	구조 변경	Pelvic diaphragm 재건술 (PD. reconstruction)	○	○	X
		PR / PC / IC / 근육거상술 (P.muscle elevation)	All	PR / PC 단계	PR
		PR / PC / IC / 근육성형술 (R-spot 성형술)	All	PR / PC 단계	PR
	자극	(PR) R-ring 성형술 (R-ring plasty)	○	X	X
		Wave 질점막성형술 (Vaginal mucosal plasty)	○	X	X

귀, 골반장기탈출증, 성감저하, 성관계 불만족을 초래하므로 치료가 필요한 질환이다.

RIZ vaginal relaxation Grading System

- Grade 1 : 골반압력 검사 정상
- Grade 2 : 1/3 정도의 질 이완, 골반 압력 경도 저하
- Grade 3 : 2/3 정도의 질 이완, 경도의 직장탈, 골반 압력중등도 저하
- Grade 4 : 완전한 질이완, 중등도의 직장탈, 골반압력 고도 저하
- Grade 5 : 요실금과 동반된 골반이완

		WVR (웨이브질성형) (Wave, 3step Multilayer)	LVR (레이저질성형) (3step, 2layer)	P.P (이쁜이수술)
수술내용	마취과	○	○	X
	다이오드레이저	○	○	X
	Step / layer	Multy	3~2	질 입구
	T.F.O	○	X	X
	Wave	○	X	X
	R-ring	○	X	X
	R-Spot	○	X	X
수술후효과	이완율	없음	낮음	높음
	흉터	X	X	○
	통증	△	△	○
	긴장성 요실금 개선	○	△	X
	변비 개선	○	△	X
	힙업(hipup) 효과	○	△	X
	직장탈(rectal prolapse) 예방	○	X	X
	탈자궁(Prolapse ut.) 예방	○	X	X
	치질 개선	○	X	X
	변실금 예방	○	X	X
	교감성	Ⅲ Positive	Ⅰ positive	X
	탄력성	Ⅲ Positive	Ⅰ positive	X
	성감도	Ⅲ Positive	Ⅰ positive	X
	파트너 성감도	Ⅲ Positive	Ⅰ positive	X
	kegel exercise(골반근육운동)	X	X	○

LVR 수술의 종류

- PP(Posterior Perineoplasty) : 이쁜이수술
- Petit(Miss) Laser Vaginal Rejuvenation : 쁘띠(미스) 레이저 질성형수술
- Miss Laser Vaginal Rejuvenation : 미스 레이저 질성형수술
- Laser Vaginal Rejuvenation : 레이저 질성형수술
- Wave Vaginal Rejuvenation : 웨이브 질성형수술

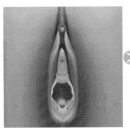

LVR 수술 전   LVR 수술 후

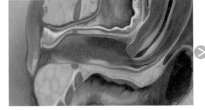 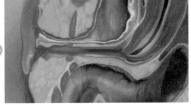

LVR 수술 전   LVR 수술 후

TIP_LVR 수술정보

수술시간	마취방법	입원여부	회복기간	체류기간
1시간 30분	수면마취	입원없음	45~60일	3~5일

DLV(Designer Laser Vaginoplasty) : 디자인레이저여성성형수술(레이저소음순성형수술)

소음순비대를 가지고 있는 대부분의 여성들은 옷에 끼거나 관계 시 말려들어 가는 불편을 호소하고 있으며, 소음순 사이에 끼어 있는 세균에 의한 질염을 유발하게 된다. 또한 모양, 색깔에 대한 고민, 자신감 결여로 성관계 시 문제점을 호소하고 있다. 그래서 소음순의 모양을 편하고 위생적이며 아름답게 성형하는 것이 DLV이다.

RIZ labia minor hypertrophy Grading System

- Grade 1 : 정상
- Grade 2 : 소음순 늘어남

  2a_ 한쪽의 이상(unilateral) / 2b_ 양쪽의 이상(bilateral) / 2c_ 두터워진 형태(lipodystophy)
- Grade 3 : 소음순 늘어남을 동반한 클리토리스 주변 비대

  3a_ 한쪽의 이상(unilateral) / 3b_ 양쪽의 이상(bilateral) / 3c_ 두터워진 형태(lipodystophy)
- Grade 4 : 소음순 늘어남을 동반한 소음순 비후 혹은 음순 후대의 비후

  4a_ 한쪽의 이상(unilateral) / 4b_ 양쪽의 이상(bilateral) / 4c_ 두터워진 형태(lipodystophy)
- Grade 5 : 소음순 늘어남, 비후, 클리토리스 주변 비대를 모두 가진 형태, 소음순 기형

  5a_ 한쪽의 이상(unilateral) / 5b_ 양쪽의 이상(bilateral) / 5c_ 두터워진 형태(lipodystophy)

기존 수술과의 차이점

기존 소음순절제술은 비후된 소음순을 절제하여 크기를 줄여주는 간단한 수술이라 한다면 레이저소음순성형수술은 비후되거나 기형화된 소음순을 아름다운 원하는 모양으로 조각하는 수술이다. 기존 소음순 절제술은 단순히 잘라내는 시술로 출혈의 부담 때문에 미용 성형이 거의 불가능하였다. 이러한 한계를 극복하기 위해 새롭게 고안된 레이저소음순성형수술은 레이저를 이용하여 출혈 및 통증이 거의 없고, 수술의 흔적이 남지 않는다. 그리고 나이프나 가위로는 곡선과 두

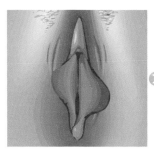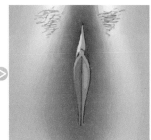

DLV 수술 전   DLV 수술 후

TIP_DLV 수술정보

수술시간	마취방법	입원여부	회복기간	체류기간
1~3시간	수면마취	입원없음	25~60일	1일

께조절이 불가능하기 때문에 날렵하고 원하는 모양을 디자인할 수 없었다. 하지만 surgical laser를 이용하면 곡선의 아름다움을 살릴 수 있으며 두께조절이 용이하므로 소음순을 아름다운 모양으로 성형할 수 있게 되었다. 레이저미세지방제거술, 레이저주름제거술 등의 시술을 동반하여 보다 날렵하고 예쁜 모양의 소음순으로 성형할 수 있다.

LMH(Laser Micro Hymenplasty) : 레이저미세처녀막재생수술

처녀막은 질 입구 초입을 감싸고 있는 얇은 조직이며 첫 관계 시 혈흔이 발생하므로 처녀성을 입증하는 상징성을 가지고 있다. 나라마다 처녀막의 의미 부여를 달리하고 있는데, 일부 나라에서는 결혼 전 지켜야 할 가장 중요한 가치로 인정하고 있다. LMH는 손상된 처녀막을 손상되기 전의 상태로 레이저로 재생시켜 주는 수술로 리즈(RIZ) 방법으로 수술을 할 경우 99% 이상 첫날 밤에 혈흔을 확인할 수 있다.

RIZ hymenal rupture Grading System

- Grade 1 : 처녀막 손상 없음
- Grade 2 : 경도 혹은 중등도의 처녀막 파열
- Grade 3 : 심한 처녀막 파열 혹은 경도의 질 손상
- Grade 4 : 처녀막 파열과 심한 질 손상
- Grade 5 : 3시나 9시 방향으로의 처녀막 파열 또는 처녀막을 이루는 링이 늘어나 있으며, 전체적으로 질 입구가 늘어난 형태, 처녀막 기형

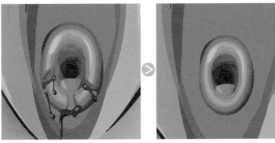

LMH 수술 전   LMH 수술 후

PVT(Personal Vaginal Training) : 개인맞춤형질관리시스템

이형근 박사가 레이저를 산부인과 영역에 처음으로 도입하여, 수많은 레이저수술 데이터를 축적하고 그것을 바탕으로 비수술적으로 질이완을 교정하는 새롭게 개발된 개인맞춤형질관리치료시스템이다.

최근에는 수술해야 할 환자들의 경우 수술 전에 개인맞춤형질관리치료시스템을 먼저 받으시고 수술을 할 경우 수술 후 효과가 더욱 높아진다. 리즈레이저센터에서는 8년 전부터 개인맞춤형질관리치료시스템을 수술 전에 실행한 결과, 수술하지 않으시고 개인맞춤형질관리치료시스템만 받으시면서 행복하게 생활하시는 분들이 80% 이상 늘어가고 있어서 무척 고무적이다.

그 개인맞춤형질관리치료시스템의 핵심은 VLT이며, VLT(vaginal laser tightening)는 특수하게 고안된 레이저나 고주파, 초음파 등을 이용하여 질 점막에 노후 된 콜라겐을 없애고 새로운 콜라겐을 형성하여 질 점막에 탄력을 불어넣는 프로그램이다. 또한 저주파바이오피드백(RadioFrequency Vaginal BioFeedback)을 통해 골반저근육의 강화와 수축력을 증대시킴으로써 질의 민감도와 탄력개선에 큰 도움을 준다. VLT는 질을 타이트하게 변화시킬 뿐만 아니라, 긴장성 요실금, 만성 질염, 방광염의 증상 완화에도 도움을 주고, 그 외로 질 방귀, 불감증, 질 건조, 질위축에도 탁월한 효과가 있다.

특히 갱년기, 폐경을 맞이하시는 여성들의 경우, 갱년기, 폐경 이후의 삶이 40~50년 이상 남아 있으므로 여성으로 행복한 삶을 영위하기 위해서는 개인맞춤형질관리치료시스템이 필수항목이다.

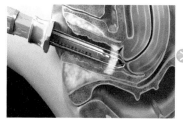 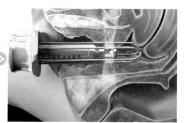

VLT 시술 전   VLT 시술 후

14 Rediscover the joys of your pre-childbirth

RIZ Cosmetic Laser Vaginal Surgery Center

RIZ Cosmetic Laser Vaginal Surgery Center is a distinguished OB/GYN clinic with a primary focus on Vaginoplasty, a specialized surgical procedure. Renowned for its exceptional medical services, RIZ Cosmetic Laser Vaginal Surgery Center has consistently delivered the highest quality surgical treatments, including Laser Vaginal Rejuvenation, Designer Laser Vaginoplasty, and Cosmetic Laser Vaginal Surgery.

Since its inception in 2001, Clients hailing from various countries, such as China, the UK, France, Dubai, the UAE, Germany, Italy, Hong Kong, Indonesia, Singapore, Japan, Brazil, Argentina, Russia, and Mongolia. Discover the transformative wonders of RIZ Cosmetic Laser Vaginal Surgery Center, an esteemed OB/GYN clinic specializing in cutting-edge Vaginoplasty procedures. Elevate your confidence and embrace a new level of intimate well-being with our signature treatments, including Laser Vaginal Rejuvenation, Designer Laser Vaginoplasty, and Cosmetic Laser Vaginal Surgery.

Rediscover the essence of feminine vitality with our transformative Vaginal Rejuvenation services! Regain the confidence and intimacy you deserve as we take you back to pre-childbirth days. Unleash the full potential of your sex life with our specialized treatments tailored to empower and revitalize. Join countless satisfied women who have experienced the life-changing benefits of our renowned Vaginal Rejuvenation procedures. Embrace a new chapter of enhanced sensuality and intimate well-being.

| Cosmetic Laser Vaginal Surgery

Cosmetic Laser Vaginal Surgery can be divided into LVR, DLV, and LMH.

LVR(Laser Vaginal Rejuvenation)

Laser Vaginal Rejuvenation is a surgical procedure designed to address various aspects of vaginal health and well-being:

1. Restorative Vaginal Surgery: Surgical interventions aimed at restoring functional vaginal structures to their pre-childbirth state. These procedures are intended to enhance overall vaginal functionality and address any issues that may have arisen due to childbirth.

2. Aesthetic Vaginal Surgery: Surgical treatments are tailored to recreate youthful vaginal structures typically associated with women in their 20s and 30s. The objective is to improve the aesthetic appearance of the vaginal area, offering a renewed sense of confidence and femininity.

3. Sexual Well-being Enhancement: Laser Vaginal Rejuvenation also includes procedures intended to contribute to a woman's sense of sexual attractiveness and fulfillment. While these procedures focus on sexual well-being, it is essential to prioritize the individual's physical and emotional health in the process.

At RIZ Cosmetic Laser Vaginal Surgery Center, we offer personalized solutions under each of these categories, ensuring that our patients receive the care and attention that aligns with their unique needs and aspirations. Our commitment to safety, expertise, and compassionate care makes us a trusted destination for women seeking to improve their intimate well-being through Laser Vaginal Rejuvenation procedures. Laser Vaginal Rejuvenation is a surgical procedure aimed at functionally reconstructing pelvic floor muscles that may naturally relax or sustain damage during childbirth.

Conversely, General Vaginal Rejuvenation involves an operation that elevates the perineal region, including the bulbocavernosus and superficial perineal muscles. Both procedures are designed to address specific concerns related to vaginal health and well-being, offering tailored solutions to meet individual needs.

Childbirth-related damage to the pelvic floor muscles can lead to various conditions.

The pelvic floor muscles play a vital role in supporting the pelvic organs, including the uterus, bladder, and rectum, preventing them from descending due to gravity. These muscles encompass the PR (puborectalis), PC (pubococcygeus), and IC (iliococcygeus) muscles.

During pregnancy, the uterus undergoes significant growth, up to 2000 times its original size, and during delivery, the fetus is expelled without damage to the deep part of the vagina as the cervix dilates by 10cm and the thin IC muscle relaxes.

Differences from Traditional Surgery (Chart)

			WVR (Wave Vaginal Rejuvenation) (Wave, 3step Multilayer)	LVR (Laser Vaginal Rejuvenation) (3step, 2layer)	P.P (Posterior Perineoplasty)
Surgical category	General	vaginal mucosal delamination plasty	○	○	○
		vaginal myofascial delamination plasty	○	○	○
		Recto vaginal space	○	○	○
	depth	intestines & PR / intestines & PC / intestines & IC / Muscle delamination plasty	All	intestines&PR/ intestines& PC step	intestines&PR
		PR, PC, IC	All	PR / PC step	PR
	adhesion sense of	ligament delamination plasty	III Positive	I Positive	X
		pudendal	III Positive	I Positive	X
	elasticity	blood vessel block plasty	III Positive	I Positive	X
	sexual pleasure	ligament plasty	III Positive	I Positive	X
		angioplasty	III Positive	I Positive	X
	Structural change	Pelvic diaphragm reconstruction	○	○	X
		PR / PC / IC / P.muscle elevation	All	PR / PC step	PR
		PR / PC / IC / R-spot cosmetic surgery	All	PR / PC step	PR
	stimulus	(PR) R-ring plasty	○	X	X
		Wave Vaginal mucosal plasty	○	X	X

However, the PC and PR muscles, being thicker muscles, are susceptible to damage during the passage of the fetal head, leading to perineal incisions being performed to minimize muscle damage. In cases of rapid or forceful delivery, damage to the pelvic floor muscles becomes unavoidable.

Moreover, factors such as chronic coughing, heavy lifting, intense physical activities, aging, and obesity can also contribute to the stretching and drooping of pelvic muscles.

		WVR (Wave Vaginal Rejuvenation) (Wave, 3step Multilayer)	LVR (Laser Vaginal Rejuvenation) (3step, 2layer)	P.P (Posterior Perineoplasty)
details of the operation	anesthesiology unit	○	○	X
	Laser diode	○	○	X
	Step / layer	Multy	3~2	entrance to the vagina
	T.F.O	○	X	X
	Wave	○	X	X
	R-ring	○	X	X
	R-Spot	○	X	X
postoperative effect	relaxation rate	None	Low	High
	Scar	X	X	○
	Pain	△	△	○
	Improved tension incontinence	○	△	X
	improvement of constipation	○	△	X
	hipup effect	○	△	X
	rectal prolapse Prevention	○	X	X
	Prolapse ut. Prevention	○	X	X
	improvement of hemorrhoids	○	X	X
	fecal incontinence prevention	○	X	X
	associability	III Positive	I positive	X
	Elasticity	III Positive	I positive	X
	sexual pleasure	III Positive	I positive	X
	Partner's sexual pleasure	III Positive	I positive	X
	kegel exercise	X	X	○

Damage to the pelvic floor muscles can result in conditions like incontinence and Vaginal Relaxation Syndrome (VRS). VRS is a significant concern as it can lead to vaginitis, urinary incontinence, vaginal flatulence, pelvic organ prolapse, decreased sexual sensitivity, and sexual dissatisfaction due to damage to the pelvic floor muscles surrounding the entrance or interior of the vagina.

Addressing these issues through specialized treatments like Laser Vaginal Rejuvenation can offer effective solutions to improve the quality of life and intimate well-being. At RIZ Cosmetic Laser Vaginal Surgery Center, our skilled team utilizes state-of-the-art techniques to address pelvic floor concerns, providing compassionate care and comprehensive support to each patient's unique needs.

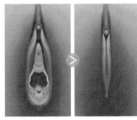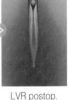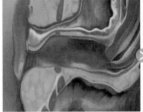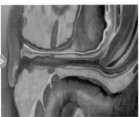

LVR preop.   LVR postop.   LVR preop.   LVR postop.

TIP_LVR(Laser Vaginal Rejuvenation) information

Procedure Time	Anesthetizing method	Hospitalization	Recovery Period	Length of Stay
1hour 30min	Sleep anesthesia	No Hospitalization	45~60 days	3~5 days

RIZ vaginal relaxation Grading System

• Grade 1 : normal   • Grade 2 : low vaginal relaxation
• Grade 3 : mid vaginal relaxation or low rectocele
• Grade 4 : high vaginal relaxation or mid rectocele)
• Grade 5 : Grade 3 or 4 combined with cystocele or stress incontinence

Types of LVR Surgery

• PP(Posterior Perineoplasty)   • Puborectalis Muscle Reconstruction
• Petit Laser Vaginal Rejuvenation   • Miss Laser Vaginal Rejuvenation

• Laser Vaginal Rejuvenation
• Wave Vaginal Rejuvenation

DLV (Designer Laser Vaginoplasty) : Labia minora Laser Cosmetic Surgery

Many women facing Labia minora hypertrophy often express discomfort due to its interference with clothing and the tendency to become displaced during sexual activity.

Additionally, this condition can lead to vaginitis, resulting from bacteria becoming trapped between the Labia minora. Furthermore, issues concerning the appearance, color, and self-confidence can arise, impacting sexual experiences adversely.

Designer Laser Vaginoplasty (DLV) offers a transformative solution, aimed at enhancing the shape of the Labia minora to achieve optimal comfort, hygiene, and aesthetic appeal. By utilizing advanced surgical techniques and laser technology, DLV ensures precise and personalized results, catering to the unique needs of each individual. At RIZ Cosmetic Laser Vaginal Surgery Center, we understand the importance of both physical and emotional well-being. Our expert team is dedicated to providing exceptional care, guiding our patients towards renewed confidence and intimate satisfaction. Join us in the journey to rediscover your self-assurance and embrace the beauty of being you with DLV

RIZ labia minor hypertrophy Grading System

• Grade 1 : noraml range
• Grade 2 : labia minora hypertrophy
        2a – unilateral / 2b - bilateral / 2c - lipodystophy
• Grade 3 : grade 2 + clitoris crus area hypertrophy
        3a - unilateral / 3b - bilateral / 3c -lipodystophy
• Grade 4 : grade 2 + fourchette hypertrophy or lipodystrophy
        4a - unilateral / 4b - bilateral / 4c - lipodystophy
• Grade 5 : grade 3 + grade 4, anomaly of labia minora
        5a – unilateral / 5b - bilateral / 5c - lipodystophy

Distinguishing itself from conventional surgery, RIZ's Laser Labia minora Cosmetic Surgery offers a superior approach to achieving desired outcomes.

While conventional labia minora resection focuses on simple size reduction by removing thickened tissue, our advanced Laser Cosmetic Surgery takes it a step further, expertly sculpting large and thickened labia minora into a beautifully desired shape.

In the past, conventional labia minora resection presented challenges due to the risk of bleeding, making it less feasible. However, our innovatively designed Labia minora Laser Cosmetic Surgery overcomes these limitations by utilizing a laser technique, minimizing bleeding and discomfort while leaving no visible scars. This cutting-edge method allows for precise curvature adjustments, resulting in stunning and natural-looking outcomes.

At RIZ Cosmetic Laser Vaginal Surgery Center, we employ state-of-the-art procedures such as laser microfat removal and laser wrinkle removal in tandem with Labia minora Laser Cosmetic Surgery, achieving sleeker and more aesthetically appealing results.

Our commitment to delivering exceptional surgical solutions ensures that each patient experiences the highest level of care and satisfaction, as we prioritize their well-being and self-confidence throughout the entire process. Embrace the transformative possibilities with our expert team and discover the beauty of a revitalized and sculpted labia minora.

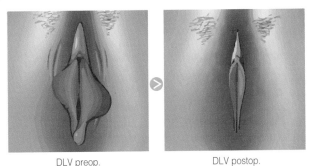

DLV preop.   DLV postop.

TIP_DVL(Laser Labia Minora Surgery) information

Procedure Time	Anesthetizing method	Hospitalization	Recovery Period	Length of Stay
1~3 hour	Sleep anesthesia	No Hospitalization	25~60 days	1 day

LMH (Laser Micro Hymenplasty)

The hymen, or virgin membrane, is a delicate tissue encircling the vaginal entrance, historically regarded as a symbol of virginity due to the occurrence of blood stains during the first sexual encounter. The significance attributed to the hymen varies across different cultures, with some countries considering it a fundamental virtue to preserve until marriage. LMH (Laser Membrane Hymenoplasty) is a sophisticated procedure that utilizes laser technology to regenerate the hymen, restoring it before any damage occurs. With the RIZ method, this surgical technique ensures that blood traces can be identified in over 99% of cases during the first night after the surgery.

RIZ hymenal rupture Grading System

- Grade 1 : hymenal ring intact
- Grade 2 : mild to moderate hymen ring rupture
- Grade 3 : severe hymen ring rupture or mild vaginal wall laceration
- Grade 4 : hymen ring rupture and moderate or severe vaginal wall laceration
- Grade 5 : 3 or/and 9 o'clock hymenal ring rupture and vaginal wall laceration or hymen intact but hymenal ring relaxation and introitus relaxation/ hymen anomaly

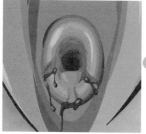

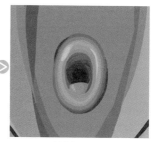

LMH preop.   LMH postop.

PVT(Personal Vaginal Therapy)

For married women, vaginal relaxation often results from pelvic floor muscle damage during childbirth, potentially impacting their sexual satisfaction and marital relationship if left untreated. Moreover, post-menopausal vaginal relaxation can lead to pelvic organ prolapse, adversely affecting both quality of life and overall health during old age. Consequently, vaginal health care becomes an essential aspect requiring attention from all women. Climecteric and post-menopause commonly present symptoms like vaginal dryness and vaginal atrophy, further emphasizing the need for comprehensive solutions.

In response to these various challenges, Dr. Lee Hyung-geun has developed Personal Vaginal Therapy (PVT) based on his extensive clinical expertise. Alongside surgical methods, PVT focuses on improving vaginal function and stimulating collagen production in the vaginal mucosa to enhance vaginal elasticity.

What is Personal Vaginal Therapy (PVT)?

Dr. Lee Hyung-geun is credited with pioneering the introduction of laser techniques in the field of Obstetrics and Gynecology, drawing upon an extensive wealth of data from numerous laser surgeries. As part of a comprehensive approach, PVT (Personal Vaginal Therapy) is thoughtfully performed prior to surgery for patients who have recently undergone or are planning to undergo surgical procedures.

At the core of PVT lies VLT (Vaginal Laser Tightening), a specialized program that skillfully employs specially designed lasers, Radio-frequency technologies, and ultrasound to remove old collagen from the vaginal mucosa and stimulate the formation of new collagen. The outcome is heightened elasticity within the vaginal mucosa. Additionally, the implementation of VBF (Vaginal BioFeedback) works to strengthen pelvic floor muscles and augment their contraction, significantly enhancing sensitivity and elasticity.

Beyond enhancing tightness, VLT serves as a comprehensive solution, effectively alleviating symptoms associated with stress urinary incontinence, chronic vaginal inflammation, and cystitis. Moreover, it proves highly effective in addressing issues like vaginal farts, insensitivity, vaginal dryness, and vaginal atrophy. Notably, for women experiencing menopause, PVT emerges as an indispensable element in fostering a happy and fulfilling life, considering that life after menopause and climecteric may span more than 40~50 years.

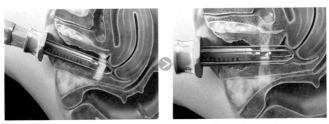

VLT pre procedure   VLT post procedure

여드름 & 여드름 흉터(Acne, Acne Scars)
과다색소침착(기미, 흑자) (Hyperpigmentation)
모공확장증(Enlarged Pores)
피부처짐 레이저 치료(Skin sagging laser treatment)

젊고 우아한 아름다움으로 나이 드는 비결 :

피부가 스펙이다

The secret to aging gracefully and maintaining youthful elegance lies in your skin condition

사람마다의 고유한 피부 특징과 문제점을 진단하여 그에 맞는 치료와 관리를 해주었을 때 개선 효과가 극대화될 수 있다.

Achieving the best results involves diagnosing individual skin characteristics and tailoring treatment accordingly.

청담은피부과의원
Eun Skin Clinic

www.eunskin.com

김태은(Tae-Eun Kim)

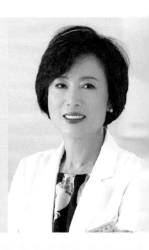

• 피부과 전문의, 의학박사(Dermatologist, PhD in Medicine)
• (전)대한피부과 의사회 부회장(Former Vice President of the Association of Korean Dermatologists)
• (전)피부과 여의사회 회장(Former President of the Association of Korean Female Dermatologists)
• (전)성균관대학 외래 부교수, (현)이화여자대학 외래 부교수, 순천향대학 피부과 외래 부교수
(Former Associate Professor at the Department of Dermatology at Sungkyunkwan University School of
Medicine, Current Associate Professor at the Department of Dermatology at Ewha Womans University
College of Medicine and Soonchunhyang University)

15 피부 속과 겉을 치유하는 메디칼 스킨케어

젊고 아름다운 피부, 치료와 미용 관리의 접목인 메디칼 스킨케어

동서고금, 남녀노소, 지역의 구분 없이 누구나 아름답고 젊게 보이고자 하는 욕망이 있다. 더욱이 100세 시대를 살아가고 있는 현대인들에게는 더욱 그러하다. 가장 먼저 피부가 아름답고 건강해야 한다. 물론 피부가 건강의 바로미터이기 때문에 평소 건강하도록 노력을 해야 함은 말할 것도 없다. 메디칼 스킨케어란 피부의 속과 겉을 '치유'의 개념으로 관리하여 젊고 아름다운 피부로 만들어주는 것이다.

이런 개념으로 필자는 1990년부터 피부의학과 피부미용, 코수메슈티컬 화장품을 접목시켜 메디칼 스킨케어의 개념으로 확대하고 접목하여 현재에 이르렀다. 그 시간을 거치면서 수많은 사람의 피부를 접해왔고 각각의 문제를 해결하면서 깨달은 건 사람마다 얼굴이 다르게 생겼듯이 피부의 특성도 다 다르다는 것이다. 따라서 각 사람마다 고유의 피부 특징과 문제점을 진단하여 그에 맞는 치료와 관리를 해주었을 때 개선 효과를 극대화할 수 있었다. 청담은피부과의 메디칼 스킨케어는 좀 더 전문적이고 정확한 개별 관리가 가능하기 때문에 그 사람에게 최적의 피부 상태가 되도록 바꾸어줄 수 있다. 그래서 꾸준히 메디칼 스킨케어를 받아온 사람은 세월이 지나도 자기 나이보다 훨씬 젊고 건강한 피부를 유지하며 우아하고 아름답게 나이 들게 된다.

토탈뷰티 MLT 프로그램

피부 겉의 문제와 피부 속의 문제까지 피부 층별로 공략하는 다양한 작용의 각기 다른 레이저를 사용하여 치료함으로써 일시적인 피부 개선이 아닌 전반적인 피부 표면의 개선과 피부 속 탄력이 복원되는 근본적인 치유 개념의 피부 개선 프로그램이다.

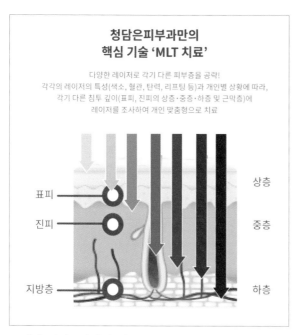

청담은피부과만의
핵심 기술 'MLT 치료'

다양한 레이저로 각기 다른 피부층을 공략!
각각의 레이저의 특성(색소, 혈관, 탄력, 리프팅 등)과 개인별 상황에 따라,
각기 다른 침투 깊이(표피, 진피의 상층·중층·하층 및 근막층)에
레이저를 조사하여 개인 맞춤형으로 치료

표피 / 진피 / 지방층
상층 / 중층 / 하층

얼굴 나이를 거꾸로 되돌리는 MLT 프로그램은 피부의 문제를 건강하고 아름답게 개선해 주는 체계적인 관리 프로그램으로서, 과도하게 활동하는 멜라닌 세포의 생산을 저하시키고 비정상적인(노화 각질, 색소낀 각질) 각질 세포를 탈락시키는 동시에 건강한 표피 세포로 재생해 준다.

거친 피부, 칙칙한 피부, 기미, 잡티, 주근깨, 검버섯, 색소침착, 탄력 없는 노화 피부, 넓어진 모공 및 여드름, 여드름 자국, 여드름 흉터, 잔주름, 붉은볼, 홍조, 아토피, 알러지 피부 등의 치료 개선에 탁월하다. 또한 피부 진피층과 근막층의 탄력을 증가시킴으로써 피부 처짐의 문제가 개선된다.

레이저 클리닉

Multi-Laser-Therapy로 Multi-Layer-Target(MLT) 요법이란?
다양한 피부문제와 깊이에 따라 선별된 레이저로 피부층별 공략

┃ 여드름 & 여드름 흉터

여드름은 생겼을 때도 골칫거리지만 자칫하면 흉터를 남기기 때문에 적절하고 빠른 치료가 매우 중요하다. 예민한 사춘기에 생기는 여드름은 심하면 대인기피증까지 이어지기도 한다.

근본적인 원인 제거와 치료 병행

성장기 여드름은 재생력이 좋은 시기라도 그 염증 정도와 깊이에 따라 흉터를 남기기도 한다. 또한 성인이 되어서도 생기는 성인 여드름은 피부 재생력이 떨어지므로 방치하면 쉽게 흉터가 생기고 거뭇거뭇하게 색소침착으로 발전하기도 한다. 사춘기에 안드로겐 호르몬이 증가하면서 모낭 피지샘에서 피지 분비가 늘어나 모낭에 존재하는 '프로피오니 박테리움 아크네' 균의 작용에 의해 분비된 피지가 유리지방산으로 바뀌게 된다. 이 지방산이 모낭벽 상피세포를 자극하고 모낭 입구를 더욱 각질화시켜 털구멍을 막으면서 염증이 유발되어 여드름의 형태로 나타나는 것이다. 최근에는 식습관과 환경변화, 스트레스, 피부에 맞지 않는 화장품의 사용으로 인해서 성인 여드름도 급격하게 늘어나고 있다.

여드름 치료는 우선 근본적인 원인이 되는 여드름균과 피지의 과다분비를 억제해 주면서 환자의 상태에 따라 내복약 복용, 약제 도포, 면포 압출이나 스킨 스케일링을 병행해 주는 것이 좋다. 더욱이 염증이 진피 깊숙한 곳에서 심하게 생긴 경우에는 후유증으로 여러 형태의 흉터를 남기는 경우가 대부분이므로 여드름 치료를 레이저로 하여 탄력섬유가 늘어나도록 유도하여 흉터가 생기는 것을 최대한 예방해 줄 필요가 있다.

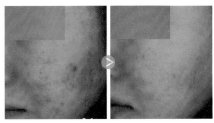

여드름 치료전후

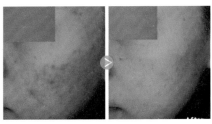

여드름, 붉은 흉터자국 치료전후

성인 여드름인 경우에는 필요하다면 내복약의 복용 및 바르는 약제(예 : 피지감소약제, 항생제, 소염제 등)과 non-comedogenic(피지형성을 유발시키지 않는 원료로 제조) 화장품을 잘 선택해서 사용하는게 매우 중요하다. 그 외에 여드름과 피지 억제 치료가 가능한 PDT(Photo Dynamic Therapy) 치료를 하게 되면 약물을 복용하지 않고도, 레블란 약제를 바른 후 그 약제가 피지선에 도달한 후 피지선을 타겟하는 레이저를 조사하면 짧은 시간에 탁월한 치료 효과를 볼 수 있을 뿐 아니라 흉터로 진행할 수 있는 것을 막을 수 있으며, 여드름 재발 방지에도 그 효과가 탁월하다. 여드름 부위에 집중적으로 흡수되는 약물(레블란)을 피부에 바르고 레이저를 쬐어 여드름균을 파괴시키고 피지선을 위축시키는 것이다.

레블란 PDT 여드름 치료는 효과가 빠르고, 피부재생효과까지 있어서 피부 톤이 개선되고 여드름 재발 및 흉터 예방에도 좋다.

여드름 흉터

남녀노소 누구나 매끄러운 도자기 피부를 갖기 원한다. 그러나 심한 염증성 여드름 혹은 여드름 관리를 소홀히 하여 패이고 얽은 피부를 가진 이들의 고민이 크다. 하지만 피부과 전문치료를 통해 얼마든지 문제성 피부를 고운 피부로 변화시킬 수 있다. 먼저, 여드름 흉터로 인하여 푹 패인 흉터 부위엔 흉터 조직을 뚫어주는 레이저(MCL31 Spot)을 이용해 흉터의 깊이와 크기에 맞게 패인 흉터를 섬세하게 뚫어준다. 여드름의 패인 흉터가 모여있는 부위의 피붓결을 우둘두둘 곱지 않고 거칠다.

이러한 부위는 MCl31 Dermablate 더마블레이트 레이저를 이용해 울퉁불퉁한 피붓결을 매끄럽게 다듬어준다 피부에 열손상을 주지 않아서 레이저 치료 시 별로 아프지 않아 바르는 마취만으로 충분하며, 레이저 치료 후 4일 정도 지나면 붉음증도 거의 남지 않는다. 또한 진피층 깊숙한 곳까지 RF 고주파 에너지를 전달해 콜라겐 재생을 도와줌으로써 흉터를 차오르게 한다. 이때 PRP를 주입하는 치료를 병행하면 더욱 효과가 크다. 이 과정을 2주일 간격으로 6~8회 진행하면 2개월 이후부터는 패인 흉터와 거친 피붓결, 넓은 모공 등이 눈에 띄게 현저히 개선되는 걸확인할 수 있다.

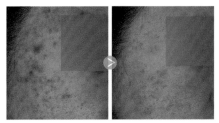

여드름 흉터 치료전후

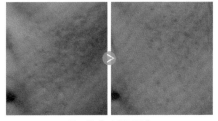

여드름 흉터 치료전후

TIP_여드름 & 여드름 흉터 시술정보				
시술시간	마취방법	회복기간	빈도	체류기간
1~1시간 30분	연고마취	4~5일	5~10회/1년	1~2일

| 과다색소침착(기미, 흑자)

기미는 주위 피부보다 특정 피부 부위가 검어진 과색소 침착증이다. 특히 이마, 뺨, 윗입술 위에 발생하는데 어두운 부위는 종종 얼굴의 양 측면에 거의 동일한 양상으로 나타나기도 한다.

기미 치료

아직까지 기미가 발생하는 명확한 원인이 밝혀지지 않았지만 자외선과 호르몬, 약물, 스트레스의 영향이 큰 것으로 알려져 있다. 임신을 하거나 경구피임약을 복

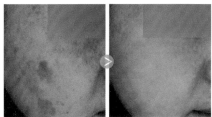

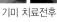

기미 치료전후

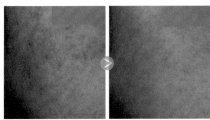

기미 치료전후

용하면서 호르몬에 변화가 생겨 기미가 발생하는 경우가 많다. 기미의 경우 오타모반 등의 다른 피부질환과 구분을 잘해야 한다. 기미는 치료가 불가능하다고 알고 있으나, 청담은피부과에서는 기미 치료를 성공적으로 하고 있다. 기미는 표피층과 진피층에 모두 분포되어 있는 혼합형인 경우가 대부분이다. 따라서 표피, 진피의 상·중·하층을 공략하는 각각의 레이저를 토닝의 방식으로 치료하게 된다.

치료방법

01 피부 색소 깊이에 따라 층별 색소 분해 치료(MLT) : 피부의 색소에 반응하는 루비레이저, 알렉산드라이트, 엔디야그, 울트라플러스 등의 레이저로 토닝방식으로 치료한다.

02 피부 표면에 겉 색소세포 탈락 및 정상 피부 세포로의 교체(청담은피부과 자체 개발한 피부에 자극없는 세이프 이지필(Safe Easy Peel) : 홈케어로 매일 밤 세안 후 미백연고제 및 가볍게 필(light peel)을 유도하는 연고제 및 색소를 품고 있는 각질이 잘 탈락되도록 각질 연화제를 바르고 자는 프로그램으로 자극이 없이 끼어있는 기미가 서서히 빠져나가도록 한다. 즉 피부과 전문 의사가 그 효능과 안전성을 약속하는 코슈메슈티컬 화장품으로 홈케어로 사용하여 정상적인 피부턴-오버 주기를 회복시켜 건강하고 깨끗한 피부로 탈바꿈시킨다.(www.mdpromise.co.kr)

흑자와 주근깨는 표피층에 위치하는 색소 문제이므로 표피층의 색소를 공략하는 KTP 레이저로 2개월 간격으로 1~2회 치료로 만족한 효과를 얻을 수 있다. 검버섯은 표피층 위로 두꺼워진 병변이므로 CO_2 레이저로 태워서 병변을 없애는 치료를 한다.

TIP_기미 시술정보

시술시간	마취방법	회복기간	빈도	체류기간
1~1시간 30분	연고마취	4~5일	2~10회/1년	1~2일

모공확장증

모공이 커지는 원인을 크게 두 가지로 분류하면 사춘기 무렵부터 성호르몬의 영향, 유전적 요인에 의해 지성, 여드름 피부인 경우와 피부 노화로 인한 탄력저하, 피부 늘어짐으로 볼 수 있다.

모공 치료

피부의 결이 좋고 매끄럽다는 건 모공이 작다는 것이다. 어릴 때는 누구나 피부가 곱고 예쁘고 모공도 보이지 않는다. 특히 사춘기 이후부터 지성피부 여드름 피부는 피지 과다 분비와 탄력 저하로 모공 확장이 된다. 또한 나이가 들면서 피부노화로 인해 모공도 커지게 된다. 여드름 지성 피부는 아이소트레티노인이라는 성분의 약제를 복용하여 피지선의 피지 분비기능을 억제시키면 여드름도 줄고 모공도 작아지는 효과가 있다.

그러나 내복약의 부작용을 걱정하여 약 복용을 원하지 않는 이들에게는 피부 손상 없이 진피층의 탄력섬유 재생을 촉진시킴으로써 넓어진 모공을 줄여주는 레이저 요법 등이 있다. 진피 재생력이 촉진되면 피부 탄력도가 높아지고 피부가 탱탱해지면서 모공도 작아지게 된다. 피부 속을 건강하게 함으로써 피부가 다시 젊어지기 때문이다.

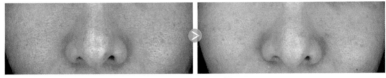

모공확장증 치료전후

TIP_모공확장증 시술정보				
시술시간	마취방법	회복기간	빈도	체류기간
1~1시간 30분	연고마취	4일	5~10회/1년	1~2일

| 피부 처짐 레이저 치료

Facial Contour 회복 : Skin Lifting, Tightening & Skin Rejuvenation with Neocollagenesis & Collagen Remodeling

01 Thermage, Oligio : 집속된 Monopolar RF(고주파)을 이용하여 콜라겐 섬유의 강화, 탄력증대, 진피 콜라겐의 리모델링으로, 피부 리프팅, 타이트닝, 피부 리쥬비네이션, 주름 완화, 늘어진 얼굴선을 올려주며, 얼굴처짐을 개선시키는데 도움이 되는 치료이다.

02 Ulthera, Thightan(High Intensity Focused Ultrasound for Skin Lifting & Tightening) : 오랜 세월 동안 노화가 조금씩 점차 진행되어 우리의 얼굴도 중력을 견디지 못하고 근육까지 처지게 된다. 울세라, 타이탄의 초음파는 근육의 근막층을 공략하는 집속 초음파 치료로 턱선 처짐, 팔자주름, 이중턱, 눈썹처짐, 눈밑 처짐 등을 완화하는데 도움이 되는 치료이다.

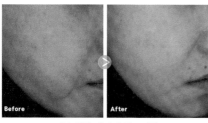
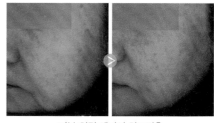

피부 처짐 레이저 치료전후   피부 처짐 레이저 치료전후

TIP_피부 처짐 레이저 치료 시술정보

시술시간	마취방법	회복기간	빈도	체류기간
1~1시간 30분	연고마취	0~1일	3~4회/1년	1~2일

에스테틱 클리닉

01 Promise Skin Care

다이오드 레이저를 이용한 피부 재생 케어로 피부의 진피층을 관리하는 스킨케어다. 다양한 피부과 치료의 연장선으로 이어지는 최고급 안티에이징 재생 유지를 위한 피부관리 프로그램이다.

02 Corage Skin Care

QMR Technology(유럽 Telea사의 특허기술)로 16가지의 멀티파장으로 피부에 어떠한 손상 없이 부드럽게 타이트닝, 리프팅, 볼륨감을 높여주는 피부세포재생 치료 및 관리 프로그램이다.

03 Home Care 요법

민감한 피부, 트러블 피부도 안전하게 피부과 전문의 처방의 코슈메슈티컬(Cosmeceuticals, 치유 개념의 화장품)으로 피부전문의 즉 의사(M.D.)가 그 효능과 안전성을 약속하는 MD Promise 화장품으로 홈케어로 치료 효과를 유지시킨다.

15 Medical Skin Care : Healing from Within

Integrating treatment and cosmetic care for youthful, radiant skin

Regardless of Eastern or Western ancestry, gender, age, or region, everyone desires to look beautiful and young. In the modern era, where many live to be 100, maintaining vibrant and healthy skin is more crucial than ever. The skin is a natural reflection of one's overall well-being, highlighting the significance of skin care. Medical skin care emphasizes "healing" both the internal and external layers of the skin to attain a youthful glow. Since 1990, I have integrated dermatology, cosmetic skin care, and cosmeceutical products under the concept of medical skin care. My extensive experience with diverse skin types and concerns has revealed that, just as every individual has a unique face, their skin characteristics are equally distinct. Therefore, personalized diagnosis and treatment of skin issues is crucial in achieving optimal improvements. Eun Skin Clinic's medical skin-care approach provides specialized and precise individual care, elevating your skin to its peak condition. Those who consistently invest in medical skin-care treatments experience aging with grace and beauty, with skin that looks and feels younger than their age.

| Total Skin Beauty Care:MLT Program

Addressing both surface and deep skin issues, the multilayer-target (MLT) program uses various lasers with different functions to offer holistic solutions that restore skin elasticity from within rather than providing temporary enhancements.

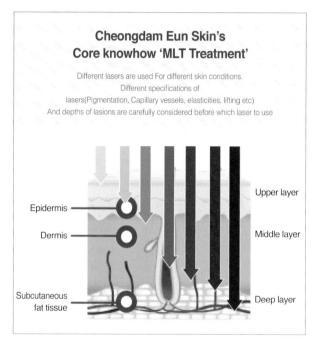

Cheongdam Eun Skin's Core knowhow 'MLT Treatment'

Different lasers are used For different skin conditions.
Different specifications of
lasers(Pigmentation, Capillary vessels, elasticities, lifting etc)
And depths of lasions are carefully considered before which laser to use

Epidermis — Upper layer
Dermis — Middle layer
Subcutaneous fat tissue — Deep layer

The MLT program reverses the signs of skin aging by offering a systematic management program that reduces the overproduction of melanin cells, eliminates abnormal (aged or pigmented) skin cells, and regenerates healthy epidermal cells. This program is highly effective for treating a range of skin issues, including rough skin, dull complexion, freckles, blemishes, melasma, sunspots, hyperpigmentation, aged skin lacking elasticity, enlarged pores, acne, acne scars, fine wrinkles, redness, rosacea, eczema, and sensitive, allergy-prone skin. It also enhances the elasticity of the skin's dermis and fascia layers, reducing skin sagging.

Laser Clinic

Multilaser Therapy and Multilayer Target (MLT) Approach

Targeting various skin issues and layers with selected lasers.

Acne and acne scars

Acne can be quite bothersome, and if not treated correctly, it can leave scars. During sensitive adolescence, it can even lead to social anxiety.

Addressing the root cause and providing concurrent treatment

During adolescence, acne can leave scars depending on the severity of inflammation and depth, despite the skin's natural regenerative abilities during this period. Even after adolescence, acne can develop, which will result in scars and hyperpigmentation if neglected, as the skin is less able to regenerate.

The increase in androgen hormones during puberty triggers increased sebum production within the hair follicles. When acted upon by the Cutibacterium acnes bacteria, this sebum transforms into free fatty acids. These acids stimulate the epithelial cells of the follicle walls, leading to further keratinizing of the follicle's entrance.

This blocks the hair opening, causing inflammation and resulting in acne. Recent changes in dietary habits, environmental factors, stress, and the use of inappropriate cosmetics have contributed to the surge in adult acne cases. Acne treatment should primarily focus on suppressing the acne-causing bacteria and excessive sebum secretion.

Depending on the patient's condition, treatment options may include oral medication, topical medication, comedone extrusion, or skin scaling. In particular, when inflammation occurs deep within the dermis, it often leaves various scars. Therefore, laser treatment for acne becomes necessary to stimulate the growth of elastic fibers

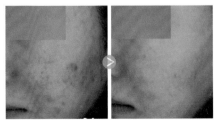

Before and after acne treatment

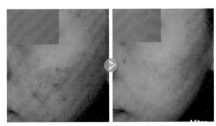

Before and after acne treatment

and prevent scarring. For adult acne, it is crucial to select and use noncomedogenic cosmetics (products that do not induce sebum production) and, if necessary, consider oral medications and apply topical medications, such as sebum-reducing drugs, antibiotics, and anti-inflammatory drugs.

Moreover, photodynamic therapy (PDT) treatment, which can suppress acne and sebum production, offers excellent therapeutic outcomes without needing medication. Laser irradiation on the sebaceous glands where the Levulan medication was applied yields excellent results in a short timeframe, as well as preventing scarring and acne recurrence.

The procedure involves applying medication (Levulan) in the acne-affected areas of the skin, followed by laser treatment that destroys acne bacteria and atrophies the sebaceous glands. Levulan PDT acne treatment has a fast-acting nature and regenerative effects on the skin, improving skin tone and preventing acne flare-ups and scarring.

Acne scars

Regardless of gender or age, everyone desires smooth, porcelain-like skin. However, those with severe inflammatory acne or who neglected their care, resulting in scarred and rough skin, face significant challenges. Now, with specialized dermatological treatments, problematic skin can be restored to a healthy and beautiful state. To address depressed scars caused by acne, an MCL31 spot laser is employed to precisely target and treat the depth and size of the scar.

Areas marked by clustered acne scars often exhibit an uneven and rough skin texture.

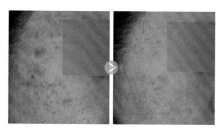

Before and after acne treatment

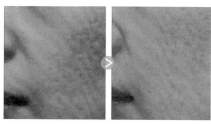

Before and after acne treatment

Such areas are smoothed out using the MCL31 Dermablate laser. This treatment ensures minimal discomfort and requires only topical anesthesia without causing thermal damage to the skin. Most of the redness subsides around four days posttreatment. Moreover, radio frequency (RF) energy is delivered deep into the dermis to promote collagen regeneration, effectively covering the scar.

This approach enhances the overall effect when combined with platelet-rich plasma (PRP) injections. Undergoing this process every two weeks for 6–8 sessions results in noticeable improvements in depressed scars, rough skin texture, and enlarged pores after two months.

TIP_Acne & Acne Scar Procedure information

Procedure Time	Anesthesia	Recovery Period	Frequency	Length of Stay
1~1.5 hrs	Topical	4~5 days	5~10 times/yr	1~2 days

Hyperpigmentation
lentigines, seborrheic keratosis, and melasma

Melasma is characterized by hyperpigmented spots that appear darker than the surrounding skin. These spots typically manifest on the forehead, cheeks, and above the upper lip.

Freckles Treatment

Melasma is characterized by hyperpigmented spots that appear darker than the surrounding skin. These spots typically manifest on the forehead, cheeks, and above the upper lip. They symmetrically appear on both sides of the face. While the exact cause of melasma remains unclear, it is believed to be influenced by factors such as UV rays, hormonal changes, medications, and stress.

Many individuals develop melasma during pregnancy or when taking birth control pills because of hormonal fluctuations. It is essential to differentiate melasma from other skin conditions, such as Nevus of Ota. Despite the belief that melasma is untreatable, Eun Skin Clinic has achieved success in treating this condition. The majority of melasma cases involve a combination of epidermal and dermal types. Therefore, toning treatments utilizing lasers that target the skin's upper, middle, and lower layers are employed.

Treatment strategy

01 Multilayer target (MLT) approach based on the depth of skin pigmentation

Toning treatments involve using lasers such as the Ruby laser, Alexandrite, Nd:YAG, and UltraPlus, specifically targeting skin pigmentation.

02 Removal of outer pigment cells from the skin surface and replacement with normal skin cells (Eun Skin Clinic's own Safe Easy Peel without causing skin irritation) : As a home care regimen, it involves applying a whitening ointment or ointment that induces light peeling with an exfoliant to remove dead skin cells every night after cleansing, followed by a sleep program that allows the melasma to gradually fade away without causing irritation. This cosmeceutical cosmetic, recommended by dermatologists for its efficacy and safety, can be used at home to restore the skin's normal turnover cycle, revealing healthy and clear skin. (www.mdpromise.co.kr)

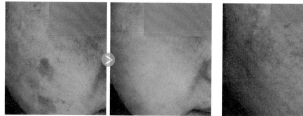
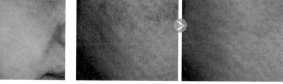

Before and after treatment for melasma

TIP_Hyperpigmentation (Freckles) treatment information				
Procedure Time	Anesthesia	Recovery Period	Frequency	Length of Stay
1~1.5 hrs	Topical	1~7days	2~10 times/yr	1~2 days

Freckles and lentigines, which are epidermal pigmentation issues, can be effectively treated with 1~2 sessions of the KTP laser every two months. Seborrheic keratosis, a raised lesion on the epidermis, can be treated by removing the lesion using the CO2 laser.

| Enlarged pores

The primary causes of enlarged pores can be categorized into two: hormonal influences and genetic factors leading to oily, acne-prone skin during puberty, loss of skin elasticity, and skin sagging due to aging.

Pore Treatmnt

A smooth skin texture is indicative of tiny pores. As a child, everyone has fine, beautiful skin with nearly invisible pores.

However, after puberty, those with oily or acne-prone skin may experience enlarged pores due to excessive sebum production and decreased skin elasticity. Aging also results in larger pores.

For those with acne-prone oily skin, taking medication containing isotretinoin can reduce both acne and pore size by suppressing sebaceous gland function. However, for those concerned about the side effects of oral medication, there are laser treatments that stimulate collagen regeneration in the dermis without damaging the skin.

As the dermis regenerates, skin elasticity improves, resulting in firmer skin and smaller pores. This rejuvenation leads to younger-looking skin.

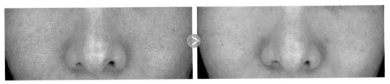

Before and after pore enlargement treatment

TIP_Enlarged pores treatment information				
Procedure Time	Anesthesia	Recovery Period	Frequency	Length of Stay
1~1.5 hrs	Topical	1~7 days	5~10 times/yr	1~2 days

| Skin sagging laser treatment

Facial Contour Recovery : Skin lifting, tightening, and skin rejuvenation through neocollagenesis and collagen remodelingt

01 Thermage and Oligio : These treatments use focused monopolar RF technology to strengthen collagen fibers, enhance elasticity, and remodel dermal collagen. This approach aids in skin lifting, tightening, reducing wrinkles, and improving facial sagging.

02 Ulthera and Tightan (high-intensity—focused ultrasound for skin lifting and tightening) : As aging gradually progresses, our facial skin becomes loose because of gravitational effects. Ulthera and Tightan offer focused ultrasound treatments that target the muscle fascia layer, helping alleviate sagging jawlines, nasolabial folds, double chins, drooping eyebrows, and under-eye sagging.

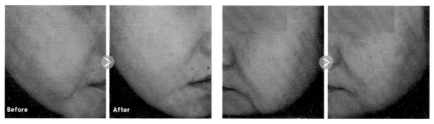

Sagging skin before and after laser treatment

TIP_Skin tightening and lifting treatment information				
Procedure Time	Anesthesia	Recovery Period	Frequency	Length of Stay
1~1.5 hrs	Topical	1~7 days	3~4 times/yr	1~2 days

01 Promise Skin Care

This skin rejuvenation treatment employs diode lasers to manage the dermal layer of the skin. It is a premium anti-aging maintenance program that complements various dermatological treatments.

02 Corage Skin Care

This treatment uses quantum molecular resonance (QMR) technology, a patented technology from Europe's Telea Medical, with 16 multiwavelengths that gently provide skin tightening, lifting, and volume enhancement without causing damage. It serves as a skin cell regeneration treatment and management program.

03 Home Care Therapy

Even sensitive and troubled skin can be safely treated with cosmeceuticals (healing concept cosmetics) prescribed by dermatologists. MD Promise cosmetics, guaranteed for efficacy and safety by dermatologists (MD), ensure effective home care for your skin.

여성헤어라인교정(Female hairline correction)
남성헤어라인교정(Male hairline correction)
여성눈썹이식(Female eyebrow transplant)
남성눈썹이식(Male eyebrow transplant)
현미경모발이식(Microscopic hair transplant)

동안모발이식 – 또다른 성형수술!

모발이식, 눈썹이식으로 젊고 어려보일 수 있다

Hair Transplant & Rejuvenescence- Another Plastic Surgery!

Rejuvenate with hair transplant and eyebrow transplant

남들이 알아보지 못할 정도로 자연스러운 헤어라인모발이식과 눈썹이식으로 또렷한 헤어라인과 선명한 눈썹을 갖게되면 자신감을 되찾을 수 있다.

Natural hairline restoration and eyebrow correction can restore Your Confidence.

홍성철성형외과
Dr Hong's Plastic Clinic Hairgraft Center

www.hairgraft.co.kr

홍성철(Sung-Chul Hong)

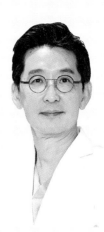

• 성형외과 전문의, 의학박사(Specialist plastic surgeon Doctor of Medicine)
• 대한성형외과학회 정회원(Regular member of the korean society of plastic surgery)
• 대한미용성형외과학회 정회원(Regular member of the korean society of aesthetic plastic surgery)
• 고려대학교 외래교수/ 대한모발이식학회 회장
Korea University adjunct professor/Former President of the Korean Society of Hair Transplantation)

16 스마트한 느낌의 동안모발이식

가장 효과적인 미용성형 – 동안모발이식

요즘 미용성형에서 동안수술이 대세인데, 사실 모발이식이야말로 어떤 미용성형 수술보다 어려 보이는 얼굴을 만드는 가장 효과적인 방법이다. 여성에서는 넓은 이마나 앞머리숱이 적은 경우에 헤어라인교정으로, 또한 눈썹숱이 적거나 눈썹의 모양이 마음에 들지 않을 때 이를 교정하는 눈썹 이식의 빈도가 점차 늘고 있다. 남성에서도 나이가 들면서 빠지는 앞머리를 자연스럽게 채워주거나, 적은 눈썹을 교정함으로써 좀 더 또렷한 인상과 비율에 맞는 젊은 얼굴을 가질 수 있다.

자신의 뒷머리카락을 옮겨 심는 자가모발이식은 미세현미경을 이용한다. 발전된 수술법인 비절개 혹은 절개로 모발이식수술을 통해 많은 양의 모발을 모낭의 손상을 최소화하면서 이식을 진행하게 되며, 절개를 통한 모발이식도 트리코파이틱수술법(trichophytic closure)으로 흉터가 거의 눈에 띄지 않는 방법으로 수술한다. 이런 모발이식은 수술한 티가 나지 않고, 남이 모를 정도로 자연스럽게 이식하는게 가장 중요하다.

여성헤어라인교정

선천적으로 이마가 넓은 여성. 나이가 들면서 앞머리카락이 가늘어지는 중년여성들이라면 헤어라인모발이식으로 작은 얼굴과 젊은 얼굴을 되찾을 수 있다.

작은 얼굴을 만드는 여성헤어라인교정

넓은 이마를 성형수술로 해결하기는 쉽지 않다. 이마피부를 잘라내고 두피를 아래쪽으로 끌어내리는 이마축소술이 있긴 하지만, 여성스럽고 동그란 이마선을 만들거나 옆얼굴의 폭을 줄여주는 건 불가능하다.

이마가 너무 넓거나 사각이마인 여성은 헤어스타일에 제약이 많고, 이마를 남에게 드러내는 걸 싫어한다. 이를 섬세한 모발이식으로 작고 자연스러운 이마를 만들 수 있다. 헤어라인을 둥글게 디자인하여, 이마에서 미간, 미간에서 코밑, 코밑에서 턱까지 길이가 1/3씩 분할되도록 한다. 여기에 얼굴형과 나이에 따라 자연스럽게 디자인에 변화를 준다.

모발을 지그재그로 불규칙하게 배열하고, 앞머리 부분은 가급적 가느다란 모발을 골라 심어서 잔머리 같은 느낌이 나도록 자연스럽게 이식한다. 때에 따라서는 잔머리모발이식을 병행하기도 한다. 보통 3,500모 이상을 1모, 2모짜리 모발로만 심으며, 관자놀이나 귀앞머리를 앞쪽으로 전진시켜서 이식함으로써 얼굴이 작아 보이고 어려 보이는 동안효과를 줄 수 있다.

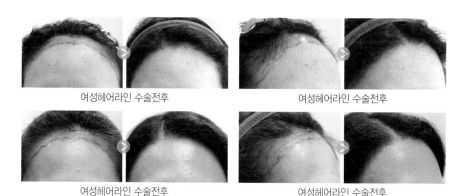

여성헤어라인 수술전후

여성헤어라인 수술전후

여성헤어라인 수술전후

여성헤어라인 수술전후

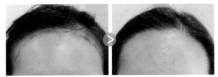
여성헤어라인 수술전후

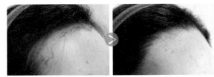
여성헤어라인 수술전후

헤어라인교정이 필요한 경우

- 사각이마 / 선천적으로 넓은 이마
- 옆얼굴이 넓은 경우
- 관자놀이 모발이 빈약하거나 안쪽으로 들어간 경우
- 헤어라인이 부분적으로 올라갔거나 어색하여 헤어라인 수정을 원하는 경우
- 미용수술 등으로 인해 생긴 머릿속 흉터

넓은 이마가 주는 여성의 이미지

- 얼굴이 길어 보임
- 실제나이보다 들어 보임
- 남성적인 이미지
- 대머리 같다는 느낌
- 나이가 들면서 눈썹이 처지므로 이마가 더 넓어 보임

여성헤어라인을 디자인하는 기본원칙

- 이마에서 미간, 미간에서 코밑, 코밑에서 턱까지 길이가 1/3씩 분할되도록 디자인
- 얼굴형에 따른 균형 있는 디자인
- 너무 좁은 이마는 답답해 보이므로 이마를 좁지 않게 디자인
- 여성분의 미용적인 욕구를 고려

자연스런 여성헤어라인 만들기 전략

- 내츄럴한 헤어라인으로 촘촘히 이식함
- 가급적이면 한 번의 수술로 마무리
- 수술의 공포와 통증을 최소화
- 공여부 흉터를 최소화하기 위해 비절개나 특수봉합법

TIP_여성헤어라인교정 수술정보

수술시간	마취방법	입원여부	회복기간	체류기간
5시간	수면, 국소마취	입원없음	5일	2일

| 남성헤어라인교정

탈모로 인해 앞이마가 무너지는 남성, 선천적으로 이마가 높거나 옆으로 넓어서 고민하는 남성이 많다. 동안모발이식을 통해 선명한 이마선을 만들어, 멋지게 머리를 올리는 헤어스타일로 자신감을 찾을 수 있다.

자신있는 이마선을 위한 남성헤어라인교정

남성형탈모에서 M자형으로 빠지거나 앞이마가 올라가는 경우, 그리고 진행된 탈모에서도, 모발이식으로 우선 자연스런 헤어라인을 만들어 주는게 중요하다. 만약 탈모가 계속 진행되더라도 이식된 앞머리카락으로 탈모부위를 가리기 용이하기 때문이다. 보통 1회에 3,000~4,000모를 이식하는데, 필요하다면 추가로 1~2회 비슷한 양을 더 이식할 수 있다. 공여부 모발채취는 비절개, 절개와 혹은 그 둘을 병행해서 시행할 수 있다.

남성형탈모는 유전적 배경이 있는 경우가 많으므로, 가족의 탈모유형과 탈모시기를 참고하여 모발이식수술의 시기와 이식부위를 결정해야 한다. 남성에서도 미용성형수술이 많이 성행하는 요즘, 탈모가 아닌 선천적으로 이마가 넓은 남성에서도 모발이식을 통해 이마의 높이와 폭을 줄여줄 수 있다. 지그재그 패턴의 헤어라인으로 촘촘히 이식한다면, 넓고 큰 얼굴을 아담한 얼굴로 바꿀 수 있는 얼굴축소 효과를 볼 수 있다.

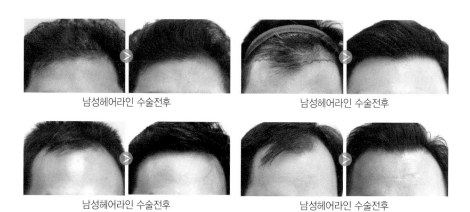

남성헤어라인 수술전후   남성헤어라인 수술전후

남성헤어라인 수술전후   남성헤어라인 수술전후

수술시간	마취방법	입원여부	회복기간	체류기간
5시간	수면, 국소마취	입원없음	5일	2일

여성눈썹이식

매번 눈썹을 그리기 귀찮거나 반영구나 문신이 부자연스런 여성에서는 눈썹이식으로 또렷한 인상의 영구적인 눈썹을 가질 수 있다.

눈썹콤플렉스를 극복하는 눈썹이식

눈썹도 심을 수 있다는 걸 아는 사람은 많지 않다. 탈모증에서 모발이식을 하듯이 눈썹도 이식할 수 있으며, 이식한 눈썹의 생착률은 90% 이상이다. 눈썹은 얼굴의 중앙에 있기 때문에 생착률도 높아야겠지만 자연스러운 결과를 만드는 게 가장 중요하다.

여성은 남성에 비해 빈약한 눈썹에 대해서 스트레스를 덜 받는다. 눈썹을 그리기도 하고 문신을 하기도 한다. 하지만 눈썹을 그리는 데 아침마다 많은 시간을 투자해야 하며, 땀이 나면 그린 눈썹이 쉽게 지워져서 수시로 화장을 고쳐야 하는 번거로움이 있다. 눈썹이 앞부분만 있다가 뒤로 희미한 반쪽 눈썹이나 처진 눈썹으로 스트레스를 받기도 하는데, 사진을 찍으면 더 어색해 보인다. 반영구화장이나 문신으로 커버하기도 하지만 영구적이지 않고 부자연스럽다는 단점이 있다.

보통 한쪽 눈썹에 200~300모 정도를, 자연스러운 달팽이 문양으로, 눈썹의 흐름을 살려 기존의 눈썹 사이사이에 하나씩 심는다. 특히 눈썹 앞머리는 위를 향하도록 이식하여 자연눈썹과 가깝도록 만든다. 눈썹문신이 있거나 화상이나 교통사고 등의 눈썹 흉터에도 이식이 가능하다.

눈썹이식 후에 눈썹이 풍성해지는 건 물론이고, 전체적인 얼굴의 느낌도 좋아져서 대부분의 환자는 결과에 만족한다. 하지만 이식한 눈썹은 자라므로 일주일에 한두 번은 다듬어 주어야 하는 불편함은 감수해야만 한다.

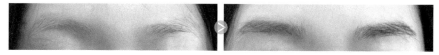

여성눈썹이식 수술전후 - 흐린눈썹

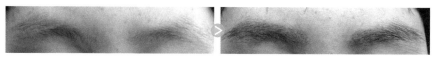

여성눈썹이식 수술전후 - 흐린눈썹

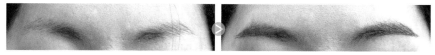

여성눈썹이식 수술전후 - 반쪽눈썹

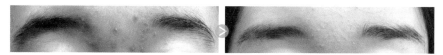

여성눈썹이식 수술전후 - 처진눈썹

눈썹이식이 필요한 경우

- 선천적으로 눈썹이 전체적으로 빈약한 경우
- 눈썹 앞부분은 있는데 뒷부분이 없는 경우
- 눈썹이 아래로 처진 경우, 팔자눈썹
- 눈썹 앞부분 숱이 적은 경우
- 눈썹 흉터

자연스런 눈썹만들기 전략

- 수술 전 세심한 눈썹 디자인
- 이식 마무리 단계에서의 여러 번 세심한 교정
- 눈썹결을 맞춰서 입체적인 눈썹이식
- 자연스럽도록 하나짜리 털로만 이식
- 눈썹 앞머리는 가느다란 털을 골라서 위를 향하도록 이식
- 한쪽에 200~300개 정도를 최대한 눕혀서 이식
- 반쪽눈썹에서는 눈썹중간부터 연결하여 뒷부분까지 이식

눈썹흉터를 가리는 눈썹이식

- 눈썹흉터는 대개 흉터축소술보다는 눈썹이식을 하는게 효과적이다.
- 주변 기존 눈썹에 잘 어울리도록 방향과 각도를 맞춰 심는다.
- 세심히 시술한다면 흉터에도 생착률이 높다.

● 흉터이식에서는 뒷머리를 절개하지 않고 비절개로 시술한다.

TIP_여성눈썹이식 수술정보

수술시간	마취방법	입원여부	회복기간	체류기간
3~4시간	수면, 국소마취	입원없음	3일	2일

│ 남성눈썹이식

눈썹이식을 통해 강한 인상은 부드럽게 그리고 너무 연약해 보이는 사람은 또렷한 인상으로 바꿀 수 있다.

얼굴의 균형을 잡아주는 눈썹이식

흐린 눈썹을 가리려고 머리카락을 아래로 내리는 헤어스타일을 고수하기도 하고, 간혹 관상 때문에 눈썹이식을 받기도 한다. 남성은 반영구나 문신이 어색하므로 눈썹이 없어서 고민인 경우에는 눈썹이식이 가장 효과적인 방법이다. 남성의 눈썹디자인은 여성과 약간 다를 뿐 이식의 전체적인 과정은 유사하다. 남성눈썹은 좀 더 힘있게 굵은 디자인을 선택하며, 일자형보다는 약간 눈썹산을 만들어 주는 경향이 있다. 눈썹이식을 통해 강한 인상은 부드럽게 그리고 너무 연약해 보이는 사람은 또렷한 인상으로 바꿀 수 있다.

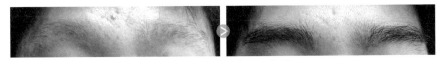

남성눈썹이식 수술전후 - 흐린눈썹

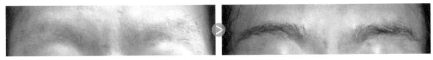

남성눈썹이식 수술전후 - 흐린눈썹

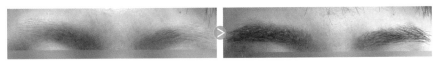

남성눈썹이식 수술전후 - 반쪽눈썹

TIP_남성눈썹이식 수술정보

수술시간	마취방법	입원여부	회복기간	체류기간
3~4시간	수면, 국소마취	입원없음	3일	2일

현미경모발이식

눈썹이식을 통해 강한 인상은 부드럽게 그리고 너무 연약해 보이는 사람은 또렷한 인상으로 바꿀 수 있다.

홍성철모발이식센터 현미경모발이식 과정

홍성철모발이식센터는 1993년부터 시작되어, 성형외과 전문의가 전문화한 모발이식전문병원으로 성장되어 왔다. 지난 20년 넘는 기간동안 100% 미세현미경을 이용한 자체 모발분리팀을 보유하고 있으며, 기존의 시술법에만 안주하지 않고 활발한 연구와 학회활동을 통하여 새로운 모발의료기술을 발전시키고 있다.

요즘 병원들이 대형화되는 추세지만, 홍성철모발이식센터는 홍성철원장이 처음부터 끝까지 직접 챙겨서 수술을 진행한다.

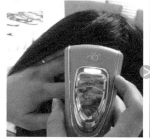
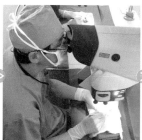
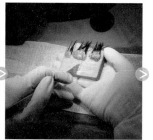

1. 제공여부 모발밀도 측정　　2. 현미경으로 모낭분리하는 모습　　3. 전과정 현미경으로 모낭분리

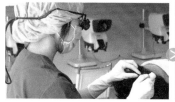
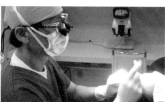

4. 이식된 모근의 깊이를 조절하는 작업　　5. 확대경으로 모발이식하는 모습

16 Hair transplant that makes you look smart and young

Rejuvenescence with hair transplant - The most effective cosmetic surgery

Hair transplantation is becoming one of the cosmetic surgeries. It is the most effective way to achieve a younger-looking effect than other plastic surgeries. Hairline correction is possible not only for women with a wide forehead or thinning bangs, but also for those with thin eyebrows or narrow eyebrow shapes.

The frequency of eyebrow transplantation to correct unwanted eyebrows is gradually increasing. For men, this is a way to fill hairs that fall out with age or to correct sagging eyebrows.

By using this, you can have a younger-looking proportions.

Autologous hair transplantation is a method of transplanting hair follicles harvested from the back of one's scalp. Advanced fue(follicular unit extraction), or strip hair transplant surgery allows large amounts of hair follicles to be harvested from a donor's scalp.

Even in the case of strip surgery, the trichophytic closure method is used so that the scar is barely noticeable.

| Female Hairline Correction

Women with naturally wide foreheads or middle-aged women whose frontal hair becomes thinner as they age can achieve a smaller and younger face with hairline hair transplantation.

Female hairline correction to create a small face

It is not easy to correct a wide forehead with plastic surgery. Forehead reduction surgery can reduce the forehead by cutting off the forehead skin and pulling the scalp downward. However, it is not easy to create a feminine, round forehead line, and it is impossible to reduce the width of the profile of the face.

Women with foreheads that are too wide or square have many restrictions on hairstyles, and they do not like their foreheads exposed to others. You can have a small, natural forehead with this delicate hair transplant. It is designed to be balanced so that the length from the forehead to the eyebrows is divided by 1/3, the length between the eyebrows to the bottom of the nose is divided by 1/3, and the length from the bottom of the nose to the chin is divided by 1/3. Here, the design naturally changes depending on the face shape and age of the patient.

The hair is deliberately arranged irregularly in a zigzag pattern. In the area in front of the hairline, thin hair is selected and transplanted to give the appearance of fine hair.

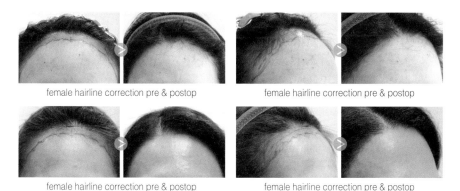

female hairline correction pre & postop   female hairline correction pre & postop

female hairline correction pre & postop   female hairline correction pre & postop

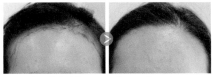
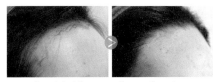

female hairline correction pre & postop   female hairline correction pre & postop

Usually, more than 3,500 hairs are planted with only one or two hairs. Also, by advancing the temples or front of the ears forward and transplanting them, the face looks smaller. It can give you a youthful appearance.

When hairline correction is needed
• Squaro forohoad / Naturally wide forehead
• If the side face is wide
• If the temple hair is sparse.
• Scalp scars caused by cosmetic surgery
• If you want to modify the shape of your hairline

The image of a woman given by a wide forehead
• Face looks longer
• Looks older than actual age
• Masculine image
• Feeling like I'm bald
• As you age, your eyebrows droop, making your forehead look wider

Basic principles of designing female hairlines
• Designed to divide the length from the forehead to the eyebrow, from the eyebrow to the bottom of the nose, and from the bottom of the nose to the chin by 1/3 each.
• Balanced design according to facial shape
• A forehead that is too narrow looks stuffy, so design the forehead so that it is not narrow.
• Considering women's cosmetic needs

Strategies for creating a natural female hairline
• Natural hairline and dense transplantation
• If possible, complete with one surgery.
• Minimize the fear and pain of surgery
• Non-incision or special suture method to minimize scarring at the donor site.

TIP_Female hairline correction surgery information				
Operation time	Anesthesia	Admission	Recovery period	Stay duration
5 hours	Sedation&Local anesthesia	No	5 days	2 days

| Male Hairline Correction

There are many men whose forehead line is receding due to hair loss, and many men who are concerned about their foreheads being naturally high or wide on the sides. You can create a clear forehead line through a youthful hair transplant and gain confidence with a stylish hairstyle that puts your hair up.

Men's hairline correction for a confident forehead line

Even in advanced male pattern baldness, it is important to first create a forehead hairline through hair transplantation. Even if hair loss continues, it is easy to cover the bald area with the transplanted front hairs.

About 3,000 to 4,000 hairs are transplanted at a time, and if necessary, a similar amount can be transplanted one to two additional times. Hair collection from the donor area can be performed through non-incision, incision, or a combination of the two.

Since male pattern baldness often has a genetic background, the timing and location of hair transplant surgery should be determined by referring to the hair loss type and

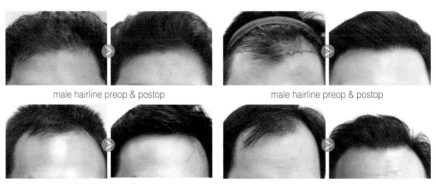

male hairline preop & postop

male hairline preop & postop

male hairline preop & postop

male hairline preop & postop

timing of hair loss in the family history. Plastic surgery is very popular among men these days, and even men with naturally wide foreheads without hair loss can reduce the height and width of their foreheads through hair transplantation.

If you transplant closely with the hairline in a zigzag pattern, you can see the facial reduction effect that change a wide and large face into a small face.

TIP_Male hairline correction surgery information

Operation time	Anesthesia	Admission	Recovery period	Stay duration
5 hours	Sedation&Local anesthesia	No	5 days	2 days

| Female Eyebrow Graft

Women who find it difficult to draw eyebrows every time or who are reluctant to get semi-permanent tattoos can have permanent eyebrows with a clear impression through eyebrow transplantation.

Eyebrow transplant to overcome eyebrow complex

Not many people know that eyebrows can also be implanted. Just like hair transplantation for alopecia, eyebrows can also be transplanted, and the survival rate of transplanted eyebrows is over 90%. Eyebrows are easily visible because they are located in the center of the face. So the grafts survival rate must be high, but the most important thing is to create natural results.

Women are less stressed about their sparse eyebrows than men. They often wear eyebrow makeup and even have tattoos. However, they have to invest a lot of time every morning to draw eyebrows, and when sweating, the drawn eyebrows are easily erased, so having to frequently retouch your makeup, which is a hassle.

Some people get stressed out by having eyebrows that are only in the medial side and then faint at the back, or half eyebrows or droopy eyebrows, and they look even more awkward when taken in pictures. It can be covered with semi-permanent makeup or tattoos, but it has the disadvantage of being not permanent and unnatural.

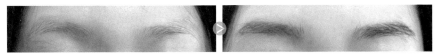

female eyebrow graft pre & postop - blurred eyebrows

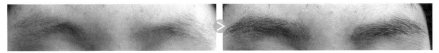

female eyebrow graft pre & postop - blurred eyebrows

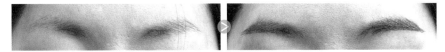

female eyebrow graft pre & postop - half eyebrows

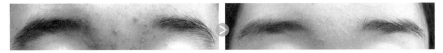

female eyebrow graft pre & postop - drooping eyebrows

Approximately 200 to 300 hairs are transplanted into each eyebrow, one in a natural snail pattern, using the eyebrow flow between existing eyebrow hairs. In particular, the medial eyebrows are transplanted to face upward to make them closer to natural eyebrows. Transplantation is also possible for eyebrow scars such as eyebrow tattoos, burns, and traffic accidents.

After eyebrow transplantation, not only do the eyebrows become fuller, but the overall feel of the face also improves, and most patients are satisfied with the results. However, as the transplanted eyebrows grow, you have to endure the inconvenience of having to trim them once or twice a week.

When eyebrow transplantation is needed
- If the eyebrows are congenitally thin overall.
- If there is a front part of the eyebrow but no back part.
- If the eyebrows droop down
- If there is thinning in the front part of the eyebrows
- Eyebrow scar

Strategies for creating natural eyebrows

• Careful eyebrow design before surgery
• Multiple careful corrections at the final stage of transplantation
• Three-dimensional eyebrow transplant by matching the eyebrow texture
• Transplant only one hair follicle for a natural look
• For the front eyebrows, select thin hairs and transplant them facing upwards.
• Transplant about 200 to 300 hairs on one side, lying down as much as possible.
• In half eyebrows, connect from the middle of the eyebrow and transplant to the back.

Eyebrow transplant for eyebrow scars

• For eyebrow scars, eyebrow transplantation is usually more effective than scar reduction surgery.
• Impant in the correct direction and angle so that it matches well with the surrounding existing eyebrows.
• It is mainly performed using fue, a non-incision method.
• If the procedure is performed carefully, the survival rate in scars is high.

TIP_Female eyebrow transplant surgery information

Operation time	Anesthesia	Admission	Recovery period	Stay duration
5 hours	Sedation&Local anesthesia	No	5 days	2 days

| Male eyebrow transplant

Through eyebrow transplant, a strong impression can be changed to a softer one, and a person who looks too weak can be changed to a clear impression.

Eyebrow transplant to balance the face

Some people stick to a hairstyle with their hair down to hide their blurry eyebrows, and sometimes they get eyebrow transplants for cosmetic reasons.

For men, semi-permanent tattoos are awkward, so if you are concerned about having no eyebrows, eyebrow transplantation is the most effective method. Men's eyebrow designs are slightly different from women's, but the overall transplantation process is similar. Men's eyebrows tend to have a more powerful and thick design, with a slight ridge rather than a straight shape. Through eyebrow transplantation, a strong impression can be softened and those who look too weak can be given a clear impression.

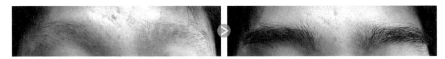

male eyebrow graft pre & postop - blurred eyebrows

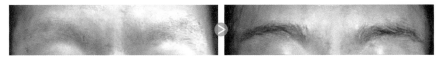

male eyebrow graft pre & postop - blurred eyebrows

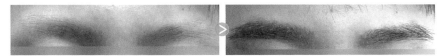

male eyebrow graft pre & postop - half eyebrows

TIP_Male eyebrow transplant surgery information

Operation time	Anesthesia	Admission	Recovery period	Stay duration
3~4 hours	Sedation&Local anesthesia	No	3 days	2 days

| Microscopic hair transplant

Through eyebrow transplant, a strong impression can be changed to a softer one, and a person who looks too weak can be changed to a clear impression.

Microscopic hair transplant process of Hong's Hair Transplant Center

Dr Hong's Hair Transplant Center has grown into a hair transplant hospital specializing in plastic surgery for over 20 years. We have our own hair follicle dissection team who have been using 100% microscopy. We are not satisfied with existing treatment methods and are developing new hair medical technologies through research and academic activities.

Hospitals are getting bigger these days, but at our hair transplant center, director Dr Hong is personally responsible for the surgery from start to finish.

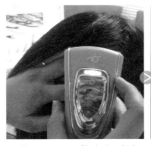

1. Measurement of hair density in donor area

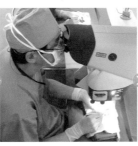

2.Hair follicle dissection under a microscope

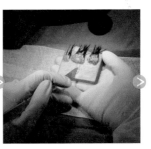

3. Hair follicle separation under a microscope throughout the process

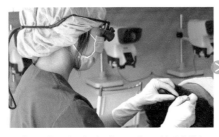

4. Controlling the depth of transplanted hair follicles

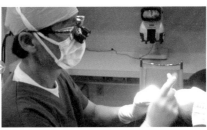

5. Hair transplant using a loupe

림프부종(Lymphedema)
하지정맥류(Varicose veins)

세계 어디에서도 고칠 수 없는 불치병 – 림프부종

림프부종은 영원히 고칠 수 없는 질환인가? 아니다!!!

Incurable lymphedema : nobody can not cure completely in the world

Can't really cure lymphedema forever? No!!!

심영기 박사는 타 병원과 비교해서 끊임없이 림프부종 치료에 대해 연구하고 독보적인 치료법을 개발해서 여러 가지 시술을 통해 풍부한 경험을 쌓았다. 수술 전 림프부종의 심한 정도 및 상태에 따라 차이가 있지만 시술 후 1년 림프부종은 80%에서 110% 정도 감소하였다.

Dr.Young Ki Shim has researched lymphedema over than 20 years and developed his own therapeutic method with good experiences. By his operation method, the average patient's volume reduction rate was 80~110% after one year.

연세에스의원
Yonsei S clinic

www.yssh.kr

심영기(Young-Ki Shim)

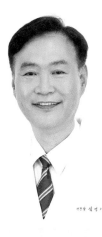

- 연세에스의원 대표원장(Director of Yonsei S clinic)
- 성형외과 전문의(Certified Board of the plastic and reconstructive surgery)
- 연세대학교 의과대학 의학박사(D.M.Sc., Ph.D Yonsei University Medical college)
- 중국 대련병원 설립(Set up Dalian varicose vein clinic. China)
- 대한정맥학회 창립(Founder the Korean Society of Phlbology)
- 중국 북경병원 설립(Set up Beijing varicose vein clinic. China)
- 림프부종, 하지정맥류 전문치료(main care: lymphedema, varicose vein)

17 불치병 림프부종에 도전한다!

림프부종은 영원히 고칠 수 없는 질환인가? 아니다!!

심영기 박사는 타 병원과 비교해서 끊임없이 림프부종 치료에 대해 연구하고 독보적인 치료법을 개발해서 여러 가지 시술을 통해 풍부한 경험을 쌓았다. 수술 전 림프 부종의 심한 정도 및 상태에 따라 차이가 있지만, 시술 후 1년 림프부종은 80%에서 110% 정도 감소하였다. 현재까지 개발된 방법보다 심영기 박사의 치료법이 임상적 결과가 더 좋았다.

치료 자체가 덜 침습적이며 흉터가 적고 통증도 적으며 회복기간이 짧다. 수술결과가 다른 치료법보다 빨리 나타난다. 세계 최초로 림프흡입수술 및 줄기세포 치료를 병합사용하였으며 성공적인 결과를 얻었다.

줄기세포치료는 신생혈관 및 신생림프관 형성 작용이 있어 림프부종 및 하지 허혈성 괴사에 효과가 좋았다. 이 치료는 안전한 치료이며 2~5년에 1회 반복 시술이 가능하며 2010년 심영기식 수술을 시작한 이래 100%의 성공률을 보이고 있다. 줄기세포는 배양하지 않고 수술실에서 즉시 분리하여 환자 본인에게 이식해 줌으로써 줄기세포로 인한 암 발생이나 돌연변이로 발전될 가능성이 없다.

| 림프부종

림프부종이란 림프액이 순환계로 배액되지 못하고 피부 및 피하지방 안에 비정상적인 고농도 단백질로 구성된 림프액의 축적으로 생긴 부종을 말하며, 합병증으로 피부 만성염증, 조직 섬유화 등이 수반되는 질환이다.

림프계

림프계는 심혈관 계통과는 다르게 인체의 체액순환을 담당하는 계통으로 세포, 조직, 기관에 "림프"라고 불리는 액체 상태로 존재하면서 정화 및 영양공급을 하는 작용을 한다. 혹자는 림프계통을 신데렐라 같다고 말한다. 림프계는 신데렐라처럼 묵묵히 체내에서 생성된 노폐물을 치우고 조직의 재생과 치유역할을 한다. 림프계는 동시에 영양분, 무기질, 비타민 등도 공급하며, 박테리아, 노폐물, 독성 물질을 효과적으로 여과시켜 혈액 순환계로 보내서 배출되도록 하는 작용을 한다.

림프계의 기능

· 순환기능
· 해독기능
· 영양공급
· 면역작용

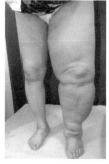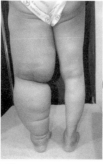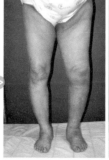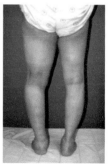

수술 전   수술 후 13개월

▲ 좌측 하지에 발생한 2차성 림프부종 : 62세 여자 환자. 자궁암 수술 후 발생한 림프부종 10년간 투병. 다리 무게 때문에 무릎관절에도 퇴행성 관절변형 발생. 점점 림프부종 악화. 연세에스병원 심영기 원장 집도후 무릎 관절운동 및 통증이 호전됨. 수술 후 림프선염 염증 발생안함. 면역력이 향상됨. 체중 84kg에서 66kg으로 수술 13개월 동안 18kg 감소. 종아리 쪽 직경 22.5cm 감소.

림프부종 증상

　림프부종 환자들은 사지에 만성적으로 부종이 생기면서 림프부종으로 진행되는데 처음에는 팔 또는 다리가 비대칭이 되고 평소에 잘 맞던 옷이 꼭 끼게 되며 부종이 심해지면 부종으로 인해 무게가 늘어나면서 만성피로, 외모에 대한 콤플렉스가 생겨 사회 활동의 위축 등 삶의 질이 떨어지고, 세균이나 진균의 감염이 자주 발생하게 된다. 림프부종 80%의 환자가 다리에 생기는 데 팔, 얼굴, 외음부, 체간부에도 림프부종이 생길 수 있다. 부종 초기에는 원위부에서부터 붓지만 진행되면 점점 근위부까지 붓게 된다. 환자분들은 보통 통증이 없는 부종 및 무게감을 호소한다.

　발열, 오한, 전신쇠약 등의 증상이 있으며 반복감염, 피부가 갈라지거나 궤양이 생기고 사마귀가 생기기도 한다. 환자들은 세균이나 진균의 감염 위험이 높다.

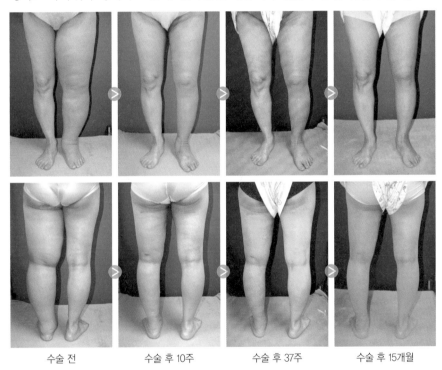

| 수술 전 | 수술 후 10주 | 수술 후 37주 | 수술 후 15개월 |

▲ **좌측 하지 2차성 림프부종** : 53세 여성. 좌측 하지 림프부종 2기. 8년전 자궁암수술. 방사선 치료 10회. 암 완치 판정 받음. 다리에 반복적인 림프선염. 심영기 박사 집도 후 37주에 거의 정상 다리크기가 됨.

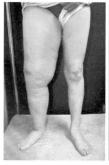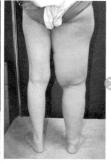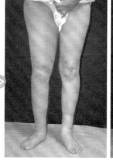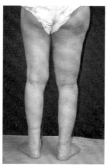

수술 전   수술 후 8개월

▲ 우측 하지에 발생한 2차성 림프부종 : 66세 여자 환자. 38년전 자궁암 수술 후 발생한 림프부종 20년간 투병. 점점 림프부종 악화. 심영기 원장 집도후 8개월 : 14cm감소. 수술 후 림프선염 염증 발생안함.

림프부종의 가장 좋은 치료는 초기부터 철저히 압박요법을 잘해 주는 것이 중요하다. 피부 섬유성 변화 및 피하 지방세포비대가 생기기 전에 물리치료사의 도움을 받는 것이 좋다. 림프부종의 진행을 늦추기 위해 가급적 많은 방법을 동원하는 것이 좋고 특히 암수술을 받은 환자에게서 림프부종 발생이 가능하므로 주의 깊게 관찰하고 조기 압박치료를 해주는 것이 좋다.

림프부종의 종류

• 일차성 림프부종 :   – 선천성 림프부종 : 단순성. 유전성 림프부종
                         – 조발성 림프부종 : 14세 전후 발생
                         – 완발성 림프부종 : 35세 전후 발생

• 이차성 림프부종 :

   – 원인   ① 감염 : 기생충. 세균. 진균 등
            ② 외상 : 수술. 방사선치료. 화상 등
            ③ 암수술 이후
            ④ 기타 : 전신질환. 임신 등

림프부종의 치료

대부분의 림프부종 환자들은 의사로부터 외면을 당한다. 의사들은 림프계통에 대해 배우지도 못했고 눈에 잘 보이지도 않아서 거의 치료가 불가능하기 때문이다.

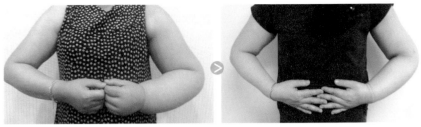

수술 전   수술 후 5개월

▲ 좌측 팔 2차성 림프부종 : 56세 여성증례, 11년전 좌측 유방암수술, 화학요법 및 방사선 치료, 8년간 부종으로 고생. MCS+ EBW 수술 후 팔 슬리브 및 붕대요법으로 관리.

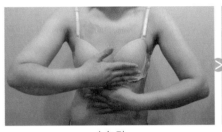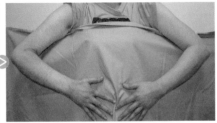

수술 전   수술 후 8개월

▲ 우측 팔에 이차성 림프부종 : 지방줄기세포를 이용한 복합치료법 시술. 붕대요법을 하지 않아도 됨.

림프부종의 진행 정도에 따라서 치료원칙은 다르다. 초기에는 체류된 림프액을 배출 배액 시켜주는 것이며 림프오니가 쌓이지 않도록 해주는 것이다. 말기에는 재생 회복이 불가능한 병변 조직을 절제해 주거나 국한적으로 림프관이 막힌 부분을 연결시켜주는 것이다.

- **초기 림프부종의 치료** : 비수술적 치료가 위주가 된다.
- **거상치료** : 30~40cm 하지를 거상하면 림프의 순환이 좋아지고 부종이 경감된다.
- **압박요법** : 의료용 압박 스타킹, 압박붕대, 공기압펌프
- **감염예방**
- **말기 림프부종의 치료** : 주로 수술 치료를 사용한다. 일차성 림프부종 환자의 약 15%에서는 하지 절단 수술 등 절제수술은 한다. 현재 존재하고 있는 수술방법으로 림프부종을 치료하기는 것은 불가능하지만 수술을 하면 증상이 개선된다.
- **현재 전 세계적으로 사용되고 있는 림프부종의 수술법**

- 유리 피판수술(Free Flap)
- 미세 림프정맥문합술(LVA)
- 미세 자가림프절 이식술(VLNT or ALNT)
- 도수 림프배액술(MLD)
- 외과적 절제술(excision)

심영기 박사의 치료법

- 최소 침습수술이며 병합요법을 사용한다.
- 림프흡입술 + 지방흡입술 + 줄기세포 + 미세림프수술
- 경구약, 복합물리치료, 해독요법, 주사요법은 수술 후 정기적으로 방문하여 치료받는다.
- 압박붕대 및 의료용 압박양말은 수술 후 12~24개월 착용하며 더 이상 붓지 않을 때는 착용하지 않는다.

TIP_림프부종 수술정보

수술시간	마취방법	입원여부	회복기간	체류기간
3~4시간	국소정맥마취	2~3주	2주	3~4주

하지정맥류

선천적으로 혈관 판막이 얇고 약하거나, 움직이지 않고 같은 자세로 오래 있는 경우, 하지에 혈액이 축적되게 된다. 정맥압이 높아지게 되고 정맥 판막이 파손되어, 피부표면에 혈관이 돌출되는 현상이 생긴다. 하지정맥류의 가장 중요한 특징은 피부 표면으로 혈관이 지렁이처럼 구불구불 돌출된다는 것이다.

하지정맥류의 진단

하지정맥류는 일단 생기면 스스로 치유되지 않고 점점 나빠지는 질환이다. 일단 하지정맥류가 있다고 진단되어지면, 혈관을 전문으로 보는 외과계 전문의에게 진찰을 받아서 수술 적기를 놓치지 않는 것이 좋다.

- 1기 : 모세혈관 확장증, 거미상 정맥
- 2기 : 직경 2mm의 푸른색 세정맥이 돌출된 것
- 3기 : 직경 2~4mm의 푸른색 정맥 세줄기 이상이 돌출된 것
- 4기 : 직경 4~8mm의 푸른색 정맥이 돌출된 것

- 5기 : **직경 8mm의 푸른색 정맥이 돌출된 것**
- 6기 : 혈전성 정맥염, 피부궤양, 피부 색소침착 등 합병증이 있는 경우

하지정맥류는 어떻게 치료할까?

하지정맥류는 흔히 볼 수 있는 질환으로 발병원인에 따라 두 가지로 분류할 수 있다.

1. 원발성 하지정맥류는 가장 많이 생기는 형태이며 제일 좋은 치료는 근본 수술이다.
2. 속발성 하지정맥류는 심부정맥의 판막의 이상에 의해서 생기는 것으로 보존적 치료를 받는 것이 좋다.

정확한 진단이 하지정맥류 치료 성공의 중요한 열쇠이다. 여러 가지 치료 방법 중에 외과의사가 직접 초음파를 보면서 소절개를 통해 하지정맥류를 수술하는 것이 국제적인 추세이며 대부분의 환자에게 적합한 방법이다. 이와 같은 방법은 정확한 진단으로, 소 절개, 입원하지 않고 통원치료, 수술 후 즉시 걸을 수 있는 장점으로 환자 및 가족들에게 매우 편리한 방법이다. 하지정맥류는 유전성향이 있는 질환이므로 가족 중에 하지정맥류가 있다면 주의 깊게 살펴볼 필요가 있다. 그리고 조기에 발견하여 조기 예방하는 것이 좋다.

하지정맥류 치료 후 재발의 원인

최근 하지정맥류 치료법은 매우 많아졌다. 하지만 전통적인 외과 수술법뿐만 아니라 레이저치료도 어느 정도의 재발률이 있다. 실제로 하지정맥류 치료 후 재발되는 것은 막을 수 있다. 수술 후 하지정맥류 재발되는 가장 많은 이유는 부정확한 진단과 수술을 철저하게 하지 않았기 때문이다. 그러므로 하지정맥류 치료는 수술적 정확한 진단과 풍부한 경험이 있는 외과계열의 전문의가 집도해야 하고 완전히 철저하게 필요 없는 정맥혈관을 제거해야 하지정맥류의 재발을 최소화할 수 있다.

하지정맥류를 수술하지 않고 방치할 경우 정맥의 혈전, 피부염, 피부궤양 등의 합병증이 생길 수 있다. 그러므로 하지정맥류는 조기 진단, 조기 치료를 받는 것이 재발률을 최소화하는 길이다.

■ 하지정맥류 1기 : 모세혈관 확장증, 거미상 정맥

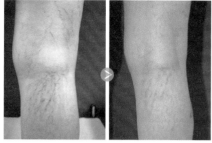
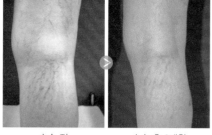

수술 전   수술 후 2개월

■ 하지정맥류 2기 : 직경 2mm 푸른색 세정맥 돌출

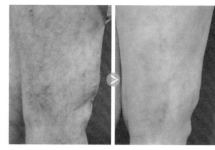

수술 전   수술 후 7개월

■ 하지정맥류 3기 : 직경 2~4mm의 푸른색 정맥 세줄기 이상 돌출

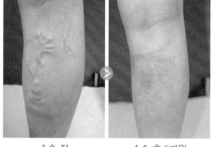

수술 전   수술 후 5개월

■ 하지정맥류 4기 : 직경 4~8mm의 푸른색 정맥 돌출

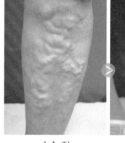
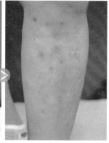

수술 전   수술 후 4개월

■ 하지정맥류 5기 : 직경 8mm의 푸른색 정맥 돌출

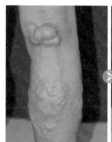

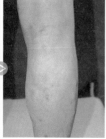

수술 전   수술 후 7개월

■ 하지정맥류 6기 : 합병증

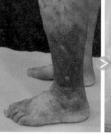

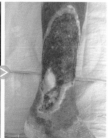

피부착색   피부궤양

TIP_하지정맥류 수술정보

수술시간	마취방법	입원여부	회복기간	체류기간
1시간	국소정맥마취	당일	1주	7일

17 Challenge against incurable lymphedema

Challenge against incurable lymphedema

Dr. Young Ki Shim has researched lymphedema over than 20 years and developed his own therapeutic method with good experiences. By his operation method, the average patient's volume reduction rate was 80~110% after one year. His clinical results are comparable to old conventional methods. The world first his lymphosuction and stem cell graft method is less invasive, less scar, fast recovery, short down time, visible reduced extremities immediate after operation, high overall success rate. He can get very good successful results after stem cell graft to the necrosed leg ulcer, and revealed its function of neoangiogenesis & neolymphangiogenesis. This stem cell graft is very safe no side effects, no risk of cancer development and very good success rate since 2010. The stem cells are harvested from patient's own adipose tissue mostly at the belly. And cells are immediately grafted to the patients. This stem cell graft can repeat every 2~5 year.

| Lymphedema

Lymphedema means abnormal collection of lymph fluid at subcutaneous tissue of affected limb. Lymph fluid becomes thicker and thicker by time as it is not circulated well and does not drained properly. Its composition is high protein contained fluid. The common complications are lymphangitis, tissue fibrosis, skin necrosis.

Lymph system

Lymph system is different from cardiovascular system, it has 3 functions i.e., circulation, detox, immune function. It gives nutrients such as mineral, oxygen, vitamins to the cells, tissues, organs where the blood vessels does not reach and its volume is 4~5 folds more than blood plasma. And it removed waste material, toxins from them to lymph drainage ducts. It also has immune functions fight against the bacteria, virus, fungus, etc. by filtration.

Functions of lymph system :

• circulatiom
• detoxification
• Nutrition
• Immune function

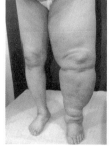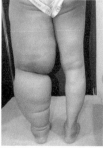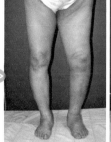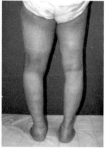

preoperative view   postoperative view 13 months after

▲ Secondary lymphedema on left leg : a 62-year-old female patient. lymphedema was developed after uterine cancer operation for more than 10 years. Degenerative change on knee joint due to heavy leg. Lymphedema was aggravated by time. After lymphedema operation, the pain on knee and range of motion was improved. Body weight was reduced from 84Kg to 66 Kg. Diameter on calf also reduced 22.5cm.

Symptoms of lymphedema

Lymphedema is characterized as chronic swelling of limb and aggravated. Due to asymmetry of limb, the imbalance of posture, the patients can not wear their own clothings that fit before, heavy limb makes fatigue. Frequent attack of bacterial and fungal inflammation named lymphangitis restrict the normal life. And due to the complex of appearance, reduced social activities and depressed. The most common site about 80% of lymphedema is upper limb after breast cancer operation, and lower limb after uterine cancer operation. Face, body trunk, pelvic area can be affected by lymphedema, too.

The lymphedema develops in distal part at first such as hands or feet in most cases, however sometimes it develops in proximal part of limb. Many patients do not complain

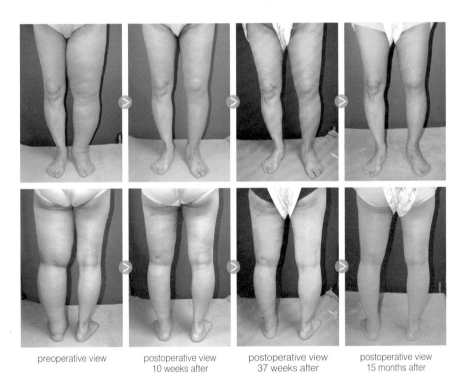

| preoperative view | postoperative view 10 weeks after | postoperative view 37 weeks after | postoperative view 15 months after |

▲ Secondary lymphedema 2nd stage on left lower limb : a 53-year-old female patient. Uterine cancer operation 8 years ago. Radiotherapy 10 times. Repeated lymphangitis. Nearly normalized leg size after 37 week.

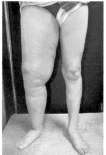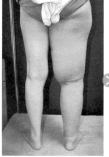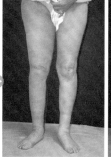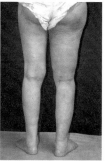

preoperative view   postoperative view 8 months after

▲ Secondary lymphedema on right lower limb : a 66-year-old female patient. Uterine cancer operation 38 years ago. Aggravated lymphedema for 20 years. After operation 8 month, diameter 14 cm reduced. No more lymphangitis.

pain, only just heaviness. As lymphedema progresses, repeated lymphangitis, fever, pain, increasing swelling, and finally complications such as skin necrosis, ulcer, wart like skin change can be developed.

The kinds of lymphedema

- Primary lymphedema
  - Congenital lymphedema
  - Lymphedema praecox: develop around 14 year old
  - Lymphedema tarda: develop around 35 year old
- Secondary lymphedema
  - Infection by filariasis, parasites, bacteria, fungi
  - Trauma: operation, radiotherapy, burn, accidents
  - After cancer operation
  - Others : generalized disease, pregnancy, etc.

Treatment of lymphedema

There are few doctors concerned about lymphedema, because the study for lymph system is still underdeveloped and can not see easily as this system is transparent nature. The lecture about lymph system in very short just few hours through the whole curriculum of medical college. The principle of lymphedema treatment can be different according to the lymphedema stage. The early stage, lymph drainage is important by detoxification, manual lymph drainage, compression therapy and prevention of accumulation of lymph sludge. At later stage of lymphedema, excision of fibrotic tissue is required. Microlymphatic anastomosis is not recommended as this operation has no effects at all.

- The early stage of lymphedema: non surgical conservative therapy
- Limb elevation 30~40 degree could be helpful.
- Compression therapy : medical compression stockings, elastic bandage wrapping, pneumatic compression
- Prevention of infection
- Later staged lymphedema : Mainly excisional surgery. Among the primary lymphedema, 15% of patients are necessary to cut off hypertrophied fibrosed tissue.

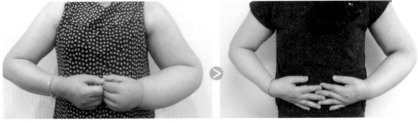

preoperative   postoperative view 5 months after

▲ Secondary lymphedema 2nd stage on left upper limb : a 56-year-old female patient. Left breaste cancer operation 11 years ago. Radiotherapy Chemotherapy were done. Suffered from lymphedema for 8 years. After operation, compression therapy: medical compression stockings and elastic bandage wrapping

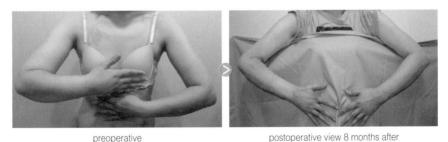

preoperative   postoperative view 8 months after

▲ Secondary lymphedema on right upper limb : stem cell graft, no need compression therapy

- The operation methods of lymphedema in the world
  - Microvascular free tissue transfer(free flap)
  - Lymph vein anastomosis(LVA)
  - Vascularized lymph node transfer
  - Manual lymph drainage
  - Surgical excision

Dr. Shim's lymphedema treatment method (DECOBEL therapy)

DECOBEL: DEtox + COmpression + elastic Banage + Elcure

- Combination therapy by noninvasive therapy
- Lymphosuction + liposuction + stem cell graft
- Oral medication, complex physiotherapy, detox therapy, during follow up period
- Compression therapy: medical compression stockings, elastic bandage wrapping should be done at least 12~24 months after operation.
- Elcure therapy: high voltage microcurrent therapy for iontolysis of lymph sludge invented by Dr. Shim.

TIP_Guide of lymphedema operation

Operation time	Anesthsia	Admission	Recovery time	Stay in Korea
3~4 hours	Local and intravenous anesthesia	2~3 weeks	2 weeks	3~4 weeks

| Varicose veins

When the venous valves are failed to close completely, the venous blood flow falling down(= venous reflux) and this cause venous hypertension. As the time pass, reflux flow become severe and veins are protruded outside skin and become tortuous. This is called as varicose veins

Diagnosis of varicose veins

Varicose veins does not subside by themselves, and it aggravated by time. Early diagnosis by specialists, phlebologists or vascular surgeon and early treatment is highly recommended.

- 1st stage : telangiectasia, spider veins
- 2nd stage : diameter 2 mm reticular veins. No protrusion
- 3rd stage : diameter 2~4 mm. protruded, Ramen noodle size
- 4th stage : diameter 4~8 mm. protruded, Udon noodle size
- 5th stage : diameter over 8 mm. protruded, finger size
- 6th stage : complication stage thrombophlebitis, hyperpigmentation, skin ulcer

How to treat varicose veins?

Varicose veins are very common disease. There are 2 kinds of varicose veins.

1. Primary varicose veins—reflux at superficial vein. Control of reflux is necessary.
2. Secondary varicose veins---reflux at deep vein. Conservative therapy only

Exact diagnosis is utmost important. The surgeon should examine thoroughly where the venous valve function failed and its size, degree of reflux. And precise operation for block the reflux is also very important to get the best postoperative results. Small incision, no admission, least postoperative pain, fast recovery, short down time, best cosmetic results are factors of successful treatment . those are depending on surgeon's wisdom and experience. Dr.Shim has operated varicose veins over 40,000 cases since 1995 in Korea and in China.

Varicose veins has a tendency of inheritance. It will be good if there are varicose veins patients in your family, periodic early diagnosis after adolescent period is highly recommended.

Why the varicose veins are recurred after treatment?

Recently, there are so many treatment methods are invented and developed. Despite conventional stripping method, radiofrequency electric coagulation, endovenous laser

■ 1st stage : telangiectasia, spider veins

■ 2nd stage : diameter 2 mm reticular veins. No protrusion

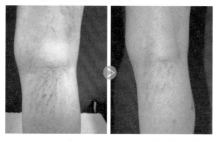

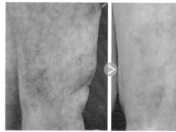

| preoperative | postoperative 2 months | preoperative | postoperative 7 months |

■ 3rd stage : diameter 2~4 mm. protruded, Ramen noodle size

■ 4th stage : diameter 4~8 mm. protruded, Udon noodle size

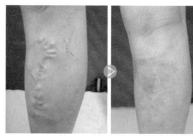

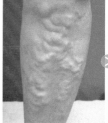
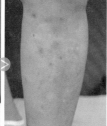

| preoperative | postoperative 5 month | preoperative | postoperative 4 month |

■ 5th stage : diameter over 8 mm. protruded, finger size

■ 6th stage : complication stage thrombophlebitis, hyperpigmentation, skin ulcer

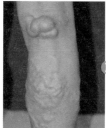
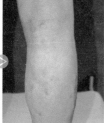

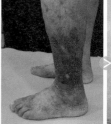
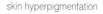
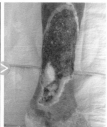

| preoperative | postoperative 7 month | skin hyperpigmentation | skin ulcer |

TIP_Guide of varicose vein operation

Operation time	Anesthsia	Admission	Recovery time	Stay in Korea
I hour	Local intravenous anesthesia	Outpatient dispensary	1 week	7 days

vein ablation, cyanoacrylate injection, mechanical injury of venous epithelium, Duplex guided sclerotherapy, etc.

And advantages and disadvantages and side effects are different according to the treatment.

The common people does not know in these special medical area, there it will be clever to choose best surgeon with good experience for the patients.

The reason why the recurrence, the poor experienced surgeon. Improper diagnosis. Inacuurate treatment.ad did not follow up in time.

If let varicose veins left untreated long time, varicose veins are aggravated and finally leads to complication such as thrombophlebitis, hyperpigmentation, skin ulcer. Therefore periodic early diagnosis and proper treatment are highly recommended.

안면필러성형(Dermal filler surgery)
각 부위별 필러를 이용한 개선 사례(Examples of improvement using fillers for each part)
보톡스(Botox)

수술없이
얼굴의 라인을 살리다

Rejuvenate facial lines
without surgery

필러(filler)란 단어는 '채우다'라는 뜻으로 필러시술은 '피부 속을 채워주는 물질'을 이용한 주름 및 안면 볼륨을 개선하는 방법이다. 현재는 이러한 필러를 이용한 시술이 대중화되어 환자들도 회복의 걱정 없이 안전한 쁘띠성형을 받을 수 있다.

The word "filler" means "to fill up," and filler procedure is a method to improve wrinkles and facial volume by using "substances that fill the inner part of the skin." Currently, procedures using these fillers have become popular, and patients can have petit surgery safely without worrying about recovery.

코디성형외과
KODI Plastic Surgery

www.kodips.com

홍현준(Hyun-Jun Hong)

• 성형외과 전문의(Plastic Surgeon)
연세대의과대학 성형외과 외래교수(Adjunct Professor of Plastic Surgery, Yonsei University College of Medicine)
• 대한성형외과학회 종신회원(Lifetime member of the Korean Society of Plastic and Reconstructive Surgeons)
• 대한미용성형외과학회 정회원(Regular member of the Korean Society for Aesthetic Plastic Surgery)
• 대한두개악안면학회 정회원(Regular member of the Korean Cleft Palate-Craniofacial Association)
• 대한미세수술학회 정회원(Regular member of the Korean Society for Microsurgery)

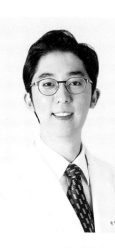

18 비수술적인 방법으로 숨겨진 아름다움을 발견

쁘띠 성형의 대중화

10년 전만 하더라도 성형수술이라는 단어는 준비, 수술 일정, 수면의 방법, 회복 기간 등 계획을 잘 세워서 진행해야 하는 매우 스케일이 큰 일종의 행사 같은 느낌이었다. 또한 수술이 잘되었는지를 알기 위해서는 부기가 빠지고 나의 얼굴 또는 몸에 완벽하게 적응한 자연스러운 모습이 되기까지 상당한 시일이 소요되었다.

최근에는 생명과학의 발달과 시간이 부족한 현대인들의 트렌드로 인해 편리하고 곧바로 시술의 결과를 확인할 수 있는 쁘띠 시술이 각광받고 있는 추세이다. 반면 시술의 부작용은 수술에 비해 비교적 적다고 볼 수 있다.

적은 비용부담과 짧은 시술시간으로 성형수술 효과를 기대할 수 있는 성형용 필러 주사 시술이 관심을 받고 있다. 입체감을 살리거나 주름을 채우는 등 미용 목적으로 사용되는 성형용 필러는 안면부의 시각적인 개선을 위해 피하에 주입해 볼륨감을 채워준다.

안면필러성형

필러 성형은 주로 인체 동일 성분으로 구성되어 무해한 히알루론산 필러를 사용하여 수술 없이도 얼굴의 볼륨감을 얻고 윤곽을 살리는 시술 방법이다

인체에 안전한 히알루론산(HA) 필러

일반적으로 필러는 이마나 팔자주름 등 간편하게 꺼진 부분을 채우는 시술로 많이 알려져 있다. 주사를 이용한 시술이기 때문에 통증이나 회복에 대한 부담이 적은 편이며, 시술 결과도 바로 확인이 가능하다. 또한 추가 시술을 통해 모양을 다시 잡거나 녹이는 주사를 활용하여 모양이 마음에 안 들 경우에는 이전의 모습으로 되돌리는 것도 가능하다.

이에 함께, 보톡스는 미간, 눈가, 이마 등의 잔주름을 완화하는 데 주로 사용되며 사각턱이나 종아리, 얼굴윤곽 개선에 적용되기도 한다. 모두 시술 시간이 짧고 간단하기 때문에 바쁜 직장인들이 많이 선호하는 시술이다.

이처럼 필러, 보톡스는 비침습적인 시술로 부담을 최소화하는 가운데 빠르고 간편하게 받을 수 있지만 엄연한 의료시술이기 때문에 시술의 안전성과 전문성을 충분히 확인하고 진행하는 것이 중요하다. 무엇보다 적당한 양의 필러와 보톡스를 사용하는 것이 인위적이지 않고 자연스러우며 만족스러운 시술 결과를 얻을 수 있다.

필러의 경우 단순히 얼굴의 한 부위에 볼륨감을 주는 것을 목적으로 하기보다

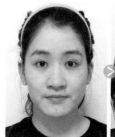 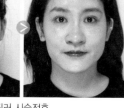

필러 시술전후

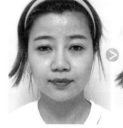 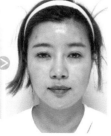

필러 시술전후

전체적인 이목구비의 조화와 균형을 고려해 디자인하는 과정이 필요하다. 특히 얼굴은 미세한 차이만으로도 전반적인 이미지의 변화가 생길 수 있기 때문에 전문 의료진의 시술 기술뿐만 아니라 미적 감각 또한 중요한 부분이다.

구분	반영구 필러	히알루론산 필러	보형물
장점	• 반영구적인 효과 • 시술직후 일상생활 바로가능 • 자연스러운 볼륨감 형성	• 시술직후 일상생활 바로가능 • 자연스러운 볼륨감 형성 • 섬세한 볼륨 시술 가능 • 인체와 비슷한 히알루론산 성분으로 피부 개선 • 체내 콜라겐 생성으로 주름과 탄력 개선 • 부위별 맞춤 필러 선택 가능 • 유지 기간에 따른 필러 선택 가능 • 모양교정(몰딩)과 수정 및 제거가 용이	• 영구적인 효과
단점	• 수정 및 제거가 어려움 • 체내의 이물반응 가능성	• 반영구 필러에 비해 짧은 유지 기간	• 별도의 회복기간 필요 • 수정 및 제거 시 재수술 필요 • 체내의 이물반응 가능성
부위	• 얼굴의 제한된 부위 시술 가능	• 얼굴의 거의 모든 부위 시술 가능	• 얼굴의 제한된 부위 수술 가능

히알루론산 필러 비교

필러의 장점

• 빠른 효과 및 시술 직후 일상생활 바로 가능
• 주름 및 흉터의 시각적 개선
• 비교적 적은 부담
• 자연스러운 볼륨감

그러나 각 부위의 부족함을 채우는 것과 동시에 풀페이스 필러 시술로 얼굴 전체의 모양, 형태를 잡아 주는 것도 가능하다.

우리 얼굴은 한 부위의 시술만으로도 전체적인 인상에 변화를 줄 수가 있는데 풀페이스 시술은 각 부위에 적정한 용량과 제품을 사용하여 얼굴이 밋밋하거나 입체감이 없는 환자들에게 윤곽수술 없이도 얼굴의 조화를 살려 원하는 얼굴의 라인을 보정하고 전체적인 이미지의 개선을 기대할 수 있다.

예를 들어, 이마와 광대 쪽은 볼륨을 주어 좀 더 생동감 있게 해주고 턱선은 갸름해 보이는 V라인으로 보이게 한다.

풀페이스에 사용되는 필러는 입자의 특성에 따라 풍부한 볼륨을 위해 사용되는 필러 제품군과 코필러와 같이 입체감을 주는 필러 제품군으로 구분하여 사용하여야 한다. 무조건 비싼 제품을 택하기보다는 부위별로 본인에게 적합한 필러를 권하는 전문의의 추천을 받아 시술하는 것이 모양 면에서나 유지 기간 면에서 도움이 된다.

또한 풀페이스 시술을 할 경우 HA필러의 성분으로 인해 전체적인 얼굴 피부에 수분감을 주어 촉촉한 듯한 느낌을 줄 수 있다.

대표적인 히알루론산 필러

현재 시장에는 수많은 필러들이 다양한 제약회사를 통해서 생성이 되고 수입이 되고 있는 상황이다.

안면부의 필러 시술을 함에 있어서는 안전성과 유지력 등 여러 요소가 고려된다.

각 부위마다 피부의 상태가 다르고 필러마다 입자의 크기나 밀도, 탄성, 점도 등 특성이 각각 다르기 때문에 필러를 다루는 기술과 노하우가 매우 중요하다 할 것이다. 그래서 필러 시술은 필러의 성질에 대한 이해와 기술을 가진 성형외과 전문의에게 받는 것이 중요하다.

TIP_필러 시술정보

시술시간	마취방법	입원여부	회복기간	체류기간
10~20분	국소마취	입원없음	당일	당일

각 부위별 필러를 이용한 개선 사례

필러는 꺼진 부위에 원하는 만큼의 볼륨을 채울 수 있는 시술이다. 필러 성형은 얼굴전체에 시술이 가능하며 윤곽의 볼륨을 보충해 줄 뿐만 아니라 연부 조직의 볼륨을 보충하는 부위까지 시술이 가능하다.

이마필러

    이마필러의 경우 동안을 완성시켜주는 볼륨 있는 이마로 가꿔주는 시술 중 하나이다. 이마가 평평하고 납작한 경우 강한 인상을 주게 된다. 이에 볼륨 조절로 한 듯 안 한 듯 자연스러운 이마를 만들어 주기 때문에 평소 푹 꺼지고 좁은 이마가 콤플렉스였던 이들 사이에서 선호도가 크게 증가하고 있다. 측면에서 볼 때 앞부분이 동그란 모양으로 볼륨감을 충분히 살려주어 수술을 하지 않고도 이마의 볼륨을 높여주고 실제 나이보다 더 어려 보이는 효과를 볼 수 있다.

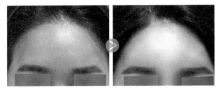 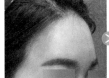 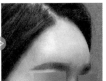

이마필러 시술전후   이마필러 시술전후

턱필러

    무턱필러는 얼굴 뼈를 건드리는 안면윤곽수술 없이도 간단한 주입을 통해 V라인의 갸름한 얼굴형을 만들 수 있어 관심을 모으고 있다.

    입술에 비해 턱끝이 앞으로 충분히 나오지 않은 무턱은 얼굴 하관의 볼륨감이 없어 입이 부각되는 얼굴형으로, 턱선이 거의 없어 인상이 흐릿하거나 이중 턱이나 돌출 입 등으로 오해받는 경우도 많다.

    이러한 무턱을 해소하는 무턱필러(Filler)는 턱끝 라인을 V라인을 만들어 얼굴이 전체적으로 갸름해 보이는 인상을 준다. 무턱 필러는 전체적인 얼굴 윤곽선에 영향을 미치는 만큼, 일반적인 필러시술에 비해 시술법이 비교적 섬세한 편이다.

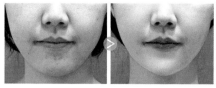
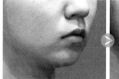

무턱필러 시술전후   무턱필러 시술전후

입술필러

입술이 빈약하고 입꼬리가 처진 경우에는 우울하면서도 차가운 인상을 주기 쉽다. 이에 반해, 볼륨 있는 입술과 기분 좋게 올라간 입꼬리는 긍정적인 인상과 더불어 사랑스러운 이미지를 갖게 한다.

입술에 볼륨이 없고 처진 입꼬리를 가진 사람들이 이미지를 바꾸기 위해 찾는 방법으로 입술필러와 입꼬리필러가 있다. 또한 입술에 주름이 많으면 나이 든 느낌을 줄 수 있기 때문에 입술 필러로 볼륨을 보충하며 팽팽하고 촉촉한 입술로 만들어 줄 수 있다. 이와 함께, 보톡스를 이용 입꼬리를 올려 웃는 인상을 만들어 주는 시술도 여성들에게 인기가 많다.

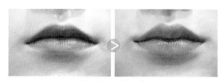
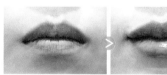

입술필러 시술전후   입술필러 시술전후

눈밑/애교필러

눈밑이 꺼지면 퀭하니 건강하지 못하고 사나워 보이는 인상을 주게 된다. 눈물꺼짐으로 움푹 패이면서 어두워 보이는 다크서클은 눈밑 필러가 도움이 되며, 그림자가 지던 눈밑에 필러를 주입해 볼륨감을 살려주는 이 시술은 다크서클 없애는 법으로 알려져 있다.

최근에는 다크서클의 개선을 위해 성형외과를 찾는 남성들도 상당히 늘고 있다. 눈밑 필러는 수술에 비해 비용이 저렴하며 시술과정 역시 간단한 편이다.

애교필러는 눈매의 분위기를 바꿔줄 수 있을 뿐 아니라 눈 밑이 꺼지면서 퀭한 이미지가 나타나는 것을 개선해 줄 수 있어서 마니아층이 형성되어 있는 시술이다. 속눈썹 바로 아래 자연스런 애교살 볼륨을 만들어 눈매가 또렷하고 생기있게 한다. 시술 시간이 10~15분 정도로 짧고 사용되는 필러의 용량도 상당히 적은 편이라 붓기나 멍이 거의 나타나지 않고, 흉터 또한 작은 주사 자국으로 나타나서 회복 기간에 대한 부담도 매우 적다.

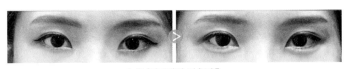

눈밑/애교필러 시술전후

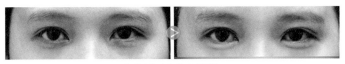

눈밑/애교필러 시술전후

보톡스

보톡스는 이마와 코, 콧등, 미간, 눈가 주름 등 탄력 저하로 주름선이 생긴 부분을 개선 시키고, 턱근육, 승모근, 종아리근육의 크기를 줄이는 목적으로 많이 사용된다.

주름을 예방하고 근육 크기도 줄이다

보톡스는 보툴리늄 독소가 주성분인 주사약의 상품명으로 보툴리늄이라는 세균에서 분비되는 신경독소를 정제, 희석하여 인체에 안전하게 사용할 수 있게 제조된 약품이다. 이 신경차단 물질을 이용한 약물을 주성분으로 미간이나 눈가, 이마 등 주름이 잘 생기는 부위의 표정 주름에 효과적이다.

특히 최근에는 안티에이징 시술로 '보톡스'를 선호하는 경우가 많은데, 이는 비교적 간단한 주사시술로 잔주름을 개선을 기대할 수 있기 때문이다. 주름 보톡스는 근육의 움직임을 조절하는 신경자극을 직접적으로 막기 때문에 주사 부위의 근육만 마비시켜 근육 움직임에 의한 주름을 개선시킨다.

또한 전문가의 진단에 따라 근육 보톡스도 함께 시술받을 수 있다. 턱뼈를 감싸는 저작근이 과도하게 발달한 경우 이 부위에 보톡스를 주사해 근육의 두께와 부피를 줄일 수 있다. 이러한 보톡스는 사각턱뿐만 아니라 승모근과 종아리 등 비대한 근육을 줄일 수 있는 시술로 알려져 있다.

승모근은 부위 특성상 운동이나 식이조절로 빼기가 어려워 의학적인 도움이 필요하다. 발달된 승모근 개선에는 승모근 보톡스가 도움이 될 수 있다. 보툴리눔톡신 성분을 주입해 근육의 부피를 선택적으로 줄여주는 방식으로, 가느다란 목과 어깨선이 길게 뻗어 보이고 쇄골까지 돋보여질 수 있다. 평소 어깨 결림으로 고생한다면 어깨 통증이 완화되는 부가적인 효과도 기대할 수 있다.

종아리에 근육이 발달하게 되어 알처럼 볼록 튀어나오는 근육을 종아리 알이라고 한다. 종아리 알은 발생하게 되면 쉽게 제거가 불가능하며, 운동을 하게 되면 계속해서 발달한다. 여성들 사이에서는 종아리 근육의 발생을 미용에 맞지 않다는 이유로 제거하려는 경우가 많으며, 최근 들어서 승모근과 종아리 보톡스의 문의가 급격히 늘고 있다.

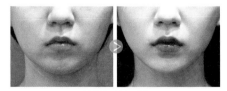

보톡스 시술전후

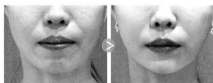

보톡스 시술전후

TIP_보톡스 시술정보

시술시간	마취방법	입원여부	회복기간	체류기간
10~20분	국소마취	입원없음	당일	당일

18

Discover the hidden beauty in non-surgical ways

Popularization of petit plastic surgery

Even 10 years ago, the word plastic surgery sounded like a kind of very large-scale event that had to be planned well in advance, from preparation, surgery schedule, sleeping position/method to recovery period. Furthermore, in order to see if the surgery really went well, it took a considerable amount of time for the swelling to subside and become a natural appearance that perfectly adapts to one's own face or body. Recently, due to the development of life science and the trend of people who are lacking time, petit surgery, which is convenient and allows you to check the results of the procedure right away, has been in the limelight. On the other hand, the side effects of the procedure can be seen as relatively minor compared to surgery.

Cosmetic filler injections, which can expect the effects of plastic surgery with lower cost and shorter time of procedure, have been attracting attention. Cosmetic fillers, used for cosmetic purposes, such as to create a three-dimensional effect or filling in the wrinkles, are injected subcutaneously to fill up the sense of volume in order to visually improve the facial area.

| Dermal Filler Surgery

Using harmless hyaluronic acid fillers, mainly composed of the same ingredients as the human body, filler procedure is a procedure that allows you to get a sense of volume while improving the contours of your face without surgery,

Hyaluronic Acid (HA) filler which is safe for the human body

In general, fillers are widely known to be used for a procedure that conveniently fills in the hollow parts, such as the forehead or nasolabial folds. As it is an injection procedure, there is little pain or less burden on recovery, and the results of the procedure can be confirmed immediately. Moreover, if you are not satisfied with the results, you can go through reshaping process through additional procedures or return back to the previous appearance by using dissolving injections.

Along with this procedure, Botox is mainly used to alleviate fine between the eyebrows, around the eyes and forehead, and is also applied to improve the square jaw, calves, and facial contours. These procedures take short time and are relatively simple, so they are preferred by busy office workers.

As such, filler procedures and Botox are non-invasive procedures that people can get quickly and conveniently while minimizing the burden, but it is important to fully confirm the safety and expertise of the procedure before proceeding, since it is undoubtedly a medical procedure. Above all, using the right amount of fillers and Botox leads you to be satisfied with the natural and non-artificial results.

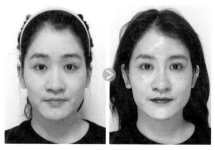
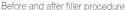

Before and after filler procedure

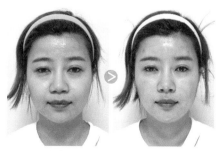

Before and after filler procedure

In the case of filler, it is necessary to come up with a facial design, considering the harmony and balance of the overall features, rather than simply giving a sense of volume to one part of the face. In particular, since the overall image of the face can change even with slight differences, not only the treatment skills of professional medical team but also the aesthetic senses are very important.

Strength of filler

- Rapid effect and daily life available immediately after the procedure
- Visual improvements in wrinkles and scars
- Relatively less burden
- Natural sense of volume

Category	Semi-Permanent Filler	Hyaluronic Acid Filler	Implants (Prosthesis)
Strength	• Semi-permanent effect • Enables daily life immediately after the procedure • Creates a natural sense of volume	• Enables daily life immediately after the procedure • Creates a natural sense of volume • Delicate procedure for volume available • Improves skin with hyaluronic acid, similar to the human body • Improves wrinkles and skin elasticity by producing collagen in the body • Can select filler, customized for each part • Can select filler according to the maintenance period • Easy to correct shape (molding), modify and remove	• Permanent effect
Weakness	• Difficult to modify and remove • Possibility of foreign body reaction in the body	• Short maintenance period compared to semi-permanent fillers	• Requires a separate recovery period • Requires reoperation for modification or removal • Possibility of foreign body reaction in the body
Parts	• Can only be applied to the limited parts of the face	• Can be applied to almost any part of the face	• Can only be applied to the limited parts of the face

Comparison of Hyaluronic Acid Fillers

However, it is also possible to fill in each hollow part of the face while adjusting the shape and form of the entire face with a full face filler procedure at the same time.

The overall impression of our face can be changed with just one procedure.

The full face procedure uses the appropriate amount and product on each part for the patients with a flat face (without volume) or lacking a three-dimensional effect, and this procedure can improve the overall image of a person as it corrects the desired facial line by bringing the harmony of the face without contouring surgery.

For example, it gives volume to the forehead and cheekbones to make them look more lively, and makes the jawline look slimmer with V-line.

Fillers used for full face procedure should be categorized according to the characteristics of the particles: a filler group used for rich volume and a filler group that gives a three-dimensional effect, such as a nose filler. Rather than unconditionally choosing an expensive product, it is helpful in terms of appearance and maintenance period to get a recommendation from a specialist who suggests a filler suitable for each part. In addition, in case of the full face procedure, the ingredients of the HA filler may provide moisture to the entire facial skin, presenting a moist feeling.

Representative hyaluronic acid filler

In the current market, a lot of fillers are produced and imported through many different pharmaceutical companies.

When performing dermal filler procedure, various elements, such as safety and maintenance, are considered.

Since the condition of the skin is different for each part, and each filler has different characteristics, such as particle size, density, elasticity, and viscosity, skills and know-how of the medical doctor who handle the fillers are very important. This is why it is important to get filler procedure from a plastic surgeon who has a good understanding of the properties of fillers with the professional skills.

Procedure Time	Anesthetizing method	Hospitalization	Recovery Period	Length of Stay
10~20 minutes	Local anesthesia	No hospitalization	The day of procedure	The day of procedure

Examples of improvement using fillers for each part

Fillers are used for the procedure that fills in the desired amount of volume in facial areas that have become hollow. Filler surgery can be performed on the entire face, and it is possible to supplement the volume to the contour of face as well as to the area where the volume of soft tissue needs to be supplemented

Forehead Filler

Forehead filler is one of the procedures to create a voluminous forehead that leads to complete the baby face. When your forehead is even and flat, it gives a strong impression. Since this procedure creates a natural forehead as if it had not been touched by adjusting the amount of volume, preference for this procedure has greatly been increasing among those who usually have a complex with a hollow and narrow forehead. When viewed from the side, the front part is round in shape and gives a sense of volume enough to increase the volume of the forehead without surgery, thereby making you look younger than your actual age.

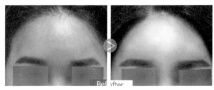

Before and after forehead filler procedure

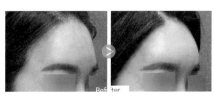

Before and after forehead filler procedure

Chin Filler

Filler on a short chin is attracting attention as it can create a slim face with V-line through simple injection without facial contouring surgery that may touch the facial bones.

A short chin, where the tip of the chin does not protrude far enough compared to the lips, is a face type in which the mouth stands out because there is no sense of volume in the lower part of the face, and people with short chin are often misunderstood to have a blurred impression due to lacking jaw line, or to have double chin or protruding mouth.

Chin filler, which is to eliminate such a short chin, creates a V-line at the tip of the chin, giving the overall impression of a slimmer face. Since chin filler affects the overall facial contour, the procedure is relatively delicate compared to other general filler procedures.

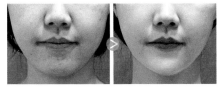
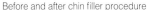
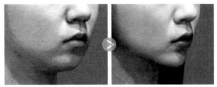

Before and after chin filler procedure   Before and after chin filler procedure

Lip Filler

When the lips are weak and the corners of the mouth are drooping, it is easy to give a gloomy and cold impression. On the other hand, voluminous lips and pleasantly raised corners of the mouth give a positive impression with a lovely image.

There are fillers for lips and the corners of the mouth as a way for people with no volume on their lips and sagging lip corners to change their image. In addition, you can

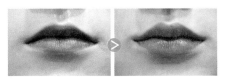
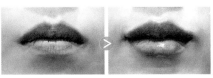

Before and after lip filler procedure   Before and after lip filler procedure

add volume to your lips with lip fillers and make them plump and hydrated, because wrinkles on your lips may give you an aged look. A procedure which uses Botox to lift the corners of the mouth to create a smile is also popular among women.

Filler on Fat under Eyes called Aegyo-sal

When your under-eye areas are hollow, it tends to give unhealthy and ferocious impression. Fillers on under-eyes are helpful for dark circles that look dark due to the hollow under-eyes, and this procedure which injects filler under the eyes to restore volume, is known as a way to get rid of dark circles.

Recently, the number of men seeking plastic surgery to improve dark circles is significantly increasing. Fillers on under-eyes are less expensive than surgery and the procedure is also simple. Filler on fat under eyes called Aegyo-sal is a procedure that attained a group of mania because it can not only change the mood of the eyes, but also improve the appearance of a dull image when the lower eyes are hollow. It creates a natural volume right under the eyelashes, making the eyes clear and lively.

The procedure takes only 10 to 15 minutes and the amount of filler used is quite small, so there is almost no swelling or bruising after the procedure. In addition, scars appear as very small injection marks, so the burden on the recovery period is very small as well.

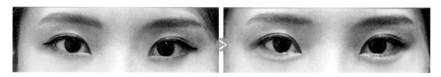

Before and after filler procedure on fat under eyes

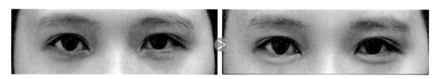

Before and after filler procedure on fat under eyes

| Botox

Botox is widely used for the purpose of improving wrinkles on the forehead, nose, bridge of the nose, middle of the forehead, and wrinkles around the eyes, and reducing the size of jaw muscles, trapezius muscles, and calf muscles.

Prevents wrinkles and reduces size of muscle

Botox is the product name for an injectable drug, containing botulinum toxin, and is a drug manufactured by refining and diluting a neurotoxin secreted by a bacterium called botulinum so that it can be safely used in the human body. This nerve-blocking substance is used as the main ingredient of this drug, and it is effective for wrinkles in areas, used when making facial expressions, where wrinkles are common, such as between the eyebrows, around the eyes, and on the forehead.

In particular, recently, many people prefer 'Botox' as an anti-aging procedure, because a relatively simple injection procedure can be expected to improve fine wrinkles. Wrinkle Botox directly blocks nerve stimulation that controls muscle movement, thereby paralyzing the muscles where Botox is injected and improving wrinkles caused by muscle movement.

Furthermore, Botox can also be injected to muscles depending on the diagnosis of the expert. If the masticatory muscles surrounding the jaw bone are overdeveloped, Botox can be injected into this area to reduce the thickness and volume of the muscle. In this regard, Botox is known as a procedure that can reduce hypertrophy of muscles, such as trapezius muscles and calves as well as square jaws.

Due to the nature of the trapezius muscle, it is difficult to remove muscle volume in this body part through exercise or diet control, so medical help is necessary. Trapezoid

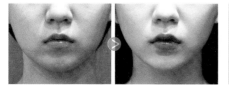 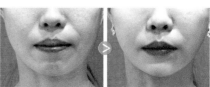

Before and after Botox procedure

Botox can be helpful in improving such developed trapezius muscles. By injecting a botulinum toxin component to selectively reduce muscle volume, you may have slender neck and shoulder stretched out along with the collarbones that may stand out as well. If you suffer from stiff shoulders on a regular basis, you can expect an additional effect to relieve shoulder pain.

Muscles develop in the calves, and these muscles that protrude like eggs are called muscle knots in the calves. These cannot be easily removed once they occur, and they continue to develop if you keep exercising. Among women, there are many cases of trying to remove the development of such muscles, because it does not look beautiful, and as a result, inquiries about Botox injection on trapezius muscle and calves are rapidly increasing in recent years.

TIP_Information on Botox

Procedure Time	Anesthetizing method	Hospitalization	Recovery Period	Length of Stay
10~20 minutes	Local anesthesia	No hospitalization	The day of procedure	The day of procedure

mnckorea.kr

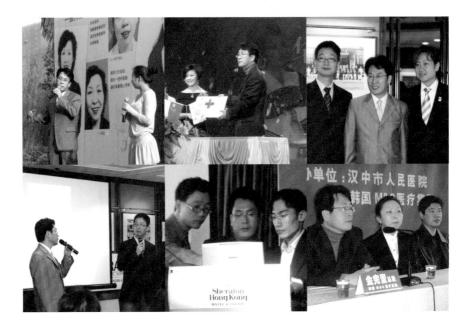

• Korea plastic surgery seminar and VIP consultation
  (Hong Kong, China, Mongol etc)

• K-AURA FILLER domestic sales and overseas exports

• Collaborative medical treatment consultation of Korea and China

• Registered company for foreign patient attraction business in Seoul

• Marketing and consultation of national and international plastic surgery and dermatology

M&C Korea e-mail. mnc_korea@naver.com
Unit 549, 202 Jagok-ro Gangnam-gu Seoul Republic of Korea(Zip 06373)
Tel : 82-2-459-7060

18 experts in Korean cosmetic plastic surgery publish English version

It has already been 10 years since the publication of the master book of Korean cosmetic surgery.

In 2014, we made a total of seven books from the Korean-Chinese version to this English version. There have been many books with a similar concept to the master of Korean cosmetic surgery, but I think the reason why we have been able to publish series for such a long time is due to our differentiated planning ability and in-depth contents of excellent writers in each field.

First, I would like to express my deepest gratitude to the directors who provided in-depth cosmetic surgery information. While 20 directors participated in the writing of one volume, many directors graced the page with a variety of relevant clinical cases, the best surgical techniques, detailed explanations, and photos and illustrations to aid understanding. I am truly grateful.

It takes the hands of many people to create a book, but writing it in a foreign language seems to be an even more complicated and difficult process. Nevertheless, I would like to thank those involved in the production department for their hard work in editing and design.

The English version of Gosu 18 of Korean Aesthetic Plastic Surgery, to be published this time, is planned to be distributed not only to the United States and English-speaking countries, but also to non-English-speaking countries. Online era!! Separately, we plan to produce and service an Android version of the app so that people who cannot obtain the book can view it on their smartphones.

With the advent of an aging society, plastic surgery trends seem to be changing with a tendency to look even one year younger. I put a lot of effort into creating a book, so I always think this is the last time, but I want to do my best to serve as a navigator to provide correct plastic surgery information to countless people who are thirsty for advanced Korean plastic medicine.

December 2023

$M_{\&}C$ Korea **Wan-Gyu Kim**

The 18 Korean Masters in Plastic Surgery
한국 미용성형의 고수 18

18 Korean cosmetic surgery experts, guidelines you need to know before plastic surgery
한국 미용성형의 고수 18, 성형수술 전 알아야할 지침서

초판 인쇄(First printing) December 15, 2023
초판 발행(First edition published) December 15, 2023

지은이(Author) 양동준 외 19인(Dong-Jun Yang and 19 others)

펴낸이(Publisher) 김완규(Wan-Gyu Kim)
펴낸곳(Place of publication) M&C KOREA
출판등록(Publication registration) November 20, 1991(No. 301-1991-101)
표지/디자인(Cover design) 김유경(Yoo-Kyoung Kim)
인쇄(Print) 현대원색문화사(Hyundae color printing Co.)
기획(Plan) M&C KOREA 김완규, 신동호(Wan-Gyu Kim, Dong-Ho Shin)
주소(Address) 06373 서울특별시 강남구 자곡로 202 강남 힐스테이트 에코 549호
　　　　　　　　Unit 549, 202 Jagok-ro Gangnam-gu Seoul Republic of Korea
전화(Phone call) 02)459-7060   이메일(email) mnc_korea@naver.com

ISBN 978-89-97029-22-8

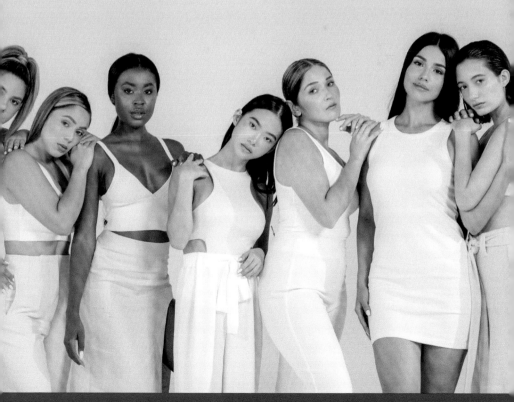

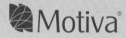

What do you dream about?

#motiva #womenhealth #committedtowomenshealth

moeava

MONOÏ OIL

A French beauty secret 🔍

A timeless French beauty secret, used by Queen Pommare IV and by the French for centuries - in daily rituals and treasured for its medicinal and remedial qualities.

MADE IN TAHITI
DISTRIBUTED IN AUSTRALIA

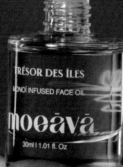

TRÉSOR DES ÎLES
MONOÏ INFUSED FACE OIL
moeava
30ml | 1.01 fl. Oz

www.moeavabeauty.com

info@moeavabeauty.com

K-AURA HA FILLER

| Beauty | Safety | Pleasure |

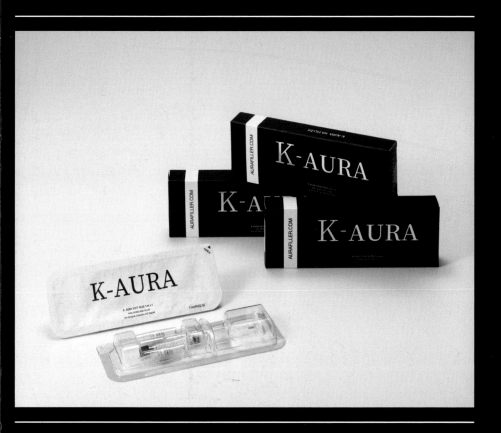

aurafiller.com

M&C Korea

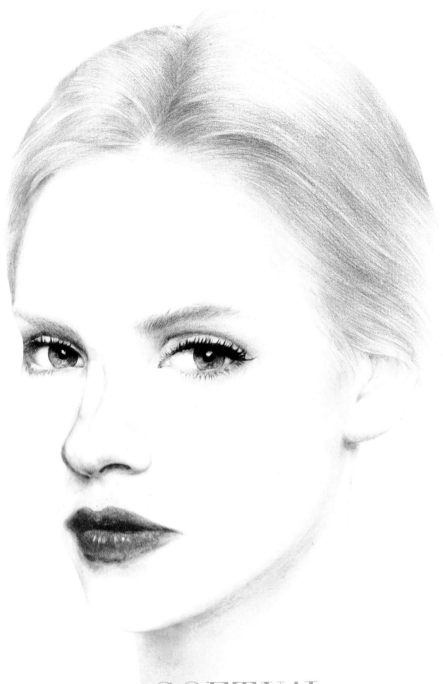

SOFTXiL

High soft silicone / Facial implants

BISTOOL | 3, 5 FL.,Deokseong–bldg., 9, Gwangnaru–ro 6gil, Seongdong–gu, Seoul, Korea
T.+82 2 3446 7688 www.bistool.com